The Psychophysical Measurement of Visual Function

The Psychophysical Measurement of Visual Function

Thomas T. Norton, Ph.D., F.A.A.O.
Professor of Physiological Optics, School of Optometry, University of Alabama at Birmingham

David A. Corliss, O.D., Ph.D.
Associate Professor of Physiological Optics, School of Optometry, University of Alabama at Birmingham

James E. Bailey, O.D., Ph.D., F.A.A.O.
Professor of Basic and Vision Sciences, Southern California College of Optometry, Fullerton

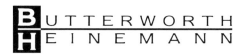

An Imprint of Elsevier Science

Amsterdam • Boston • London • Oxford • New York • Paris
San Diego • San Francisco • Singapore • Sydney • Tokyo

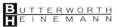

An Imprint of Elsevier Science

225 Wildwood Avenue
Woburn, MA 01801

Notice

Every effort has been made to ensure that the drug dosage schedules within this text are accurate and conform to standards accepted at time of publication. However, as treatment recommendations vary in the light of continuing research and clinical experience, the reader is advised to verify drug dosage schedules herein with information found on product information sheets. This is especially true in cases of new or infrequently used drugs.

The Publisher

Library of Congress Cataloging-in-Publication Data
Norton, Thomas T.
    The psychophysical measurement of visual function / Thomas T. Norton, David A. Corliss, James E. Bailey.
        p. ; cm.
    Includes bibliographical references and index.
    ISBN 0-7506-9935-3
        1. Vision—Testing. 2. Psychophysics. I. Corliss, David A. II. Bailey, James E., OD. III. Title.
        [DNLM: 1. Vision Tests. 2. Psychophysics. 3. Vision—physiology. WW 145 N888p 2002]
    RE76 .N674 2002
    617.7'15—dc21

2001052908

Publisher: Susan F. Pioli

Printed in the United States of America

Last digit is the print number: 9 8 7 6 5 4 3 2 1

To our students and those they will serve

Contents

Contributing Authors

Anthony J. Adams, O.D., Ph.D., F.A.A.O.
Dean Emeritus and Professor of Optometry and Vision Science, School of Optometry, University of California, Berkeley

James E. Bailey, O.D., Ph.D., F.A.A.O.
Professor of Basic and Vision Sciences, Southern California College of Optometry, Fullerton

Karlene K. Ball, Ph.D.
Professor of Psychology, University of Alabama at Birmingham

Carl J. Bassi, Ph.D.
Associate Professor of Optometry, University of Missouri-St. Louis

Harold E. Bedell, Ph.D., F.A.A.O.
Professor of Vision Sciences, College of Optometry, University of Houston

Nancy J. Coletta, O.D., Ph.D., F.A.A.O.
Associate Professor, Department of Vision Science, The New England College of Optometry, Boston

James P. Comerford, Ph.D., O.D., F.A.A.O.
Professor of Vision Science, The New England College of Optometry, Boston

David A. Corliss, O.D., Ph.D.
Associate Professor of Physiological Optics, School of Optometry, University of Alabama at Birmingham

Vasudevan Lakshminarayanan, Ph.D., F.A.A.O.
Associate Professor of Physics and Optometry, School of Optometry, University of Missouri-St. Louis

Thomas T. Norton, Ph.D., F.A.A.O.
Professor of Physiological Optics, School of Optometry, University of Alabama at Birmingham

Deborah Orel-Bixler, Ph.D., O.D., F.A.A.O.
Associate Professor of Clinical Optometry, School of Optometry, University of California, Berkeley

Wayne A. Verdon, O.D., Ph.D., F.A.A.O.
Associate Professor of Clinical Optometry, School of Optometry, University of California, Berkeley

Preface

The book you now hold in your hands is the culmination of many years of evolution that began with a set of class notes prepared by two of the editors (DC and TN) for a basic vision science course that introduces students to the fundamental sensory processes of vision. Its birth occurred during a period when there was no single book in print that covered the material at a level, or with an emphasis, that was appropriate for beginning professional students whose goal is to become clinicians. Its continuing development and maturation into a published work have been focused by consideration of the needs of these students, while simultaneously broadened by the addition of a third editor (JB) and multiple contributors representing different areas of expertise and academic environments. The result is one that blends the methods of psychophysics with the concepts of scientific measurement and our resultant knowledge of vision in a manner that, we hope, bridges the gap between basic scientific knowledge and practical clinical decision making.

This gap between basic science and its practical application in a clinical setting is familiar to anyone charged with teaching students whose primary concern will be making the right clinical decisions. There are often difficult decisions to make about what material to include and what material to exclude as there is more emphasis on selecting material that is "clinically relevant." This is usually accomplished by including descriptions of clinical conditions that represent anomalies in the particular functional areas that are being discussed. Although this is appropriate, it leaves a lot of the basic science knowledge with no direct link to any clinical entity, and we know that those concepts are important to building a student's overall knowledge base for future professional development. To address this dilemma, we focus in this book on what the basic sciences and their clinical application have in common: the concept of measurement.

Consider that psychophysical measurements are used in every clinical eye examination. For example, the simple question "Which is better, one or two?" familiar to anyone who has had or given an eye examination, requires a patient to compare the clarity of vision through two different lens configurations and make a choice. The elements of this procedure define the characteristics of any psychophysical test of the visual system. In general terms, the clinician is attempting to relate the report of a visual perception to a physical dimension of a stimulus. The report in this case is, of course, the verbal indication that vision is better through one of the two lens combinations or the same through both. The physical dimension in this case is the power of the lens combination.

Consider another, more familiar example of a psychophysical test of vision acuity. In this case, the patient is asked to read letters of decreasing size while the clinician records the size at which the patient can no longer correctly identify the letters. Here the report is the naming of the letters, and the primary physical dimension of interest is letter size.

Both of these tests measure the clarity of vision, but consider the differences. In the first case, the clinician is attempting to refine the lens power for optimum correction of a refractive error. In the second case, the clinician is determining the smallest letter size the patient can read under certain conditions. In the first case, the patient is forced to make a choice between two alternatives presented over a series of trials. In the second, the patient is presented with all of the stimuli at once and is allowed to guess the letters that may not be completely clear. These differences bring us to the primary questions addressed in this book. The first is, what scientific basis is there for choosing to perform psychophysical tests in one way and not another? The second is, given that a choice has been made regarding certain methods and the physical stimulus dimensions, what do the responses reveal about the functioning and integrity of the patient's visual system?

Although these appear to be distinct questions, this book shows that they cannot be addressed independently. This is because the normal visual system gives different answers to slight variations in the presentation of the physical dimension of a stimulus for a constant psychophysical method. It also gives different answers to variations in psychophysical methods of testing the system for a constant physical dimension. In the end, it is a matter of judgment that determines how the system is tested and what constitutes normal variation in sensory processes. The student of vision must therefore understand the scientific basis on which these judgments are made, and how they can be made in the future as new tests of visual function are developed.

Chapters 1 and 2 can be considered together as an introduction to basic measurement techniques. Chapter 1 describes the basic psychophysical measurement tools, including the basic elements of stimulus presentation. It introduces the probabilistic nature of these measurements due to stimulus fluctuations, noise in the nervous system, and observer bias. Chapter 2 introduces the student to the fundamental concept that, to obtain consistent, interpretable psychophysical measurements, one must always control the dimensions of stimulus intensity, wavelength, size, exposure duration, shape, relative locations of stimulus elements, cognitive meaning, location on the retina, and level of light adaptation. A now-classic experiment used to determine the absolute threshold of vision serves as a paradigm for how to perform psychophysical measurements of vision.

Each of Chapters 3 through 8 concentrates on measuring one characteristic of vision. Chapter 3 introduces the concepts involved in measuring thresholds of relative light sensitivity. The principles of measuring relative intensity discrimination are basic to subsequent chapters. Chapter 4 includes a further exploration of multiple stimulus dimensions as a function of time in the dark and as a function of background light levels. It introduces the fundamental neural processing that allows the eye to see over such a wide range of light intensities. Chapter 5 describes multiple measures of spatial acuity that are basic to the visual acuity measures that are so fundamental to the clinical examination of the visual system. Chapter 6 explores the importance of edges in detecting objects and the measurement of contrast sensitivity that is fundamental to the detection of edges and, hence, the identification of shapes. In Chapter 7, the effects of stimulus duration and fluctuations over time are described in more detail. Chapter 8 explores the use of single wavelength lights on discrimination and how we perceive wavelength mixtures.

Chapters 9 and 10 explore the effects of age at both extremes (infancy and aging). Because of the unique characteristics of infants and the elderly, the problems of distinguishing normal development and aging from pathologies when measuring vision in these age groups have required the invention of new psychophysical techniques.

To integrate the contributions of the multiple contributors to this book, the editors have worked to develop a consistency of style in presenting the text and graphics. One device used throughout the book is to replace the usual cryptic section headings with declarative statements. These make it immediately obvious to the reader the point of the subsequent text. They also serve as a quick study guide for students. Furthermore, it is possible to look at the statements in the table of contents for a chapter, or the book, and see how the story unfolds.

To create a consistently clean look to the figures in the book, all the graphs displaying quantitative information were digitized from the original sources and replotted by one of the editors (DC). Having the data in digital form not only enabled us to use a consistent style, it also allowed us to change scales to be consistent across related graphs, refit curves, invert axes, and perform other manipulations designed to either simplify or improve the expository value of a graph.

The resulting book, we hope, will be useful both for its descriptions of how vision is measured and for its information on visual function.

T.T.N.
D.A.C.
J.E.B.

Acknowledgments

A book such as this, designed as it is for students new to a discipline, attempts to integrate and simplify concepts as much as possible and present them at a level appropriate to what these students already know. In the bibliography, we acknowledge the work of many of the countless scientists who have contributed to our knowledge of visual function, and, here, acknowledge the work of the many more who could not be listed.

The chapter authors of this book deserve a special acknowledgment. They brought unique perspectives and expertise that ultimately melded well together and speak to the theme of this book. We thank them for their patience when it seemed as if their work would be for naught and for their forbearance as we worked to create a coherent voice throughout.

Our respective schools, deans, and department chairs also deserve an acknowledgment for their support in both resources and time. Our colleagues, too, generously supported us with critiques and served as sounding boards for our ideas. Gwendolyn Norton suggested the inclusion of glossary terms at the end of each chapter. Thanks to all.

We also acknowledge the contributions of the students in our classes who provided extremely valuable feedback as they used and critiqued the developing materials over the past several years. Their input should benefit the students who will be using this book in the future.

During the years that we have been working on this book, we have spent many evenings and weekends in front of a computer monitor or pouring over edited manuscript. We thank our families and our wives, Carol, Deane, and Marilyn, who have been very supportive of our efforts and understanding of our ups and downs through it all.

Finally, we thank the editors, Karen Oberheim in particular, and our publisher for continuing to support this project despite many missed deadlines. Thank you also to Lucinda Ewing for being so patient with us during the production process.

The Psychophysical
Measurement of
Visual Function

1   Principles of Psychophysical Measurement

David A. Corliss and Thomas T. Norton

Overview

Psychophysics is a scientific discipline designed to determine the relationship between a physical stimulus and a perceptual response signaled verbally or behaviorally. Measuring visual function, the theme of this book, requires an understanding of the available psychophysical tools. These tools include how to physically arrange a stimulus, change a single dimension of a stimulus to measure a specific aspect of vision, present a series of stimuli in systematic ways, elicit the desired response from the observer of the stimulus, and control for psychological bias that can distort the results.

Most psychophysical studies are designed to determine a threshold, which is defined as the minimum value of a stimulus required to elicit a perceptual response or an altered perceptual response. Because threshold measurements are subject to random variations in the physical stimulus, the physiological state of the observer's nervous system, attention, and psychological bias, the choice of a psychophysical method from the many available must be done carefully. Because clinical measures of visual function are derived from the scientific findings and methods, a clinician must understand how the method selected affects the outcome of any measurement. Consequently, this chapter describes the three classical psychophysical methods and their variations. It discusses ways of controlling for bias, including forced-choice methods and experimental procedures based on signal detection theory.

In addition to threshold measurements, psychophysical methods also are used to measure the magnitude of above-threshold sensations as a function of stimulus magnitude. It is important for a clinician to understand these relations and how they affect the accuracy of his or her own observational judgments and the verbal reports the patient makes during an examination.

Psychophysics

Psychophysics is the study of the relationship between physical stimuli and perceptual responses

Perception, the "appreciation of a physical situation through the mediation of one or more senses" (Hofstetter et al. 2000), occurs inside our brains and cannot be measured directly. Psychophysics (from the Greek *psyche* [soul] and the Latin *physica* [natural science]) has been developed as a way to measure the internal sensory and perceptual responses to external stimuli. To study this relationship scientifically, one must use a stimulus with well-defined physical characteristics and measure a well-defined behavioral response. For example, if an examiner turns on a light, a subject may state, "I see a light." The examiner can then determine how intense that light needs to be to elicit that response. The end result is a quantifiable relation between the physical stimulus, light intensity, and the subject's perceptual response. Note that the stimulus is always a physical entity that can be measured directly with instruments. The response can be verbal or, as in experiments with animals, it can be a criterion behavior. In all cases, the perception that occurs between the stimulus and response is inferred.

Psychophysics plays a fundamental role in the clinical examination of the eye and visual system

Any examination of the eye and visual system of a patient consists of a series of psychophysical tests. The patient indicates (verbally, or by other means) alterations in his or her perceptual response when some dimension of a physical stimulus is changed. Consider, for example, the familiar visual acuity test. The patient sits at a fixed distance from letters of varying size (the physical stimuli) and calls out the names of the letters (the perceptual response). The clinician records the accuracy of the patient's responses to determine the smallest letter size that the patient can recognize.

It is also important to note that, during an eye exam, a clinician, although not performing psychophysical self-tests, performs multiple tasks of a psychophysical nature. When examining the physical structures of the eye, it is necessary for the clinician to detect subtle variations in shape, clarity, or color that may signal the presence of an abnormality or pathology. A slight clouding of the lens may signal the beginnings of a cataract, for example, or the relative size of the arteries and veins that supply the retina with blood may signal hypertension. These tasks are psychophysical in nature, because the ability of the clinician to detect differences in lens clarity or the relative size of veins and arteries depends on the fact that the clinician's visual system produces different perceptual responses to differences in lens clarity or blood vessel diameter and color. There is the potential for more error in these kinds of psychophysical judgments than there is in simply detecting the presence or absence of a light because there is often not a simple linear relationship between the magnitude of a particular stimulus attribute and the magnitude of the corresponding perceptual response. This topic is discussed in more detail in the section Measuring the Magnitude of Sensations, later in this chapter.

Psychophysical measurements are used for descriptive and analytical purposes and to follow the course of treatment

Psychophysical measurements can be simply descriptive, providing a "specification of sensory capabilities" of the normal human visual system (Gescheider 1985). Thus, psychophysical methods have been used to establish normal levels of vision and the range of values in people with normal vision. Psychophysical measurements can also be used analytically to test hypotheses about the neural mechanisms that underlie the perceptual response of the subject (Gescheider 1985). For example, one might test the hypothesis that the relationship between the **brightness*** of an object and the light **intensity** striking the eye from the object corresponds to the relationship between the amount of light absorbed by the photoreceptors in the eye and the resulting number of **action potentials** that

*Words in bold are listed in the glossary.

reach the visual cortex. Brightness is a perceptual response that can only be measured psychophysically, and intensity can be measured with a light meter. The relationship between the amount of light absorbed and the resulting neural activity has been determined in a number of ways in humans and animal models. The results of testing this hypothesis provide scientists with an understanding of the physical basis of brightness and ultimately help a clinician to understand that, if a patient says, "The light on the left is brighter than the light on the right," the light on the left may not actually be physically more intense.

In a clinical setting, responses from patients can be used to understand the pathophysiology of abnormal conditions and monitor their response to treatment. Consider this scenario: A patient did not see a spot of light of moderate intensity because an orbital tumor that was pressing on the optic nerve prevented action potentials generated by retinal ganglion cells from reaching central visual structures and producing a perceptual response. Plotting the retinal locations where the patient could not detect the light helped to diagnose the location and extent of the tumor. Treating the tumor reduced the pressure and eventually allowed the action potentials to be conducted again to central structures, so that the subject could see the stimulus. The patient's initial loss of perceptual response to a physical stimulus helped the clinician to infer the mechanism behind the anomalous perceptual response. Monitoring the recovery of the response provided a measure of the effectiveness of the treatment.

Visual thresholds are the most common psychophysical measurement

The word **threshold** refers to a boundary separating stimulus values that elicit a response from stimulus values that do not elicit a response or elicit a different response. In vision, the **absolute threshold** is defined as the minimum amount of a stimulus required to detect the presence of that stimulus under ideal conditions. Both a **difference threshold** and an **increment threshold** are defined as the threshold for detecting that two stimuli differ in some stimulus characteristic, such as intensity. Chapter 2 discusses measurements of the absolute threshold for humans to detect light. Chapter 3 discusses increment thresholds.

A threshold measurement is not concerned with how a stimulus looks; it is of no interest that it may be pretty, large, or frightening. Rather, a threshold measurement determines whether the particular stimulus dimension that is being tested can be seen at all, or whether it is seen as different from another, similar stimulus.

The task required of a subject or patient during threshold measurements varies in complexity

The most basic question regarding vision that one can ask a subject or a patient is whether he or she does or does not see something. This is a **detection task**. An example of this task would be to find the absolute threshold for detecting a stimulus. For example, one could determine how many quanta a flash of light must contain to be at threshold for the perception of light (discussed in Chapter 2).

A second type of threshold task is a **discrimination task**. This measures the threshold for detecting that a test stimulus is different from a reference stimulus. One example of this task would be to determine how much more or less intense an already visible spot of light must be in comparison to another visible spot for the two spots to be seen as different in brightness. Alternatively, a subject might be asked whether there are one or two objects visible. The classic example of this task involves determining how far apart two point sources of light must be to be seen as two lights. Another example of a discrimination task would be to ask a subject to pick one particular object out of a field of similar objects. Examples would be to pick the "yield right-of-way" sign from a group of traffic signs or specify some aspect of the object, such as its orientation. This type of discrimination is discussed in Chapter 6.

A third kind of threshold measurement is recognition task. In this case, the object is already visible, and the person could be asked to name the object. Visual acuity tasks in which a subject says the names of letters would fall into this category.

The distinctions among these various types of tasks are not sharp. They are hierarchical in the sense that the perceptual processing required to produce a response becomes more complex as the tasks proceed from simple detection to recognition. It is not necessarily true in all cases, however, that performance on a higher level task, such as letter recognition, depends on being able to perform the task at a lower level of complexity, such as detection or discrimination. A patient might, for example, be able to recognize the letter *A* under some test conditions even if it is blurred beyond the eye's ability to discriminate its details or detect all parts of the letter.

Psychophysical Methods

Clinical psychophysical procedures evolved from laboratory examination techniques

Whether testing acuity with an eye chart, measuring a patient's visual fields with an automated perimeter, performing streak retinoscopy, or using an infrared autorefractor, an eye examination involves many psychophysical measures that have been devised using fundamental psychophysical principles that were first described in the mid-1800s by Gustav Fechner. Accomplishing tasks, such as efficiently determining acuity and refractive error or locating possible visual-field losses, requires the use of procedures that give accurate, reliable results (1) with the fewest number of stimulus presentations, (2) without requiring sophisticated judgments on the part of the patient, and (3) with minimal opportunities for psychological bias to affect the results. By the end of this chapter, it should be clear why controlling these factors is important and how that is achieved. First, however, it is necessary to consider a few of the many ways in which visual stimuli can be configured for presentation to elicit perceptual responses from subjects in psychophysical examinations.

The choice of stimulus configuration is determined by the question asked

Psychophysical measurements of visual function involve presenting visual stimuli that vary along any one of a number of possible dimensions, including intensity, wavelength, size, exposure duration, shape, relative locations of elements of the stimulus, and cognitive meaning. In addition, the location on the subject's retina and the level of light adaptation of the subject's visual system may need to be controlled. By combining these stimulus dimensions in various ways, an infinite number of possible stimuli can be presented. Later chapters show how, in any laboratory or clinical psychophysical procedure, the number of these stimulus variables to be altered should be kept as small as possible. In the ideal measurement procedure, all stimulus dimensions except one are fixed, and that one dimension is varied according to some pattern dictated by the psychophysical procedure that is used. To some extent, the type of psychophysical procedure that is used dictates the possible stimulus configurations and vice versa.

As an example of how choices are made about the stimulus configuration, consider the problem of determining how much light must be added to a stimulus or subtracted from it, before it can be detected as being different from the original intensity. Figures 1.1A, 1.1B, and 1.1C show a few of the traditional stimulus configurations that can be used to present stimuli in an increment threshold task. Figure 1.1D shows a stimulus configuration used for a difference threshold task (see Chapter 3). All are presented on a completely dark background.

In Figure 1.1A, the larger gray region represents a reference field that has a certain **luminance** L. (Luminance is a measure of light intensity; see Appendix.) The reference field surrounds a smaller test field that has a variable luminance L_T. When making a psychophysical measurement, L remains constant. L_T is varied such that the test field becomes more intense than L, as in the example in the left column of Figure 1.1A, or less intense than L, as in the right column of Figure 1.1A. The subject responds to successive presentations of the stimulus by indicating whether the brightness of L_T is the same as or different from L. With proper psychophysical procedures, the minimum value of L_T needed for it to be seen as different from L can be determined.

Figure 1.2 shows the same stimuli as Figure 1.1A and the inter-relationship between L, L_T, and ΔL (the change in L) that is of importance throughout this text. When one determines the threshold value of L_T that is seen as brighter (or dimmer) than L, one also determines the threshold amount of light, ΔL, that needs to be added to (or subtracted from) L to make L_T be seen as brighter (or dimmer). Three facts to remember are (1) L + ΔL is a luminance value, L_T; (2) L_T differs from L by the value of ΔL; and (3) there are many ΔL values, but only one is the threshold ΔL—the minimum ΔL required to make L_T appear different from L.

Figure 1.1B shows another stimulus configuration called a *bipartite field*. Again, L is the luminance of the reference field and L_T is the luminance of the test field. A bipartite field makes it easy to minimize the effects of visual adaptation by briefly presenting L and L_T simultaneously against an otherwise dark field. In determining the minimum value of L_T needed for it to be seen as brighter than L, L_T should sometimes be presented on the left and sometimes on the right. This prevents subjects from discovering a position cue, such as the brighter side being always on the left or the right.

The arrangement in Figure 1.1C is a bipartite field surrounded by an **adapting field**. The adapting field may be very large or only slightly larger than the bipartite field. The luminance of the adapting field can be used to set the adaptation level of the visual system (discussed in Chapter 4). This stimulus configu-

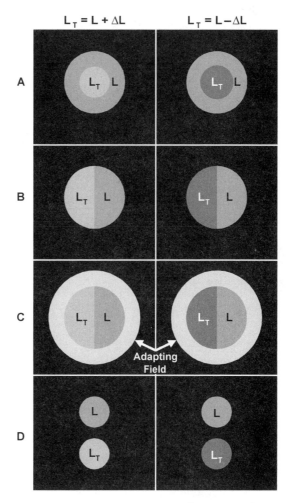

FIGURE 1.1   *Examples of stimulus configurations used in intensity discrimination tasks. The left column shows configurations in which the test fields are more intense than the reference fields. In the right columns, the test fields are less intense than the reference fields. **A–C** show stimuli used for increment threshold measurements; **D** shows separated stimuli used for difference threshold measurements. **A.** A test field of luminance L_T surrounded by a reference field of luminance L. The test field on the left has a luminance ($L_T = L + \Delta L$) that is greater than the reference field. The test field on the right has a luminance ($L_T = L - \Delta L$) that is less than that of the reference field. **B.** This configuration is called a bipartite field. **C.** A bipartite field surrounded by an adapting field. **D.** Physically separated test and comparison fields configured for measuring a difference threshold.*

ration mimics normal viewing more closely than the other two stimulus configurations because the visual system normally operates at a level of adaptation above that which would be provided by a black background.

In Figure 1.1D, the stimuli labeled L and L_T are physically separated. Although shown against a dark field, they could also be presented on a luminous adapting field. An intensity discrimination in which the stimuli that are to be compared are physically separated is called a *difference threshold task*.

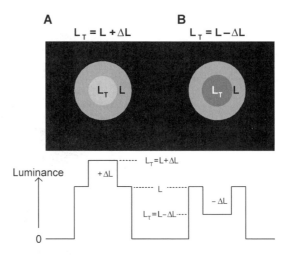

FIGURE 1.2   *Appearance of stimuli (**top**) and their luminance profiles (**bottom**). **A.** The central test field luminance (L_T) is more intense than the luminance of the reference field (L) by the value of ΔL. **B.** The central test field luminance (L_T) is less intense than the reference field luminance (L) by the value of ΔL.*

Psychophysically measured threshold values vary because of fluctuations in the stimulus, neural activity, attention, and psychological bias

It was once thought that sensory systems responded in an all-or-none fashion. This would mean that, for any given physical dimension of a stimulus, there would be one particular value below which the stimulus would never be detected and above which it would always be detected. It is now known that the threshold almost always shows some variability from trial to trial within a measurement session and across several sessions. The threshold may even depend somewhat on the type of psychophysical test that was used.

One reason for variability in the measured threshold value of a stimulus is that, under some conditions, such as testing the absolute threshold of vision (covered in Chapter 2), random fluctuations in the stimulus occur and can impact the threshold measurement.

Another reason for variability is that there are continual, random fluctuations in the activity levels of the neurons carrying visual signals from the retina to more central visual structures. Even if the identical stimulus is presented repeatedly, the neural response varies somewhat from presentation to presentation.

For example, the three rows of action potentials in Figure 1.3 are the responses of the same neuron to three separate presentations of a near-threshold stimulus. Each time the stimulus was presented, the neuron responded with a different number of action potentials during the 0.5 second period when the stimulus was presented. On a stimulus presentation trial when a strong response occurred, such as in the top row of the figure, the stimulus might be above threshold. On a trial when a weak response occurred, such as that shown in the middle row, the stimulus might be below threshold. In this example, the stimulus was the same on each trial. It was the nervous system that exhibited variability.

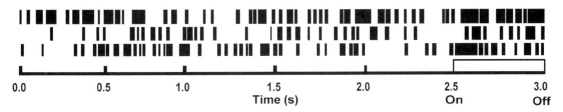

FIGURE 1.3   *Responses of a neuron in the lateral geniculate nucleus of an anesthetized cat to three presentations of a near-threshold visual stimulus. Each small vertical line represents an action potential produced by the neuron. Each row shows the responses of the neuron in a 3 second period. From 0.0 to 2.5 seconds, only a background luminance was present. The light stimulus was turned on at 2.5 seconds and turned off at 3 seconds, so the stimulus was on for only 0.5 second. (From DW Godwin, TT Norton, unpublished data.)*

Note also that the neuron produced action potentials during the period (from 0.0 to 2.5 seconds) when the stimulus was not being presented. This maintained, or spontaneous, activity was primarily due to the presence of a constant background luminance. This constitutes background noise, similar to static on a telephone line, which can make it difficult to hear what the other person says during a telephone conversation. As discussed later in this chapter, for a visual stimulus to be seen, the neurons in the visual system must respond strongly enough to the stimulus for the response to be distinguishable from the action potentials produced when the stimulus is absent. On this basis, the bottom trace is most likely to be above threshold because the response to the stimulus is most different from the spontaneous activity.

A third reason for variability in threshold values is that a person's level of alertness or attention can vary. A boring and repetitive task can decrease the level of alertness. If there is a long interval between stimuli with nothing else happening, attention may wander. Through either decreased alertness or wandering attention, stimuli that are actually above threshold may be missed.

A fourth factor that contributes to the variability of the measurements is psychological bias. One person might bias his or her threshold measurement by responding to a stimulus only when he or she is absolutely sure that it was present. Another person might adopt a strategy of responding to a stimulus whenever there is the slightest hint that one is present. These biases can creep into the clinical situation in unexpected ways. For example, a patient who is angry because she sat in a waiting room for an hour may give different threshold responses than one who is seen on time. Also, the clinician is not immune; a clinician who has just learned that he did not detect elevated blood pressure in a previous patient who then had a stroke may change his threshold for deciding whether to refer the next patient for treatment of elevated blood pressure.

As a result of these four types of variability, a carefully measured threshold really comprises a small range of stimulus values over which the probability of the perceptual response changes. Scientists and clinicians, however, want to record a single threshold value. In the mid-1800s, Gustav Fechner devised the three general psychophysical methods described in the following sections to accomplish just that. They are directed at measuring the probability of detecting the various levels of stimulus (or detecting a change in the stimulus level) to determine a single value that best describes threshold under a particular set of conditions. With these methods, quite precise estimates of threshold can be obtained.

In the Method of Constant Stimuli, the examiner randomly presents a set of stimuli with fixed, predetermined values

In Chapter 2, a psychophysical study by Hecht, Shlaer, and Pirenne is described in which they determined the least amount of light that a flashed spot must contain to be detected. They used a special case of the stimulus configuration shown in Figure 1.1A in which L was 0. They presented brief flashes (L_T) to a subject who was sitting in the dark and asked whether each flash was visible. Because they had collected some preliminary data, they had a fairly good idea of how much light would be below threshold and never be seen and how much light would be above threshold and visible all the time. Because it is considered to be the most accurate psychophysical method, they used the **Method of Constant Stimuli** (Graham 1965b; Kling & Riggs 1971). In this method, the examiner selects a fixed set of stimulus values (usually 5–9) covering a range such that the lowest values are expected to be slightly below the threshold and the highest values are expected to be slightly above threshold. Each stimulus value is then presented many times in random order. After each stimulus presentation (also called a *trial*), the subject is asked to indicate whether he or she detected the stimulus. In a simple threshold measurement, each stimulus value might be presented 50 times or more.

To determine the threshold, the percent of time that the subject detected the stimulus (the percent of "yes" responses) is plotted against the stimulus dimension (test field intensity). The result is an S-shaped (ogive) **psychometric function**,* also called a **frequency-of-seeing curve**, like the one shown in Figure 1.4. Threshold is usually taken as the point where the subject detects the stimulus 50% of the time. In this example, that stimulus value corresponds to 5.0 units of test field intensity, as indicated by the arrow in Figure 1.4. Thus, in this example, absolute threshold would be 5.0 units. The selection of the 50% point as threshold is somewhat arbitrary, and some investigators use slightly higher values.

The Method of Constant Stimuli, when used properly, gives highly accurate estimates of absolute thresholds and, with some modifications, of intensity discrimination thresholds. Many of the threshold values listed in texts were derived using this method. It is, however, subject to the effects of guessing and other biases. For this reason, methods to counteract the effects of guessing and subject biases have been devised as described later in this chapter. Also, because the Method of Constant Stimuli requires many trials using stimuli that are above and below the value that is eventually determined to be the threshold, it is rather inefficient and is rarely used in clinical measurements.

---

*In Chapter 6, it is useful to know that a psychometric function is equivalent to a cumulative normal distribution. The mean of the distribution occurs at the 50% point.

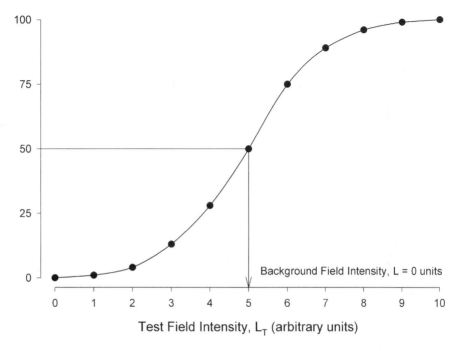

Percent "YES"
Responses

Background Field Intensity, L = 0 units

Test Field Intensity, L_T (arbitrary units)

FIGURE 1.4   *Idealized psychometric function for a threshold detection task using the Method of Constant Stimuli. The threshold stimulus value is obtained by drawing a horizontal line from the 50% value on the response axis to the psychometric function and then dropping a vertical line from the function to the test field intensity axis.*

In the Method of Limits, the examiner sequentially presents a set of stimuli with fixed values

Table 1.1 presents simulated results from a threshold examination using the **Method of Limits** (Kling & Riggs 1971). As was the case with the Method of Constant Stimuli, the examiner chooses a set of stimulus values that span the expected threshold. The stimuli are then presented sequentially starting, for instance, with values below the expected threshold. The stimulus values are listed in the first column and the subject's responses are listed for five trials in the next five columns. The intensity is increased step-by-step, until the subject detects the stimulus. Because a subject might say, "Yes, I see it" when the stimulus is still below threshold owing to any of the four types of variability discussed earlier in this chapter, it is safer to proceed to increase the stimulus until two successive "yes" responses are reported in the ascending direction, as shown in Table 1.1. The transitions, the stimulus values where the response changes from "yes" to "no" or vice versa, are noted with a dark line. In the first trial, because the subject did not detect the stimulus when its value was 5, but did detect it with values of 6 and 7, the transition value is recorded as 5.5. The examiner then reverses the order of presentation and, starting at the top of the selected range of stimulus values, decreases the value of the stimulus, until

TABLE 1.1   Example of subject's responses over five trials using the Method of Limits

Stimulus value	Trial number (stimulus presentation direction)					
	1 (ascending)	2 (descending)	3 (ascending)	4 (descending)	5 (ascending)	Average
1	N		N		N	
2	N	N	N		N	
3	Y	N	N		Y	
4	N	Y	Y	N	Y	
5	N	Y	Y	N		
6	Y	Y		Y		
7	Y	Y		N		
8		Y		Y		
9		Y				
10		Y				
Transition	5.5	3.5	3.5	5.5	2.5	4.1

N = "no" response; Y = "yes" response. Horizontal lines indicate the transition points.

the subject reports not seeing it on two successive stimulus values. The ascending and descending stimulus procedures are repeated several times. The mean value of the transitions for all the trials is the threshold L_T. The result is 4.1 in this example.

The Method of Limits is more efficient than the Method of Constant Stimuli because fewer trials are presented. Stimulus values significantly less or greater than the threshold are omitted after the transition point has been reached. There are two potential problems with this method, however. First, because stimulus intensities are presented sequentially, subjects can come to realize that, if the initial trials in a series contain below-threshold stimuli, higher stimulus values will eventually be presented. They may *anticipate* that the higher values will be detectable and respond with a "yes" for a stimulus value that is actually below threshold. Similarly, they may give anticipatory "no" responses in a descending series.

A second problem is that subjects may adopt the opposite strategy. Instead of anticipating and changing early, they may be reluctant to switch from a "no" to a "yes" (or vice versa) and *perseverate*, meaning that they continue giving the same response that they have been giving. To some extent, anticipation and perseveration can be counteracted by starting the ascending or descending series at various stimulus values, as in trial 4 of Table 1.1, so that sometimes threshold is reached after only a few stimuli have been presented, and sometimes it is not reached until after more have been presented. As long as the subject consistently perseverates (or anticipates) on ascending and descending trials, the measured threshold is not seriously affected, because it is the average of the transition points. If the subject consistently anticipates in one direction and perseverates in the other direction, the measured threshold value is affected. In some circumstances, only the ascending or descending portion of the Method of Limits is used. In such cases, the effects of anticipa-

TABLE 1.2   Example of a subject's responses over 17 trials using the staircase variation on the Method of Limits

Stimulus value	Trial number 1	2	3	4	5	6	7	8	9	10	11	12	13	14	15	16	17
1																	
2											N						
3							N			N							N
4						N			Y			N				N	
5					Y			Y					N		Y		
6				N										Y			
7			Y														
8		Y															
9	Y																

N = "no" response; Y = "yes" response. Horizontal lines indicate the transition points.

tion or perseveration are not counterbalanced, and care should be taken to learn whether these factors may have affected the measured threshold.

To avoid these limitations, two variations on the Method of Limits have been devised. One variation is called the *staircase procedure* (Cornsweet 1962). In the staircase procedure, the examiner reverses the direction of stimulus values to be presented based on some criterion sequence of responses. For instance, in Table 1.2, the stimulus values were decreased on successive trials, until the subject reported that the stimulus was not seen for two successive trials. The examiner then increased the stimulus by two steps. If the subject reported seeing the stimulus, the descending staircase then continued, until the subject again did not detect the stimulus on two successive trials. The intensity was increased again by two steps; this time the subject did not detect the stimulus, so on the next trial, the stimulus value was increased by one step. When the subject reported detecting the stimulus, the values were again decreased in a stepwise manner. As in the standard Method of Limits, threshold is taken as the mean value of the transition points (4.5 in this example).

With the staircase procedure, the stimulus values never stray far from the threshold value, making this a very efficient procedure. However, although the subject is not informed of the rule the examiner is using to raise or lower the stimulus value on successive trials, the staircase method can be affected by other strategies on the part of a subject. For instance, he or she might recognize that, after two or three failures to detect the stimulus, the stimulus is always detectable, and this information might alter his or her responses. To avoid the subject's discovery of a pattern, two (or more) simultaneous staircases are often used in which a computer keeps track of the subject's performance and randomly selects whether to present a particular stimulus value based on the performance on the first staircase or second staircase.

A second variation is called *tracking* (Békésy 1947). In tracking, the stimulus dimension of interest is gradually raised or lowered, usually by a computerized apparatus, at a smooth, constant rate. If the starting point is below threshold, the subject indicates when the stimulus becomes visible, usually by pressing a button. The apparatus then reverses the direction of change of the stimulus dimension. For example, if the stimulus was getting more intense, it then becomes less intense as a function of time. The subject indicates when the stimulus is no longer visible by releasing the button. This routine is continued until many reversals have occurred. The threshold is taken as the average of the stimulus value at the reversal points. Because the stimulus value is always changing in the vicinity of the threshold value, tracking is a very efficient procedure. This procedure can be very tiring to patients because the stimulus may frequently cross threshold in short time periods.

Other variations on the Method of Limits are still being devised. Most commercial instruments that determine threshold, such as visual field testing instruments, use staircase strategies with rules and step size changes that have been thoroughly tested so that they determine the threshold with maximum accuracy, reliability, and efficiency.

In the Method of Adjustment, the subject controls the stimulus values

In some ways, the **Method of Adjustment** is the simplest and most direct method for estimating thresholds. The examiner simply provides the subject with a dial or another device that controls the stimulus parameter being investigated and an instruction such as, "Set the dial so that the light is just visible." The examiner begins each trial by setting the initial value of the stimulus well above or below the threshold and then allows the subject to adjust the stimulus to whatever criterion is being tested. In an absolute threshold measurement, the criterion response would occur either when the stimulus disappears or appears. In an increment or difference threshold measurement, the analysis is a little more complex. The subject's task is to adjust L_T (see Figure 1.1), until it appears to exactly match the brightness of L. A trial ends when the subject decides that a match, or *point of subjective equality*, has been reached.

The result over several trials is a small range of values of L_T, where L_T is judged to be equal to L. It has been found that these values of L_T are normally distributed with a mean approximately equal to L. As shown in Figure 1.5, the frequency with which L_T is judged equal to L decreases as L_T increasingly differs from L, that is, as it becomes increasingly less than L and greater than L.

As with the other psychophysical methods, in the Method of Adjustment the threshold value of L_T is based on a frequency of seeing of 50%. In this case, however, the threshold is determined on the basis of where L_T is seen as the same as L in 50% of trials and as different from L in 50% of trials. In a normal distribution, 50% of the distribution lies between plus 0.68 and minus 0.68 standard deviation from the mean (see vertical lines in Figure 1.5). Thus, an L_T with a value that differs from the mean value, L, by ΔL of ± 0.68 times the standard deviation is detected as different from L in 50% of the trials.

The Method of Adjustment is most easily used when the stimulus can be changed in a continuous manner, rather than in steps, although it can be used in a step-wise procedure in which the subject changes the stimulus value between stimulus presentations. Subjects generally enjoy the Method of Adjustment because they actively participate. Boredom and inattention are less of a problem with the Method of Adjustment than with the other methods.

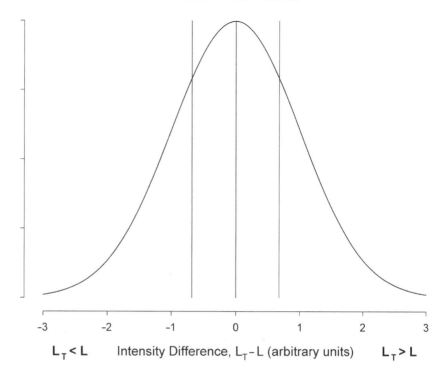

Frequency with which L_T is seen as equal to L

−0.68 SD   Mean   +0.68 SD

-3   -2   -1   0   1   2   3

$L_T < L$ Intensity Difference, $L_T − L$ (arbitrary units) $L_T > L$

FIGURE 1.5   *Hypothetical data for the frequency of seeing the test field, L_T, as equal in brightness to the reference field, L, as a function of the intensity difference between them. The mean of the normal distribution is 0.0, and the standard deviation is 1.0. The threshold ΔL is taken as the value of ΔL that, when added to or subtracted from L, is detectable on 50% of the trials. This occurs at 0.68 standard deviations (SDs) above and below the mean.*

One potential problem with the Method of Adjustment is that subjects may use the position of the dial as a cue to where threshold ought to be. If the position is obvious, the subject may move the dial from a clear subthreshold value to a clear suprathreshold value and then select an intermediate position as the threshold. In other words, the subject brackets the threshold value. This strategy can be foiled by using a dial that has no numbers and a variable amount of slip, so that turning the dial a certain amount produces variable changes in L_T.

Controlling Response Bias and Guessing

Response bias and guessing on the part of patients or subjects during psychophysical measurements have been mentioned in previous sections because they occur frequently and can seriously affect the measured thresholds. There are instances, for example, when a person may have strong bias toward saying that he or she sees something (e.g., "If I can show I see very well, I may be able to keep my driver's license, even though I'm 92 years old"). Similarly, he or she may have a bias against seeing (e.g., "If I see poorly, I might avoid combat"). As a result of bias, there are a preponderance of guesses in one direction or the other. If it is beneficial to demonstrate an ability to detect a stimulus, there are more positive responses to stimuli below threshold. If it is more beneficial to not detect the stimulus, the converse is true.

Catch trials can be used to correct for guessing

One method that psychophysicists have devised to determine the degree to which a subject is guessing is to include random *catch trials*. These are trials in which either a stimulus that should not be detected, or one that should always be detected is presented. The subject usually is not informed that catch trials are being included. A subject who has a strong bias toward a positive response responds "yes" on some catch trials when a low stimulus value is presented. A subject with a bias toward a negative response responds "no" on a fraction of catch trials with a high stimulus value. In practice, it is not necessary to use catch trials that are far below or above threshold. When the Method of Constant Stimuli is used, it is sufficient to simply ensure that the range of stimulus values used includes at least one value that can always be seen and one that can never be seen. Figure 1.6 shows such a situation.

The upper psychometric function in Figure 1.6 shows that the percent of "yes" responses did not decline to zero at low stimulus values but appeared to plateau. In this case, when no stimulus was present ($L_T = 0$), the subject reported "yes" on 30% of the trials. This indicates that the subject had a bias for responding that the stimulus was visible when it really was not. If one ignored the guessing and used as threshold the stimulus value at which the subject reported the stimulus to be visible on 50% of the trials, the threshold would be an L_T of 4.0 units. A subject with a strong bias for "no" responses would have a psychometric function with an inverse pattern: the pattern would begin at 0% "yes" for low values but would plateau at some level below 100% "yes" for high stimulus values. The problem is how to correct such curves for the subject's tendency to guess.

A basic assumption made in correcting for guessing is that the guessing rate is constant throughout the range of stimuli. In the example in Figure 1.6, it would be assumed that the subject would guess "yes" on 30% of any trial where he or she did not see the stimulus. The observed fraction of "yes" responses is therefore the sum of two components. The first component is the fraction of trials in which the subject truly saw the stimulus. The second is the fraction of trials in which the subject truly did not see it, multiplied by the guessing rate. The correction factor is thus:

$$\text{True Percent of "Yes" Responses} = \frac{\text{Observed Fractions of "Yes" Responses} - \text{Guessing Rate}}{1 - \text{Guessing Rate}} \times 100$$

Eq. 1.1

The two extremes of the curve in Figure 1.6 are helpful in understanding how this correction for guessing works. When the stimulus intensity is 0,

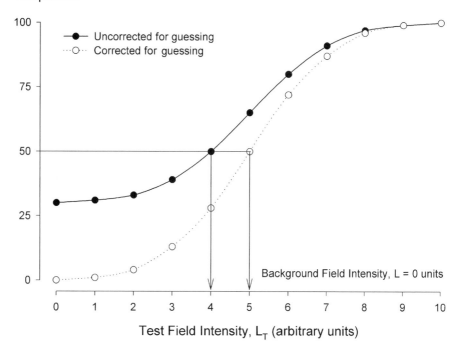

Percent "YES"
Responses

FIGURE 1.6   *Frequency of seeing curves before (**upper curve**) and after (**lower curve**) correction for guessing. Note that the amount of correction decreases as the stimulus value increases.*

the stimulus cannot ever really be seen. So, when the subject says, "Yes, I see it" 30% of the time, one can be sure that he or she is guessing. The corrected fraction of "yes" responses should be equal to zero. To achieve this, the guessing rate (0.3) is subtracted from the observed fraction of "yes" responses (0.3), giving 0 in the numerator of Equation 1.1, so the resulting **true percent of "yes" responses** is 0. When the stimulus value is 10, the subject says, "Yes, I see it" on 100% of the trials, presumably because the stimulus is visible on every trial. Thus, the corrected curve at that stimulus value should still have a value of 100%. Equation 1.1 achieves this goal. The numerator and the denominator are both equal to 1.0–0.3, so the result (0.7/0.7 × 100) is 100%. The same principle applies for all intermediate values. The lower curve in Figure 1.6 was calculated by applying Equation 1.1 to each point on the upper curve, yielding a higher threshold value of 5.0. A similar equation can be used to compensate if a subject has a bias toward saying that the stimulus was not visible when it really was. In this case, the correction equation would raise the corrected values toward 100%.

Although the correction equation works well in this example, in practice it is possible that the guessing rate is not constant across stimulus values. In addition, the guessing rate can be biased by simply telling the subject that there is only going to be a small fraction of catch trials on one set of trials and a large number of catch trials on the next set of trials.

The two-alternative forced-choice procedure sets the guessing rate at 50%

A better method of compensating for response bias and guessing is to force the subject to make choices between two or more alternatives. In the forced-choice variation (Blackwell 1953) on the Method of Constant Stimuli or the Method of Limits, the stimulus is presented either in one of two temporal intervals or in one of two spatial positions. There may, in fact, be more than two, but a two-choice situation is the one most frequently used. In a two-alternative forced-choice situation, the subject is forced to choose one of the time intervals or one of the positions in which he or she thought the stimulus appeared. One of the two choices does not contain the stimulus and the other one does, with a random assignment of the stimulus to each choice over a set of trials. The (testable) presumption is that a subject is not biased toward either of the choices.

The virtue of the forced-choice variation is that the guessing rate is established by the number of choices, not by the subject's biases, so the correction for guessing uses Equation 1.1, with the guessing rate set at a known value. In a two-alternative forced-choice procedure, the guessing rate is 0.5 for each choice. Using Equation 1.1, an observed fraction of 75% "yes" responses would convert to a true fraction of 50%, which would be used as the threshold value.

The forced-choice technique has an additional advantage: The examiner can give the subject feedback on whether he or she responded correctly on the previous trial. This can help the subject to perform at optimal levels as the testing session proceeds. Although the forced-choice procedure can help to control guessing, subject biases can still affect threshold measurements. A way to control subject bias using insights gained from signal detection theory is described after this topic has been introduced in the following section.

Using Signal Detection Theory to Understand Threshold Variability and to Control Subject Bias

At threshold, neurons must "decide" whether a stimulus is present against a background of noise

The idea was introduced, earlier in this chapter, that threshold can vary from trial to trial because there is inherent variability, or noise, in the threshold of the subject. This section describes how this noise leads to situations in which biases on the part of the subject influence the threshold.

One place in which noise is introduced is at the level of individual neurons. This is due to random variability in the firing rate of the neurons in the visual pathway whether the stimulus is absent or present. When the stimulus value is well above threshold, there are always more action potentials produced when a stimulus is present than when it is absent.* When the stimulus value is close to threshold, neural fluctuations make it difficult to set a single criterion level for the number of action potentials that accurately signal that a stimulus is present (see Figure 1.3). The neuron might randomly have produced a brief period of relatively rapid firing in the absence of the stimulus or might produce few action potentials when the stimulus is present.

In the example shown in Figure 1.7A, the number of action potentials that were produced in 30 repeated trials by a single retinal ganglion cell ranged from one to nine during a 50 millisecond sample period when only the background luminance was present. The 50 millisecond period was picked for this example because the nervous system seems to sample over approximately this time period. Most often, five action potentials occurred. When a stimulus was presented on a series of 30 trials (Figure 1.7B), the number of action potentials ranged from 6 to 14, with 10 action potentials occurring most frequently. A comparison of the distributions in Figure 1.7A and Figure 1.7B shows that when fewer than six action potentials occurred, the message is clear: No stimulus was present. Similarly, whenever more than nine action potentials occurred, a stimulus was always present. In the range of six to nine action potentials, the two distributions overlap. This means that the stimulus could have been present or absent when these numbers of action potentials occurred. In this ambiguous situation, the cells deeper in the brain that receive these action potentials must "decide" whether or not a stimulus was present based on other factors. This is where the subject's biases play a role.[†]

There is no single, optimal criterion number of action potentials that the nervous system should use to decide whether to respond as though a stimulus were present or not present. Thus, threshold is set based on other factors that constitute biases. If the neural distributions in Figure 1.7 happened to occur in a retinal ganglion cell in the eye of a mouse that was out foraging for food in an area frequented by rattlesnakes, the mouse might have the bias that detecting snakes was more important than getting that next bunch of seeds. In such a case (and presuming that the mouse depended on this one neuron to detect the snake), she might set her criterion for threshold at a low level, so that every occasion when six or more action potentials occurred during the sample period, she would decide, "Yes, a snake is there" and scamper back to the safety of her nest.

Figure 1.8A shows the *payoff matrix* that would pertain if the mouse were to set its criterion level at six. The columns in the matrix indicate whether the stimulus (the snake) is actually present or absent on a given trial. The rows indicate how the mouse can respond to the two conditions. Out of the four possible outcomes, there are two ways to be correct: by deciding that the stimulus is there when it is present (a **Hit**) and by deciding that it is not there when

---

*Although some neurons in the visual pathway reduce their activity when a stimulus is presented, the nervous system appears generally to use increases in firing rate to signal the presence of a stimulus in threshold situations (Barlow 1972).

[†]Although the central visual areas receive activity from many afferent neurons, if all afferent neurons show similar variability, the central neurons that produce a "perceptual response" receive ambiguous information when the stimulus value is close to threshold.

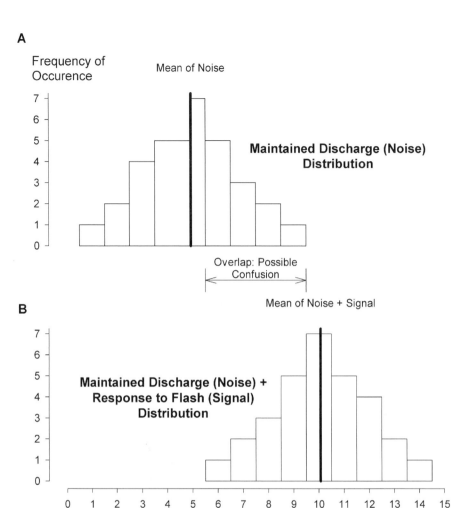

A

Frequency of Occurence

Mean of Noise

Maintained Discharge (Noise) Distribution

Overlap: Possible Confusion

Mean of Noise + Signal

B

Maintained Discharge (Noise) + Response to Flash (Signal) Distribution

Number of Action Potentials in 50 msec Period

FIGURE 1.7 *Frequency distributions of the number of action potentials produced by a retinal ganglion cell under two conditions. **A.** The maintained discharge, sampled during thirty 50 millisecond periods when only the background luminance was present. This is considered background noise. **B.** The distribution of the number of action potentials that occurred in 30 similar 50 millisecond time periods when the stimulus was present. The number of action potentials in **B** is the sum of both the noise and the additional action potentials produced by the stimulus, the signal. The difficulty faced by the nervous system is to decide whether a stimulus was present when the number of action potentials could have been produced by the noise alone.*

it is absent (a **Correct Rejection**). There are also two ways to be wrong: by deciding that the stimulus is present when it is absent (a **False Alarm**) and by deciding that it is not present when it is (a **Miss**).

As shown in Figure 1.8A, with a criterion of six, the mouse would always decide that the snake was present when one was, in fact, sitting there hidden in the bushes. However, there is a cost to setting the threshold criterion so low. Thirty-seven percent of the time she would also decide that a snake was present

A. Criterion for "seeing" = 6 action potentials

Response	Stimulus Present	Stimulus Absent
"I see it."	Hits (H) n = 30	False Alarms (FA) n = 11
"I don't see it."	Misses (M) n = 0	Correct Rejections (CR) n = 19

Hit Rate = H/(H+M)   False Alarm Rate = FA/(FA+CR)
= 30/(30+0) = 1.00   = 11/(11+19) = 0.37

Miss Rate = M/(H+M)   Correct Rejection Rate = CR/(FA+CR)
= 0/(30+0) = 0   = 19/(11+19) = 0.63

B. Criterion for "seeing" = 10 action potentials

Response	Stimulus Present	Stimulus Absent
"I see it."	Hits (H) n = 19	False Alarms (FA) n = 0
"I don't see it."	Misses (M) n = 11	Correct Rejections (CR) n = 30

Hit Rate = H/(H+M)   False Alarm Rate = FA/(FA+CR)
= 19/(19+11) = 0.63   = 0/(0+30) = 0.00

Miss Rate = M/(H+M)   Correct Rejection Rate = CR/(FA+CR)
= 11/(19+11) = 0.37   = 30/(0+30) = 1.00

FIGURE 1.8 *Hypothetical payoff matrices showing the effect of using two different criteria to decide whether a stimulus was present given the distributions of "noise" and "noise plus signal" in Figure 1.7. **A**. The criterion is "yes, the snake is present" if six or more action potentials occur. **B**. The criterion is raised to ten action potentials for the mouse to decide that the snake is present. See text for more details.*

when there was no snake. These False Alarms have a cost: The mouse expends energy scampering back to her hole and doesn't get as much food as she might. As a result, the mouse might grow hungry enough to raise her criterion so that she only decides there is a snake when ten or more action potentials occur (Figure 1.8B). This would reduce the False Alarm rate to zero, saving the mouse from interrupting her feeding to scamper back to her nest when there was no snake. However, raising the criterion to ten also means that there would be occasions (37% of the time) when the mouse would decide that there is no snake when one really is present, perhaps committing a fatal error.

In Figure 1.8, the payoff matrix is shown for only two possible criteria. The mouse could, at least theoretically, set the criterion for "yes, it is there" as low as one action potential (in which case she would starve!) or as high as 15 (in

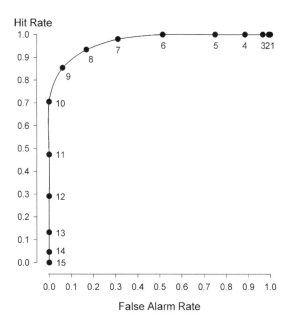

FIGURE 1.9   *Receiver operating characteristic curve derived from the distributions shown in Figure 1.7. The number beside each point is the criterion value (the threshold). If the criterion is set at 15 action potentials, there are zero Hits and zero False Alarms. If it is set at 14, there are a few Hits but zero False Alarms. As the criterion is decreased further, the Hit rate increases, but the False Alarm rate remains at zero until the criterion reaches nine, at which point the False Alarm rate begins to increase. As the threshold is further lowered, through the overlap region in Figure 1.7, the Hit and False Alarm rates increase. For criteria below six, there is no further increase in Hit rate, but the False Alarm rate climbs toward 1.0.*

which case the snake would feast!). The effect of changing the criterion on the number of Hits and False Alarms can be summarized in a *receiver operating characteristic* (ROC) curve, as shown in Figure 1.9. ROC curves originated in analyzing communications systems and have had widespread use for signal detection in a variety of fields (Tanner & Swets 1954).

Starting with a criterion of 15 (plotted as 0, 0 in Figure 1.9) and reducing the criterion toward zero, the mouse can achieve a Hit rate of 71% at a criterion of 10 before getting any False Alarms. As the criterion is lowered further, the number of False Alarms increases rapidly, while the Hit rate increases slowly to a maximum of 1 with a criterion value of 1.0. At the lowest criterion value, the Hit and False Alarm rates are 1.0. As described in the next sections, ROC curves and signal detection theory are of use in explaining threshold variability in humans and as a tool to control bias when measuring thresholds.

Signal detection theory also applies to human perceptual responses

For human subjects or patients who are in a threshold measurement situation, the combined effects of neural variability, attention, and psychological bias can produce variability in the magnitude of the perceptual response. The perceptual response when the stimulus is absent ("noise") and when a stimulus is

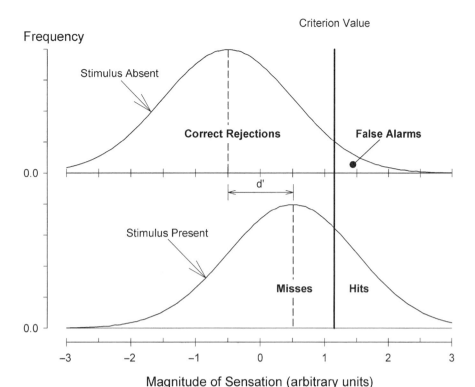

FIGURE 1.10   *Distribution of hypothetical "perceptual response" in a human subject over many trials when the stimulus was absent (**top**) and when the stimulus was present (**bottom**). The criterion value (**vertical line**) indicates the criterion a subject would adopt if Hits, Misses, False Alarms, and Correct Rejections had the rewards and costs listed in Figure 1.13.*

present ("signal plus noise") can be modeled as two normal distributions, as shown in Figure 1.10. Note the similarity to Figure 1.7. In Figure 1.10, the horizontal axis represents the magnitude of the perceptual response, increasing to the right, and the vertical axis represents the frequency with which each perceptual response magnitude occurs over many trials. The means of the two distributions in Figure 1.10 are shown as the dashed vertical lines. They have been given arbitrarily the values of –0.5 (stimulus absent) and +0.5 (stimulus present). The distance between the two means is determined by the stimulus strength because the stimulus is added to the noise. This distance is characterized by a parameter called **d'** (pronounced "**d prime**"). The value of d' is equal to the difference between the two means divided by the common standard deviation of the two distributions. In Figure 1.10, d' equals 1.0 because the difference between the means is 1.0 and the standard deviations of the two distributions are equal to 1.0 in this hypothetical example.

The strength of the stimulus used in Figure 1.10 was near threshold, which caused the distributions to overlap over almost the whole range of perceptual responses. Therefore, no single criterion perceptual response could be used to decide whether the stimulus was present or absent. In Figure 1.10, one of the many possible criterion values is shown as the thick vertical line. Whether the stimulus was absent or present, if a subject were to use that criterion, then any time the perceptual response exceeded that criterion value, he or she would decide that a stimulus was present. In the stimulus-present distribution, the area to the right of the criterion line represents the relative probability of a Hit when the stimulus is present. The area to the left of the criterion line in this distribution is the relative frequency of a Miss. In the stimulus-absent distribution, the area under the curve to the right of the criterion line represents the relative probability of a False Alarm. The area to the left of that line represents the relative probability of a Correct Rejection.

If a much stronger stimulus had been used, the lower distribution would be shifted to the right and there would be no overlap with the noise distribution. d' would be large in this case. For each value of d', there is a unique ROC curve, as shown in Figure 1.11. If the two distributions completely overlap, then the perceptual response produced when the stimulus is present is the same as when it is absent. d' equals zero, and the ROC curve is a straight diagonal line with a slope of one. With a small d' (see Figure 1.11C), the ROC curve is slightly curved. As d' increases, (see Figure 1.11A and 1.11B) the ROC curve becomes increasingly curved. For large values of d' where the distributions do not overlap (and the stimulus is always detectable above threshold), the ROC curve becomes two straight lines—one vertical, in which the Hit rate reaches 1.0 while the False Alarm rate remains at zero, and one horizontal, in which the False Alarm rate increases after the Hit rate has reached 1.0.

For any d' value in which the distributions overlap, the optimal criterion, as with the mouse and the rattlesnake, depends on what is important to the subject. Observations of birds, squirrels, deer, and other animals suggest that they normally set their criterion for deciding "a potential predator is present" at a very low level, so that there are frequent False Alarms. This is because the cost for False Alarms is a lot less than the cost of a Miss when a predator is involved. Human subjects, like the hypothetical mouse, also alter their criterion levels based on the costs and payoffs of Hits, Misses, False Alarms, and Correct Rejections. Normally, this occurs without conscious thought, and the criterion that a subject uses can be difficult to determine. It is possible, however, for the examiner to control the criterion that is selected by establishing a payoff matrix in which the costs and payoffs are made overt.

Signal detection theory can be used to control bias when measuring threshold

In psychophysical threshold measurements, a payoff matrix may be created that will cause a patient or subject to select a particular criterion so that the threshold can be measured under a situation of known bias. For instance, Figure 1.12 shows the ROC curve that is associated with all the possible criteria that could be used with the perceptual response distributions shown in Figure 1.10. Figure 1.13 shows a payoff matrix similar to the one shown in Figure 1.8. In this case, however, the subject can either win or lose money, turning the psychophysical examination into something of a game. Both Hits and Correct Rejections earn $1, whereas a Miss costs $1 and a False Alarm costs $5.

To control a person's criterion, the examiner would provide the person in advance with the payoff amounts and information on the frequency of stimu-

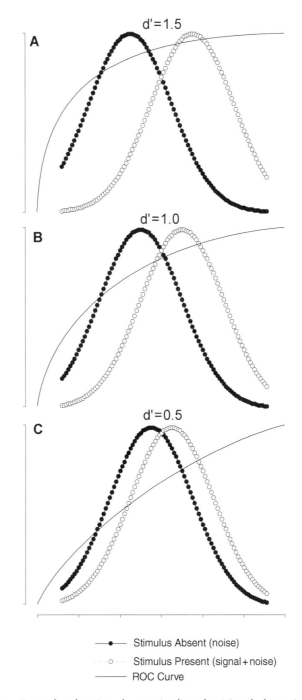

FIGURE 1.11 *Examples showing changes in d' as the "signal plus noise" distribution becomes closer to the "noise" distribution. **A.** The two distributions overlap but are relatively distinct (d' = 1.5). **B, C.** The stimulus is progressively less readily detected because there is increasing overlap of the two distributions. Also shown in each example (**thin curved line**) is the receiver operating characteristic (ROC) curve associated with each d'. As the "signal plus noise" distribution becomes closer to the "noise" distribution, the ROC curve becomes closer to a straight line.*

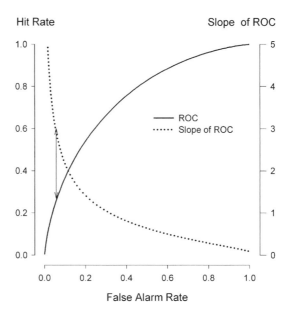

FIGURE 1.12 *The solid line is the receiver operating characteristic (ROC) curve for the distributions shown in Figure 1.10. The dotted line is the slope of the ROC curve at each point (referred to the scale at the right of the figure). The vertical line with arrows marks the criterion that a subject would select based on the payoff matrix shown in Figure 1.13.*

lus presentation (the stimulus was presented on half of the trials in this example). The only things that the subject would not know are the stimulus strength that is being presented and whether the stimulus is present in any given trial. That is controlled randomly. The subject would be informed, after each trial, whether his or her response was a Hit, a Miss, a Correct Rejection,

Response	Stimulus Present	Stimulus Absent
"I see it."	Hits (H) Reward = +$1 n = 12	False Alarms (FA) Cost = –$5 n = 3
"I don't see it."	Misses (M) Cost = –$1 n = 38	Correct Rejections (CR) Reward = +$1 n = 47
	Hit Rate = H/(H+M) = 12/(12+38)=0.24	False Alarm Rate = FA/(FA+CR) = 3/(3+47)= 0.06

FIGURE 1.13 *A hypothetical payoff matrix based on the receiver operating characteristic curve in Figure 1.10.*

or a False Alarm so that he or she could adopt a strategy that would maximize her or his winnings. The subject's strategy is simple—adopt some criterion perceptual response level for deciding whether the stimulus is present, and always say that the stimulus is present when the perceptual response value meets or exceeds that criterion.

To maximize winnings and minimize losses, a subject adopts a specific criterion based on the payoff values. Consider how the payoffs in Figure 1.13 would affect the subject's criterion. A False Alarm (–$5) is five times more costly than a Miss (–$1). Under these conditions, the subject should shift the criterion for reporting that the stimulus is present towards saying that the stimulus is present only when certainty is high (a strong perceptual response occurs). As may be seen in Figure 1.12, a higher criterion (toward the left on the ROC curve) would decrease the number of False Alarms, reduce the number of Hits, and, necessarily, increase the number of Misses and Correct Rejections relative to what they would be if costs of False Alarms and Misses were equal. In other words, for this payoff matrix, the subject shifts toward saying, "I don't see it" more often than not when uncertain. The same shift toward a high criterion could be achieved by increasing the reward for a Correct Rejection to $5 and reducing the cost of a False Alarm to –$1 while leaving the other two values at $1.

It is possible to mathematically predict the point on the ROC curve where a subject eventually should set the criterion for a given payoff matrix. The key to this is the variable, β, called the *likelihood ratio*. The equation for calculating β is

$$\beta = \frac{\text{stimulus frequency}}{1 - \text{stimulus frequency}} \times \frac{\$CR - \$FA}{\$H - \$M} \qquad \text{Eq. 1.2}$$

where the $ indicates the payoffs for Correct Rejections (*CR*), False Alarms (*FA*), Hits (*H*), and Misses (*M*).

In the example shown in Figure 1.13, given the payoff values and the stimulus frequency of 50%, β = (0.5/[1.0–0.5])×([1–(–5)]/[1–(–1)])=3.0. It has been shown mathematically that the likelihood ratio, β, is equal to the slope of the ROC curve at the point determined by the criterion that the subject selects. The vertical line with double arrows in Figure 1.12 is drawn from a value of 3.0 on the slope of the ROC curve to the point on the ROC curve where the False Alarm and Hit rates are optimal for the payoff matrix. The False Alarm rate of 0.06 and the Hit rate of 0.24 are those shown in Figure 1.13. The actual criterion value at this point is the heavy vertical line in Figure 1.10.

For a given ROC curve, it is possible to calculate the likelihood ratio that would result for any combination of stimulus frequency and payoffs and thus learn where the subject should set his or her criterion level. It has been shown empirically that subjects behave as predicted over the midrange of the ROC curve. When the payoffs or the stimulus frequencies are extreme, subjects are apparently reluctant to set their criteria to the predicted point. For example, with a high stimulus frequency, subjects generally have fewer Hits than predicted.

By using signal detection theory along with a forced-choice procedure, an examiner can manipulate the inherent biases of a patient or subject to achieve control of the subject's criterion during the measurement of threshold. In cases in which it is not possible to control biases, they can at least be measured. For instance, patients who are facing the possibility of having serious vision loss or who are simply nervous about giving the doctor the "right" answers can introduce a natural bias into many clinical tests. One such test is the examination of the increment threshold for spots of light flashed at various predetermined retinal locations with respect to the fovea. This is the visual field test or quantitative perimetry (see Chapter 3). Patients tend to use fairly strict criteria in this test, because they want to be certain that the light is present before they say that they see it. Clinical instruments now record the numbers of False Alarms and Misses and use various criteria to determine whether these values are within acceptable limits. To try to control for natural biases, patients are told the approximate location of the flash and given specific instructions about how to respond. Patients are told to respond when they think they see the light rather than just when they are certain. The clinician is constantly communicating with the patient throughout the test to try to maintain the same level of performance and keep the patient alert.

The concepts of signal detection theory form the basis of rational clinical decision making

Clinicians face detectability issues in diagnosing ocular disease. Although all clinicians wish to be 100% accurate, it is frequently the case that the patient's symptoms do not indicate unequivocally whether or not a disorder is present, a situation similar to that faced by a patient in a threshold examination. In diagnostic situations, False Alarms (False Positives in the clinical literature) occur when a diagnosis is rendered, but the patient does not have the purported disorder. Alternatively, a Miss (a False Negative, clinically) occurs when the clinician fails to detect a disorder that a patient actually has. The payoff matrix, from the clinician's (and patient's!) point of view, is determined by the relative consequences of detecting a disorder that is not there or missing one that is (Corliss 1995). If, for example, a treatment has a high risk or a high level of discomfort for the patient relative to the natural consequences of the disorder itself, the clinician is likely to try to reduce False Alarms by raising the criterion for diagnosing the disorder. On the other hand, if not detecting a disorder has a high impact on the patient's life or vision, relative to the effects of the treatment, the clinician should use a lower criterion to try to reduce Misses.

Measuring the Magnitude of Sensations

Sensations have magnitude but no obvious scale or units

The psychophysical methods that have been described thus far in this chapter have relied on simple choices between alternative stimulus values. They are used to measure one point on a sensory scale—the threshold. One can think of this point as a zero point on a sensory scale—below it there is no sensation, and above it there is. The question addressed here is "Above threshold, what is the relation between the value of the stimulus magnitude and the resultant sensation?" If, for example, the physical intensity of a light is increased to twice its original value, the perceived brightness will increase, but will it double? Because the perceptual response is the result of neural activity that is dependent on the stimulus strength, one would expect that there would be a systematic, perhaps monotonic, relation between the sensation experienced and the magnitude of the stimulus. Multiple experiments have shown that the relationship is not usually linear, however.

Sensory magnitude can be measured using scales that do not rely on any physical unit of measurement

One way to measure the relation between the magnitude of sensation and stimulus strength is to use ratio scaling. In the **Ratio Production** procedure (Stevens 1936), for example, the subject is presented with a reference stimulus and is asked to adjust the intensity, or size, or some other parameter of a test stimulus so that it appears to be some fraction or multiple of the reference stimulus. A subject might be instructed, for example, to adjust a test light so that it appears to be one-half as bright or twice as bright as a fixed reference light. Conversely, in the **Ratio Estimation** procedure, the examiner sets the physical intensities of a reference and a test stimulus and asks the subject to estimate the ratio of the test to the reference stimulus. From the subject's responses, the examiner can construct a scale relating a variety of stimulus values to the subject's responses.

A difficulty with the Ratio Production and Ratio Estimation techniques is that they are sensitive to the range of stimuli used. The **Magnitude Estimation** procedure (Stevens 1958) avoids this problem. There are two variants of Magnitude Estimation. In one, the observer is presented with a reference stimulus and told that it has a certain value (e.g., 100). A series of test stimuli are then presented, and the observer is asked to assign a number to these stimuli to indicate their perceived magnitudes relative to the reference stimulus. In the second variant, no numeric value is given to the observer. A series of stimuli that vary in some dimension (intensity is a typical dimension) are presented in random order and the observer is asked to assign a number to each. The number for the first stimulus is selected by the observer and may be fractional or whole or large or small. The numbers assigned to subsequent stimuli are expected to reflect the observer's subjective impression of the stimuli relative to the first one.

Another method is **Magnitude Production**. In this case, the observer is presented first with a reference stimulus that is given a value by the examiner. The observer is then asked to adjust a test stimulus to some value relative to the reference stimulus (e.g., "Here is a stimulus with a value of 100. Please adjust the test stimulus to a value of 25").

Sensory magnitude is proportional to the stimulus magnitude raised to some power

Using the techniques described above, S. S. Stevens, his students, and colleagues (Stevens 1975) derived the general law, known as the **Stevens' Power**

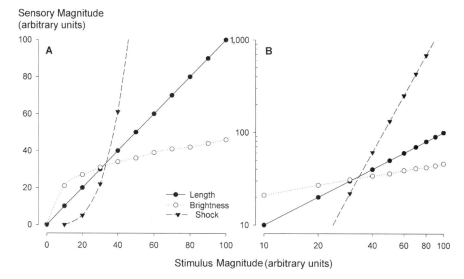

FIGURE 1.14   *Examples of sensory magnitude functions in different sensory systems plotted on linear (A) and log-log scales (B). The exponent for visual length is 1, for brightness, 0.33. The exponent for the magnitude of electric shock (current through the fingers) is 3.5. (Modified from SS Stevens. The Psychophysics of Sensory Function. In WA Rosenblith [ed], Sensory Communication. Cambridge, MA: The M.I.T. Press, 1961;1–33.)*

Law, which relates sensory magnitude to the magnitude of the stimulus. This law has the following form:

$$\psi = \kappa\phi^{\alpha}$$

Eq. 1.3

where ψ (psi) is the sensory magnitude, κ (kappa) is an arbitrary constant determining the scale unit, ϕ (phi) is the stimulus magnitude, and α (alpha) is an exponent that is characteristic of the stimulus used. As shown in Figure 1.14A, if the exponent is 1.0, then the relationship between the sensory magnitude and the stimulus intensity is a straight line. Visual length shows this relationship. If the exponent is greater than 1.0, the relationship is positively accelerating as it is for shock; if the exponent is less than 1.0, it is negatively accelerating as it is for most estimates of brightness.

Because the value of the exponent is the main determinant of the shape of these sensory magnitude functions, the main effort in sensory Magnitude Estimation and Magnitude Production studies has been to determine the exponent value. When plotted on a log-log scale, a power function becomes linear, as shown in Figure 1.14B. Because the slope of the line equals the exponent value, as shown in Equation 1.4, it is easier to discern the rate at which the magnitude of the sensation changed as a function of stimulus value.

$$\log\Psi = \log\kappa + \alpha\log\Phi$$

Eq. 1.4

Some exponent values that have been obtained in Magnitude Estimation studies for various sensory modalities are shown in Table 1.3.

TABLE 1.3 Value of some exponents in the Stevens' Power Law equation

Sensation	Exponent	Stimulus condition
Brightness	0.33	5° target in the dark
Brightness	0.50	Point source
Brightness	0.50	Brief flash
Visual area	0.70	Projected square
Brightness	1	Point source briefly flashed
Visual length	1	Projected line

SOURCE: Modified from SS Stevens. Psychophysics. New York: Wiley, 1975.

Clinicians rely on sensory magnitudes to make judgments about pathology

It is easy to see that this kind of methodology can be applied to virtually any stimulus-sensation situation, and, indeed, it has. Pain, warmth, brightness, loudness, the value of money, the depth of psychiatric illness, the effectiveness of hypnosis in reducing pain, and many other topics have all been evaluated using scaling methods. These are obviously similar to the kinds of judgments that clinicians must make all the time, such as estimating the size or location of a retinal detachment in units of disc (optic nerve head) diameters. This works because visual length (see Table 1.3) has an exponent of 1.0. Judging area would be problematic because the exponent is less that 1.0. Patients also use sensory magnitude estimates when describing such qualities as the degree of pain, the extent of eyestrain or blur, the brightness of a light, or the amount of double vision. Clinicians in this case need to understand not only that magnitude may change within a patient over time but across patients as well.

Study Guide

The following may help to learn the most important points in this chapter.

1. Define psychophysics.
2. Of what use is psychophysics to clinicians?
3. Define threshold.
4. Describe three levels of task complexity in threshold measurements.
5. Draw and label four typical stimulus configurations.
6. Explain the relationship between L, L_T, and ΔL.
7. Explain the relationship between ΔL and threshold ΔL.
8. What four factors produce variability in the measured threshold?
9. What are the three main methods used for threshold measurements?
10. Describe how threshold is measured using the Method of Constant Stimuli and the limitations of this method.
11. Describe how threshold is measured using the Method of Limits and the limitations of this method.

12. Describe how threshold is measured using the Method of Adjustment and the limitations of this method.
13. Describe two variations of the Method of Limits.
14. What is a frequency-of-seeing curve?
15. Describe how catch trials and the forced-choice procedure may be used to counteract subject bias.
16. Give the equation used to correct for guessing.
17. If a subject responds with "yes" 20% of the time when a catch trial is presented, and then says "yes" 52% of the time when a particular stimulus value is presented, what is the true percent of "yes" responses for that stimulus value? (Answer: 0.40)
18. If one uses a two-alternative forced-choice procedure and a 50% threshold, what observed fraction of "yes" responses corresponds to threshold? (Answer: approximately 0.75)
19. Draw two overlapping distributions that represent neural responses or perceptual responses in a near-threshold situation. Pick a criterion and show the location of Hits, False Alarms, Misses, and Correct Rejections.
20. Calculate False Alarm and Hit rates from a payoff matrix.
21. Draw and label a ROC curve.
22. Define d' and show how a ROC curve changes with d'.
23. Describe how a payoff matrix can control a patient's criterion response.
24. Calculate the likelihood ratio, β, expected from a given combination of frequency of stimulus presentations and payoffs.
25. How does signal detection theory apply to clinical decision making? Give examples.
26. Give the general form of Stevens' Power Law (knowing what the variables mean).
27. Show how the value of the exponent affects the shape of the curve on a linear scale and on a log-log scale.
28. Give the value of exponents of the Stevens' Power Law for several types of visual conditions (see Table 1.3).

Glossary

Absolute threshold: in vision, the minimum amount of a stimulus required to detect the presence of that stimulus under ideal conditions.

Action potential: all-or-none voltage changes that are conducted along the axon of a neuron, until they reach the synapse.

Adapting field: a visual stimulus that controls a subject's light adaptation level.

Brightness: an internal, perceptual event reflecting the neural response to the intensity of a stimulus light. Brightness can be influenced by the intensity and location of other visual stimuli.

Correct Rejection: deciding a stimulus is absent when it is absent.

d' (pronounced "d prime"): a measure of the separation of two normal distributions. d' is the difference between the means of the "noise" and "signal plus noise" distributions divided by the common standard deviation of the two distributions. d' quantifies the detectability of the signal.

Detection task: in vision, the most basic question that one can ask of a subject or a patient—whether he or she does or does not see something.

Difference threshold: threshold for detecting that two stimuli differ in some stimulus characteristic, such as intensity, when the stimuli are physically separated in space.

Discrimination task: in vision, distinguishing between two stimuli with regard to some stimulus characteristic, when each stimulus is visible by itself.

False Alarm (False Positive in clinical decision making): deciding a stimulus (or clinical condition) is present when it is absent.

Hit: deciding a stimulus is present when it is actually present.

Increment threshold: threshold for detecting that two stimuli differ in some stimulus characteristic, such as intensity, when the stimuli are immediately adjacent or superimposed.

Intensity: for visual stimuli, intensity is the amount of light energy (quanta) emitted by a stimulus (see Appendix).

Luminance: a photometric measure of the light reflected or emitted from a surface. In this text, luminance is expressed as candelas per square meter (cd/m^2). See Appendix.

Magnitude Estimation: an observer makes direct numeric estimates of the perceived magnitude of a series of stimuli.

Magnitude Production: an observer adjusts a test stimulus to a value relative to a reference stimulus (e.g., for a reference assigned a value of 10, the observer adjusts the test stimulus to 25).

Method of Adjustment: psychophysical method of threshold determination in which the subject adjusts the stimulus values.

Method of Constant Stimuli: psychophysical method of threshold determination in which the examiner presents, in random order, a variety of stimulus values predetermined to include values above and below threshold.

Method of Limits: psychophysical method of threshold determination in which the examiner presents stimulus values in an increasing and decreasing sequence.

Miss (False Negative in clinical decision making): deciding a stimulus (or clinical condition) is absent when it is actually present.

Psychometric function (frequency-of-seeing curve): The S-shaped (ogive) curve plotting the fraction (or percent) of "yes" responses as a function of stimulus value.

Ratio Estimation: the examiner sets the physical intensities of a reference and test stimulus and asks the subject to estimate the ratio of the test to the reference stimulus.

Ratio Production: a subject is presented with a reference stimulus and is asked to adjust the intensity of a test stimulus so that it appears to be some fraction or multiple of the reference stimulus.

Recognition task: recognition (providing a name or category) of a test object that is visible.

Stevens' Power Law: the law relating sensory magnitude (ψ) to the magnitude of the stimulus (ϕ) with the equation $\psi = \kappa\phi^{\alpha}$.

Threshold: the minimum value of a stimulus required to elicit a perceptual response or an altered perceptual response.

True percent of "yes" responses: the values in a psychometric function, corrected for guessing using Equation 1.1.

2 Absolute Threshold of Vision

James E. Bailey

Overview

The now-classic experiment of Hecht, Shlaer, and Pirenne (1942), which determined the minimum amount of light required to elicit a visual response, serves as a paradigm for how to measure visual function psychophysically. Because the expectation was that this would be a very small amount of light, many stimulus attributes had to be very carefully selected and controlled. This chapter describes the factors that guided the selection of the fixed and variable stimulus values, including the wavelength, size, and duration of the stimulus along with its retinal location and the state of adaptation of the subject's eye. The anatomical and physiological determinants of the choices include the distribution of rods and cones in the retina, the fact that the rods can be more sensitive than cones, the peak absorption wavelength of light by rods, spatial and temporal summation mediated by the convergence of multiple rods onto bipolar cells, and the time course of dark adaptation.

This chapter also introduces a method of analyzing the results in a way that attempts to discriminate between the effects of stimulus and subject variability. The results of the study led to the conclusion that a single quantum of light is sufficient to activate a single rod, and that 6–10 quanta must stimulate rods within a small retinal area and a brief time period to produce the perception of light. Other studies have shown that cones have a higher threshold. Approximately 5 quanta activating two cones must summate to reach minimum cone threshold.

Making threshold measurements requires choices about many fixed stimulus parameters

A basic question about human vision, "What is the minimum amount of light required to produce the perceptual response of seeing light?" was answered in a carefully controlled study by Hecht, Shlaer, and Pirenne (1942). In this study, Hecht et al. presented a series of flashes of light with various intensities to a preselected position on the retina in a dark-adapted eye and asked the subject whether he saw the light. Although there are other forms of absolute threshold in vision, such as the smallest line width that can be detected (see Chapter 5), the absolute threshold for detecting light is commonly referred to as the "absolute threshold of vision."

As was described in Chapter 1, in every psychophysical measurement of threshold, it is important that most of the stimulus parameters be set at a fixed level throughout the measurement. Only the parameter of interest (light intensity, in this case) is varied systematically to determine its threshold value. From the list of possible stimulus dimensions given in Chapter 1, there were five that needed to be set at a fixed level in this study: Wavelength, size, and duration are three characteristics of the stimulus. Two characteristics related to the observer were also fixed: the retinal location that was stimulated and the adaptive state of the observer's eye. The first section of this chapter describes the basis for Hecht et al.'s selection of specific, fixed values. The following sections describe the results they obtained and the logic they used to interpret the data.

The stimulus was presented at the retinal location with the highest density of rod photoreceptors

Because the purpose of their study was to determine the minimum amount of light required to elicit a visual response, and because it was known that the rods in the retina are the photoreceptors most sensitive to light, Hecht et al. needed to place the stimulus at the retinal location where the density of rods is the greatest. This occurs at approximately 20° (5 mm, Figure 2.1) from the center of the fovea (Curcio et al. 1990; Østerberg 1935). Because

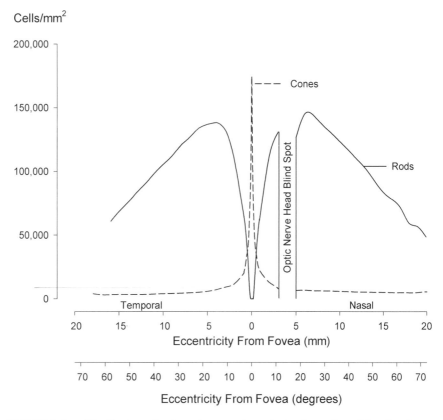

Cells/mm²

Cones

Optic Nerve Head Blind Spot

Rods

Temporal   Nasal

Eccentricity From Fovea (mm)

Eccentricity From Fovea (degrees)

FIGURE 2.1   *Distribution of rods and cones along the horizontal meridian in a human retina. (Data kindly provided by Dr. Christine Curcio.)*

the optical disc is close to this location on the nasal side of the retina, Hecht et al. chose to locate the stimulus on the temporal retina along the horizontal meridian. The results of another study (Wentworth 1930) had verified that the threshold for light detection was lowest in this region but had not measured absolute threshold.

Figure 2.2 shows a schematic diagram of the optical system used to deliver the light to the desired location on the temporal retina of the left eye. The authors took turns serving as subjects. Each sat in a totally dark room and **fixated** a low intensity red light. This positioned the eye so that the test flashes were presented on the temporal retina 20° from the fovea. The test flash passed through a 2 mm pinhole aperture that acted as an artificial pupil. Because the subject's pupil was much larger than 2 mm in the darkness, any small fluctuations in pupil diameter had no effect on the amount of light reaching the retina. The aperture in front of the fifth lens, L_5, in Figure 2.2, was at the same distance from the eye as the fixation point, and, hence, the test flash was focused on the retina when the subject viewed the fixation point. The optical system behind the aperture was used to control the other stimulus parameters.

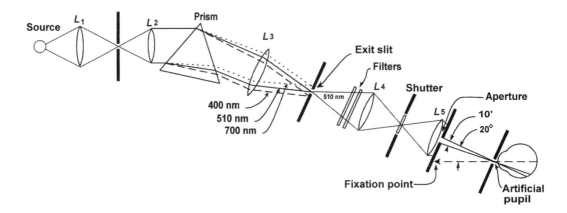

FIGURE 2.2 *Schematic representation of the optical system used by Hecht, Shlaer, and Pirenne. Light from an incandescent source was passed through a prism and exit slit to produce monochromatic light. The filters controlled the flash luminance, the shutter controlled the flash duration, and the aperture controlled the flash diameter. The artificial pupil prevented changes in pupil diameter from affecting the amount of light that reached the retina. The fixation point aimed the fovea so that the test flash was located on the temporal retina 20° from the fovea of the left eye. L_1–L_5 indicate the position of the lenses in the system. (Modified from TN Cornsweet. Visual Perception. New York: Academic, 1970.)*

The peak rod spectral sensitivity determined the stimulus wavelength

A prism, lens, and exit slit arrangement (see Figure 2.2) was used to limit the wavelength composition of the stimulus to a narrow band 10 nm wide. The band was centered at 510 nm because a prior study (Hecht & Williams 1922) had demonstrated that the threshold for detecting light at low intensities was lowest at this wavelength. Subsequent studies (Wald 1945) found that the minimum threshold for rod-mediated night vision (e.g., the wavelength at which the light quanta would be absorbed with maximum efficiency) was 507 nm, which was very close to the value used in this study. The small fixation light was comprised of long-wavelength (red) light to which rods are relatively insensitive. It had a low enough luminance and was far enough away from the location of the test flash to avoid interfering with the detection of the test flash.

The limits of spatial summation determined the stimulus size

The spot focused on the retina subtended an angle 10' in diameter.* This stimulus diameter was chosen because a previous study (Wald 1938) had found that the threshold for detection of a low-intensity flash of light, measured in number of quanta, was independent of size for spots less than approximately 15' in diameter, presented at retinal locations 5° or more from the fovea.

*A degree of visual angle can be divided into 60 minutes of arc (abbreviated as '), and each minute can be divided into 60 seconds of arc (abbreviated as "). See Appendix for a discussion of how stimulus dimensions are specified in angular terms.

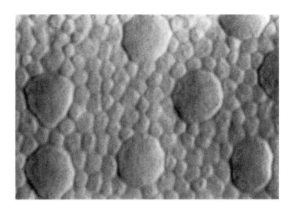

FIGURE 2.3   *Photograph of rod (small) and cone (large) outer segments in a human retina, 5 mm temporal to the fovea, close to the region stimulated by Hecht et al. This photograph shows a region approximately 40 μm wide by 25 μm high. The 10' diameter spot used by Hecht et al. would have covered a slightly larger area (approximately 46 μm in diameter). Potentially, all the rods shown in the photograph might converge onto a single bipolar cell, so that activation in the rods can summate spatially. (Reprinted with permission from CA Curcio et al. Human photoreceptor topography. J Comp Neurol 1990;292:497–523.)*

The threshold did not change when the size of the test flash was varied in this range because of a process called **spatial summation,** in which the responses of many individual receptors add together. This occurs because several photoreceptors converge through bipolar cells on to a single ganglion cell, forming a **receptive-field center**. In this part of the retina, a typical ganglion cell could have a receptive field center diameter of approximately 15'. The light quanta may be visualized as "drops of rain" falling on the retina, some of which are absorbed by the rods and some of which fall between them or on cones. Figure 2.3 shows the spatial arrangement of rod and cone outer segments in the region of the retina stimulated. If a threshold number of quanta in a 15' spot are all delivered to rods that contribute excitation to the receptive-field center of a single ganglion cell, the responses of the various rods summate at the ganglion cell and the stimulus is detected.

Spatial summation occurs regardless of where the quanta fall within that receptive-field center. If a smaller spot, 5' or 10' in diameter and containing the same number of quanta, was centered on the same retinal region, the quanta would automatically fall within the receptive-field center of the ganglion cell and, thus, would activate it to threshold. The spot size is not important as long as it is small enough so that all the quanta fall within a receptive-field center. If, however, one used a spot larger than approximately 15' that contained the same number of quanta, some of these quanta would fall outside the receptive-field center. Under this circumstance, a below-threshold number of quanta would summate within the receptive-field center and the stimulus would not be detected. One would have to increase the total number of quanta in the stimulus to assure that a threshold number would fall within the summation area. For stimuli presented farther in the periphery, the summation region can be larger than 15' in diameter.

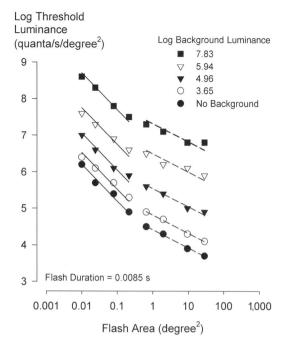

FIGURE 2.4   *Log threshold luminance versus stimulus area in degrees squared (degree²) at five different background luminance levels. The solid lines show the expected change in threshold luminance where Ricco's law holds. As the spot area increases, the threshold luminance decreases linearly on the log-log scale, up to an area of approximately 0.4 degree² (a diameter of approximately 21') where the solid lines end. The dashed lines indicate the expected change in threshold where Piper's law applies. The stimulus was located 6.5° from the fovea. (Modified from HB Barlow. Temporal and spatial summation in human vision at different background intensities. J Physiol [Lond] 1958;141:337–350.)*

Ricco's law describes a reciprocal relationship between threshold luminance and stimulus area

The constant number of quanta required to reach threshold for flashes of fixed duration and small area is expressed as a decrease in stimulus luminance with an increased stimulus area. This reciprocal relationship between luminance and area (Figure 2.4) is known as Ricco's law, which is written as

$$L \times A = C \qquad \text{Eq. 2.1}$$

where L is the threshold luminance of the stimulus, A is the area of the stimulus, and C is a constant. Because C is a constant, as one or the other of L or A increases, the other must decrease. A consequence of this summation effect is that, over the range where Ricco's law holds, each flash contains the same number of quanta. The key to understanding that a decrease in threshold luminance with an increase in area results in a constant number of quanta at threshold is expressed in the equation

$$\text{luminance} = \frac{\text{quanta (at a specific wavelength)}}{\text{duration} \times \text{area}} \qquad \text{Eq. 2.2}$$

Luminance, therefore, has the dimensions of quanta/second × degree squared. Thus, the combination of Equations 2.1 and 2.2 yields

$$\frac{quanta}{duration \times area} \times area = C \qquad \text{Eq. 2.3}$$

Because the area in the numerator and denominator cancel, and the duration is fixed, the number of quanta in the threshold flash is constant for different spot areas.

Ricco's law holds only for stimulus areas less than a certain stimulus area, called the *critical area*. The size of the critical area varies with retinal location. In the parafoveal region (4°–7° from the fovea), Ricco's law holds for spot diameters of up to approximately 30'. It also holds for spots up to 2° in diameter for stimuli presented at an eccentricity of 35° (Hallett et al. 1962). If a stimulus is slightly larger than the critical area, there still is partial summation, so that threshold luminance still declines with increasing spot area, but at a slower rate. This relationship is described by Piper's law (Equation 2.4).

$$L \times \sqrt{A} = C \qquad \text{Eq. 2.4}$$

In Figure 2.4, the threshold change for larger stimuli follows Piper's law fairly closely. Piper's law can apply for stimuli up to 24° in diameter in the peripheral visual field but often does not (Davson 1976). For stimuli with large areas, threshold depends solely on the luminance of the stimulus.

The limits of temporal summation determined the stimulus duration

Hecht et al. set the flash duration at 1 millisecond by controlling the length of time that the shutter (see Figure 2.2) remained open. This value was selected because a previous study (Graham & Margaria 1935) had found that the threshold (in quanta) did not change for flash durations of less than 100 milliseconds. This invariance in threshold quanta with changes in stimulus duration occurs because of temporal summation within the receptive-field center of ganglion cells. **Temporal summation** is defined as the adding together of events that occur at slightly different times. In the eye, temporal summation occurs within a limited time period of approximately 10–100 milliseconds. This means that if 200 quanta are delivered to the retina within 1 millisecond and stimulate it at a threshold level, then 20 quanta delivered during each millisecond for 10 milliseconds also constitute a threshold flash. One also could divide the light up into two equal groupings and deliver half within the first millisecond and half during the fifth millisecond and find the same threshold. Any combination of quanta within the temporal summation interval results in the subject reporting only a single flash.* This means that the early-arriving quanta have an effect on

---

*If the temporal integration interval were longer, then images would be built up on each other as the eyes look from one place to another. This does not occur. Thus, although a photochemical effect may be produced that lasts longer than 100 milliseconds, the neural response must not last for the same duration, or our world would be a terribly confusing place.

the photoreceptor membrane potential that persists long enough to add to the effect created by the late-arriving quanta.

Bloch's law describes a reciprocal relationship between threshold luminance and stimulus duration

The constant number of quanta required to reach threshold for flashes of fixed area and variable (brief) duration is expressed as a decrease in stimulus luminance with increased stimulus duration. This relationship is called *Bloch's law*, which is usually written as

$$L \times t = C \qquad\qquad \text{Eq. 2.5}$$

where L is the threshold luminance of the stimulus, t is the duration of the flash, and C is a constant.

By the same logic used in the explanation of Ricco's law, as flash duration (t) increases and luminance (L) decreases, the threshold number of quanta remains constant. Combining Equation 2.2 with Equation 2.5 gives Equation 2.6.

$$\frac{quanta}{duration \times area} \times duration = C \qquad\qquad \text{Eq. 2.6}$$

However, because the area value is fixed for all these flashes, quanta/area is a fixed value. The duration in the numerator and denominator cancel, so the number of quanta in the threshold flash is constant.

As is shown in Figure 2.5, Bloch's law holds only over a limited range of stimulus durations that extend to 100 milliseconds under some conditions. This means that there is an upper limit, called the **critical duration**, to the time period over which the retina can summate the arrival of quanta (discussed in more detail in Chapter 7). For flashed stimuli with durations much longer than the critical duration, threshold depends solely on the luminance of the stimulus.

A completely dark-adapted eye maximized sensitivity

It has been known for many years that when one remains in the dark for a period of time, less light is needed in a stimulus for it to reach threshold. Threshold was defined in Chapter 1. *Sensitivity* is defined as

$$\text{Sensitivity} = \frac{1}{\text{Threshold}} \qquad\qquad \text{Eq. 2.7}$$

Thus, as the threshold decreases when one remains in darkness, sensitivity to light increases. To maximize sensitivity, each subject for this study sat in a totally dark room for at least 30 minutes before beginning the measurements. This amount of time permitted a near-maximum amount of the light-absorbing rod photopigment, rhodopsin, to accumulate in the rods, so the subject was fully adapted to the dark and maximally sensitive to the light flashes. More information on adaptation and its mechanisms is presented in Chapter 4.

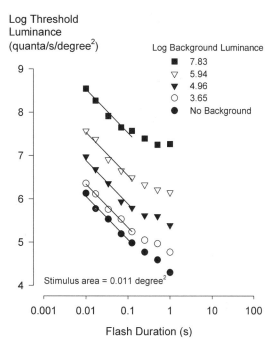

FIGURE 2.5 *Log threshold luminance versus flash duration at five different background luminance levels. The solid lines show the expected change in threshold luminance where Bloch's law holds. As the flash duration increases, the threshold luminance decreases linearly on the log-log scale up to a critical duration of approximately 0.1 second (where the straight lines end). (Modified from HB Barlow. Temporal and spatial summation in human vision at different background intensities. J Physiol [Lond] 1958;141:337–350.)*

The Method of Constant Stimuli was used to measure threshold

After adapting to the dark for at least 30 minutes, the subject was ready to begin the measurements. Before the experiment, the subject made a mold of his teeth using dental impression compound. His head was stabilized by this mold, which was mounted on a bracket connected to the apparatus. He looked at the red fixation light, and, when he felt that he was looking exactly at it and was optimally ready for the stimulus, he pressed a button to present the stimulus and reported whether he saw the flash. The subject was given control of the timing of the flash presentations so that he could look away from the fixation point periodically to avoid fatigue (boredom was another matter!). Between trials, the other investigators, who were located outside the darkened chamber, adjusted the stimulus luminance by changing the filters in the optical system (see Figure 2.2). The Method of Constant Stimuli was used to present six different intensities in random order, usually 50 times each in a session.

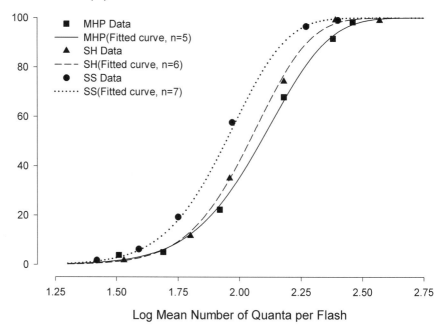

Flashes Seen (%)

- ■ MHP Data
- —— MHP(Fitted curve, n=5)
- ▲ SH Data
- – – – SH(Fitted curve, n=6)
- ● SS Data
- .... SS(Fitted curve, n=7)

Log Mean Number of Quanta per Flash

FIGURE 2.6   *Frequency-of-seeing curves for the three subjects of the Hecht, Shlaer, and Pirenne study. The data points (e.g., the circles) are the actual experimental results. The curves represent the mathematical functions that best fit the data assuming no subject variability and a threshold of (n=) 5,6, or 7 quanta as described in Figure 2.9. (Modified from S Hecht, S Shlaer, MH Pirenne. Energy, quanta and vision. J Gen Physiol 1942;25:819–840.)*

The absolute threshold for detecting light with rods was 54 to 148 quanta incident at the cornea

Figure 2.6 illustrates the resultant psychometric functions for the three subjects, Hecht, Shlaer, and Pirenne. The abscissa shows the log of mean the number of quanta incident at the cornea, which is the final location in the optical path at which they could obtain a direct measurement. The stimulus values ranged from approximately 32 ($10^{1.5}$) to 316 ($10^{2.5}$) quanta. The authors decided to set threshold at 60% of "yes" responses rather than at the 50% level described in Chapter 1. Measured on numerous occasions, the range of quanta needed to reach threshold for the authors and four additional observers ranged from 54 to 148.

Light losses reduced the number of quanta absorbed by rods to 5 to 14

If between 54 and 148 quanta incident on the cornea were required to reach threshold, the rods actually absorbed fewer quanta One reason is that there are light losses between the cornea and the retina. The cornea itself accounts for a loss of approximately 4% of the incident light. Of the amount that passed through the cornea, the authors estimated an additional 50% was lost because of internal reflection, scattering, and absorption as the light passed through the aqueous, lens, and vitreous inside the eye (Ludvigh & McCarthy 1938). Thus, if one began with 100 quanta, then approximately $100 \times 0.96 \times 0.5 = 48$ quanta actually arrived at the retina. Of the quanta arriving at the retina, Hecht et al. estimated that only 20% were actually absorbed by the photopigment molecules because the majority were either absorbed by cones (see Figure 2.3) or pigment epithelium between the rod outer segments, or passed through the rod outer segments, or without absorption. This reduced the actual number of quanta needed to produce the sensation of light to approximately 5 and 14, roughly 10% of the quanta incident on the cornea.

If one assumes that the threshold was 10 quanta, the amount of energy can be calculated using the following equation:

$$E = nh\nu \qquad \text{Eq. 2.8}$$

where n is the number of quanta, h is Planck's constant (6.625×10^{-27} erg $\times$ second), and ν is the frequency of light. The frequency of light is

$$\nu = \frac{c}{\lambda} \qquad \text{Eq. 2.9}$$

where c is the velocity of light (2.998×10^{10} cm per second) and λ is the wavelength of light. Thus, 10 quanta at 510 nm have a total energy of 3.89×10^{-11} erg. The very small magnitude of this energy can be appreciated when one considers that 1 erg is the work required to lift 1 mg against gravity to a height of 1 cm. Thus, the energy from a pea (approximately 350 mg) dropped from a height of 1 cm, if converted to light energy, could provide every human that ever lived with a faint impression of light!

Hecht, Shlaer, and Pirenne examined whether stimulus variability provided an explanation for shape of psychometric function

Hecht et al. were aware that subject variability could affect the shape of the psychometric function, as discussed in Chapter 1, and that this could affect the measured threshold value. Because the light levels in their study were extremely low, they also had to consider a second important possible source of variability—quantal fluctuations in light intensity. Therefore, they investigated whether the shapes of their frequency-of-seeing curves could be accounted for entirely by fluctuations in the number of quanta in the stimulus from trial to trial.

The number of quanta in each flash of a series of light flashes varies with predictable randomness

At low light levels, such as those used in this study, the number of quanta contained in any one short-duration flash is variable. Some flashes contain more quanta than the mean value of a series of flashes, whereas some contain fewer

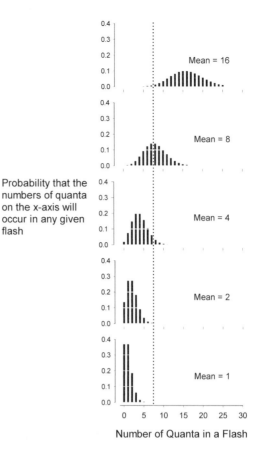

Probability that the numbers of quanta on the x-axis will occur in any given flash

Number of Quanta in a Flash

FIGURE 2.7   *Probability distributions illustrating the variability in the number of quanta contained in single flashes for five series of flashes with different mean numbers of quanta. See text for details.*

quanta. Each black bar in Figure 2.7 shows the probability that a flash contains the number of quanta indicated on the x-axis. Together, these probabilities comprise what is known as a *Poisson distribution*, which is used to describe discrete events that are distributed randomly in space or time. Five such distributions are shown in the figure. Imagine that these five distributions were created by a series of 100 flashes each and that the mean number of quanta in each series was different, ranging from 1 to 16, as shown. Because all the probabilities for one distribution add to 1.0, it is possible to say, for example, that when the mean number of quanta in a series of 100 flashes is eight, only 14 of the flashes actually contain eight quanta.

Thus, even if one sets the apparatus to produce flashes of the same intensity, the random nature of the emission process makes it impossible to know exactly the number of quanta in a given flash. It is important to note, however, that the process is not chaotic. The randomness is predictable in that when the mean is set, the numbers of quanta in individual flashes are constrained to certain limits set by the Poisson distribution.

Poisson distributions can be used to derive the shapes of the psychometric functions assuming only quantal variability

Suppose that the three subjects in Figure 2.6 were perfect observers with no subject variability and that their threshold for detecting the flashed spot was, for instance, eight quanta. This would mean that every time their retinas absorbed eight or more quanta, they would say that the light was present. The question, therefore, is: What is the probability that eight or more quanta were contained in a flash for each average flash intensity in the Hecht et al. study? The vertical dashed line in Figure 2.7 divides the distributions into regions with fewer than eight quanta and regions with eight or more quanta. Notice that when the mean number of quanta is high, the percentage of flashes that contain eight or more quanta is high. More than 97% of the flashes with a mean of 16 quanta contain eight or more quanta. For flashes with a mean of eight quanta, 54.7% contain eight or more. When the mean is two, fewer than 1% of the flashes contain eight or more quanta, and for a mean of one, virtually no flashes contain eight or more quanta. These percentages can be determined by adding up all the probabilities to the right of the vertical line in Figure 2.7 and multiplying by 100.

The previous paragraph showed how to calculate the percentages of flashes having eight or more quanta for series of flashes with different means. For a distribution with a given mean, it is possible to determine the resulting percentages for different thresholds. Consider the distribution in Figure 2.7 with a mean of eight quanta. As indicated previously, 54.7% of all the flashes contain eight or more quanta. This is equivalent to saying that 54.7% of the flashes contain more than seven quanta. Likewise, 81% contain more than five quanta, 100% contain more than zero quanta, 28% contain more than nine quanta, 11.2% contain more than 11 quanta, and so on. All similar values can be summarized in what is called an *inverse cumulative Poisson distribution*, such as that shown in Figure 2.8. Each bar in the graph shows the probability that a flash contains more than the number indicated on the x-axis when the mean of series of flashes is eight. The arrow in Figure 2.8 represents the fraction of flashes (54.7%) that would contain eight or more quanta—that is, more than seven quanta.

An inverse cumulative distribution can be constructed for a Poisson distribution of any mean. The left side of Figure 2.9 shows just such a family of curves for flashes containing mean numbers of quanta from 2 to 16. The vertical line is drawn through these curves for a threshold of eight or more quanta, that is, more than seven quanta. The curve on the right side of Figure 2.9 translates the vertical line on the left into a frequency-of-seeing curve. It shows the probability that a flash contains the threshold number of quanta (eight or more in this case) if the flash has the mean number of quanta indicated on the abscissa. This is the psychometric function that Hecht et al. would have produced if they were perfect observers who detected the flash each time it contained more than seven quanta.

One can construct a frequency-of-seeing curve for any threshold by drawing a vertical line through the family of curves on the left side of the figure and constructing the curve on the right side by plotting the intersections against the means. Three such curves are shown in the inset in Figure 2.9. They are the fre-

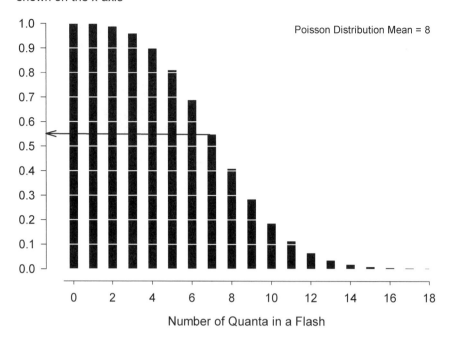

Probability that a flash
will contain more than
the number of quanta
shown on the x-axis

Poisson Distribution Mean = 8

Number of Quanta in a Flash

FIGURE 2.8   *Inverse cumulative distribution for a Poisson distribution with a mean of eight quanta per flash. See text for details.*

quency-of-seeing curves that would be obtained if a perfect observer had any of these thresholds. Note that the frequency-of-seeing curves become steeper as the threshold increases.

Because they could only calculate the number of quanta absorbed by the retina and did not know the actual number, Hecht et al. matched the shape of theoretical frequency-of-seeing curves to the data shown in Figure 2.6 by sliding the curves along the abscissa. The curves in Figure 2.6 were, in fact, generated in that manner. Based on the shape of the best fitting curves, Hecht et al. concluded that the threshold was between five and seven quanta, if they were perfect observers.

Hecht et al. realized they were not perfect observers, so they considered how the curves would be affected if most of the shape of the curve were due to stimulus variability, with some variability on the part of the observer. As noted in Chapter 1, subject variability would tend to flatten a frequency-of-seeing curve. Thus, if subject variability were a factor, the real threshold would be slightly higher than the apparent threshold. Because they felt that there had to be at least some subject variability, Hecht et al.'s conclusion was that between 6 and 10 quanta, rather than between five and seven quanta, were required to reach threshold.

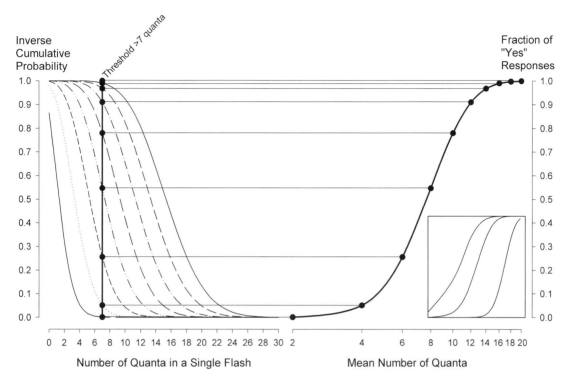

FIGURE 2.9   *Method of generating a theoretical frequency-of-seeing curve (**on the right**) from several inverse cumulative frequency distributions (**on the left**), assuming a threshold of eight quanta. The inset shows three such frequency-of-seeing curves for threshold values greater than four, seven, and 16 quanta, from left to right, respectively.*

One quantum can excite a rod

Because the number of quanta required for threshold is 6–10, it must be the case that a single quantum can excite a rod and that several individual rod responses must occur in close temporal proximity to elicit a visual response. Hecht et al. estimated that there were between 300 and 500 rods within an area 10' in diameter, 20° from the fovea. The probability of any individual rod absorbing one incident quantum is on the order of 8 to 40 in 1,000. The probability of a single rod absorbing two quanta is even smaller. Thus, a single quantum of light must be capable of exciting a single rod. Subsequent studies (Baylor et al. 1979) have confirmed, by measuring the potentials generated in individual rods, that a single absorbed quantum, regardless of wavelength, triggers a consistent response (Figure 2.10).

If a single rod can be stimulated by a single quantum absorption, why does it take more than one quantum to elicit a visual response? The answer is that sufficient spatial and temporal summation must occur in the receptive-field center of at least one ganglion cell to raise its firing rate to a level that can be communicated to the visual cortex and produce sufficient activity there to cause the perception of light. Spontaneous quantum-like activation of the pho-

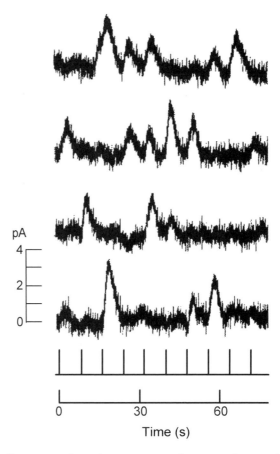

pA
4
2
0

0   30   60

Time (s)

FIGURE 2.10   *Responses of a rod outer segment from a toad to a series of 40 consecutive low-intensity flashes. Ten flashes were presented in each row. Each vertical mark on the abscissa indicates when the flash was presented. In most cases, the rod did not respond. When rod hyperpolarization occurred, the response was either small (approximately 1.5 picoampere [pA]) or large (approximately 3 pA). The flash response was quantized and Poisson-distributed. The quantal events resulted from either a single or pair of light quanta being absorbed by the rod. (Reprinted with permission from DA Baylor, TD Lamb, KW Yau. Responses of retinal rods to single photons. J Physiol [Lond] 1979;288:613–634.)*

topigment can occur and cause the release of neurotransmitters along the visual pathway. As discussed in Chapter 1, these events produce a level of noise in the visual system to which a real signal must add to be reliably identified as being present. The noise has been called the *dark light, self light,* and *intrinsic light* of the visual system. Thus, there is a limit set on the absolute threshold by the intrinsic noise in the system. The requirement that there be summation offers some protection against False Alarms.

The threshold for practical vision is higher but still low

The absolute threshold study described above determined the smallest value of light that can produce a visual sensation. This measurement was made at a fixed retinal location, however. A slightly different but related issue is to determine the lowest value of retinal **illuminance** (see Appendix) required for visual situations in which the observer can freely move the eyes and change the retinal location. To answer this question, Pirenne (1962) used a white test stimulus spread out over many degrees on the retina and viewed with both eyes for a 15 second duration. The threshold for detecting this stimulus was determined to be 0.75×10^{-6} **candelas per square meter** (cd/m^2) (see Appendix). This is on the order of 5–30% of the luminance of the darkest night sky measured by the National Physical Laboratory (Pirenne 1962). Thus, even the darkest night provides sufficient light for some visual function. This threshold intensity corresponds to the illuminance provided by a source of 1 **candela** illuminating a perfectly diffusing (white, matte surface) object 650 m away from the source. This is the illuminance that an automobile headlamp could produce on the same surface from a distance of 70 miles!

Another determination of the threshold for useful vision involved using spots of small diameter (point sources), so that Ricco's law held, but allowing the subject to detect the stimulus with free eye movements during a 15 second period. The threshold, in this case, was found to be approximately equivalent to a source of 1 candela of luminous intensity (see Appendix) at a distance of 16 km (approximately 10 miles) (Pirenne 1962). This corresponds to 100–150 quanta per second entering the pupil of the eye.

Determining cone thresholds requires using a different retinal location, stimulus intensity, and adaptation state

Most retinal locations include a mixture of rods and cones, and at most locations, the number of rods exceeds the number of cones (see Figure 2.1). An exception is the fovea. As shown in Figure 2.1, only cones, which are specialized for vision in high-luminance conditions, are found at this location. These provide the best visual acuity but have a much higher threshold for light.

To determine the threshold for light perception using cones, small spots of light were presented on the fovea for brief durations (Vimal et al. 1989). The threshold using cones is approximately five quanta per cone, with summation needed over two cones to elicit a visual response. The higher threshold of cones compared to rods has been attributed to higher levels of thermal noise in cones than in rods (Baylor et al. 1979). These researchers also suggested that cones may be cone-shaped to help to compensate for this higher thermal noise. The taper of cones may concentrate light into a smaller space than is possible in a rod, thereby increasing the likelihood of absorption.

Any accurate and reliable measurement of visual function must adhere to the principles presented in this chapter

This chapter has provided a case study in the care that must be taken to obtain valid, reliable, psychophysical measurements. The stimulus wavelength, size, duration, retinal location, and the subject's adaptive state were carefully chosen based on anatomical considerations, the wavelength sensitivity of the photoreceptors, and spatial and temporal summation. Similar care has been taken in the design of many clinical instruments. It is important to understand the conditions under which these need to be used and, when first using them in a new setting, such as a new practice location, to consider whether aberrant results might be due to incorrect stimulus conditions. If, for example, no one measured in a new office can detect a spot of light during visual field testing, it might be suspected that something has been set up incorrectly.

Study Guide

1. List the three stimulus characteristics and two observer characteristics that were fixed in the study of Hecht, Shlaer, and Pirenne.
2. Where on the retina was the flash presented, and why was that location selected?
3. What wavelength of light was used, and why?
4. What stimulus size was selected, and why?
5. What stimulus duration was selected, and why?
6. What was the subject's adaptation state, how did he get that way, and why?
7. What is the equation given for luminance?
8. Define sensitivity.
9. Define spatial summation.
10. What is the neural explanation for spatial summation?
11. Write Ricco's law. (Define each variable.)
12. Explain how Ricco's law means that the threshold number of quanta is constant.
13. Define temporal summation.
14. Write Piper's law. (Define each variable.)
15. Write Bloch's law. (Define each variable.)
16. Define critical duration.
17. Explain how Bloch's law means that the threshold number of quanta is constant for durations shorter than the critical duration.
18. What are quantal fluctuations of light energy?
19. Explain how the frequency-of-seeing data obtained by Hecht, Shlaer, and Pirenne might have been due to quantal fluctuations.
20. How does one know that one quantum of light must be able to excite one rod?
21. How does one know that "seeing" at absolute threshold must be due to summation across several rods?
22. Give two estimates of the threshold for useful vision.
23. Why is the threshold for cone vision higher than for rod vision?

Glossary

Candela (cd): a measure of luminous intensity equivalent to 1 **lumen**/steradian (see Appendix).

Candela per square meter (cd/m²): a measure of the intensity of reflected or emitted light expressed as the number of candelas per unit area of the surface (see Appendix).

Critical duration: the longest flash duration for which Bloch's law holds.

Fixate: to aim the fovea (region of highest cone density and best spatial acuity) at a target.

Illuminance: the measure of the amount of light incident on a surface (see Appendix).

Lumen: a measure of luminous flux equal to a rate of energy flow of 4.07×10^{15} quanta per second at 555 nm wavelength (see Appendix).

Receptive-field center: the region on the retina that, through direct, sign-inverting connections of photoreceptors to bipolar cells, produces a depolarizing response in an on-bipolar cell and, consequently, the on-center ganglion cells that receive excitatory input from the on-bipolar cell. Similarly, sign-conserving synaptic connections from photoreceptors to off-bipolar cells produce hyperpolarization in the bipolar cell and a decrease in the rate of action potential production in the center of off-center ganglion cells. Lateral geniculate nucleus cells also have a receptive-field center due to the connections from retinal ganglion cells.

Spatial summation: the adding together of responses that occur in different photoreceptors. Also known as *pooling*.

Temporal summation: the adding together of events that occur at slightly different times.

3   Intensity Discrimination

James P. Comerford, Thomas T. Norton, and James E. Bailey

Overview

The ability of the visual system to determine whether one luminous stimulus differs in intensity from another is of fundamental importance for seeing and is the basis for many clinical tests. As will be seen in Chapter 5 and Chapter 6, this ability, refered to as *intensity discrimination*, is the basis for spatial visual acuity and for detecting the boundaries of objects. The basic psychophysical paradigm presented in this chapter is the measurement of how much the intensity of a test stimulus must differ from the intensity of a reference stimulus before it can be seen to be different. Often, the reference stimulus is presented as a background luminance against which a test spot with a different luminance is viewed. The task is to determine the threshold change in luminance (ΔL) that must be added to, or subtracted from, the background luminance to be seen as having a different brightness. These thresholds vary considerably with the choice of stimulus parameters and the adaptive state of the eye.

As the background luminance is increased from zero over a small range of scotopic luminance levels, quantal fluctuations set a lower limit on intensity discrimination thresholds. At these low background levels the human visual system can act like an ideal detector in that, as the background luminance level increases, the threshold change in luminance (ΔL) needed to detect that the test stimulus differs from the background luminance, increases approximately as the square root of the background luminance (the deVries-Rose law applies). For higher levels of the background luminance, the visual system does not behave like an ideal detector because of neural interactions. The result is that the threshold ΔL of the test spot increases approximately in direct proportion to increases in the background luminance (Weber's law applies). At high intensities, neither relationship holds because the rod and cone systems saturate. As a result, the test spot luminance must differ greatly from the background luminance in order to be seen as differing in brightness. Both the deVries-Rose law and Weber's law are useful in predicting visual performance.

Intensity discriminations form the basis for visual field testing, an important clinical tool for detecting the presence or absence of pathological conditions that cause an increased intensity discrimination threshold in part of the visual field. Isopters define points in the visual field with similar increment thresholds and provide a topographic map of retinal sensitivity.

Glare affects intensity discrimination thresholds by reducing the contrast. Glare can be introduced by adding a constant amount of light to both the background and the test stimulus or by the scattering of light by the ocular media, such as occurs in a cataract.

Intensity discrimination is the process of distinguishing one stimulus intensity from another

The absolute threshold of vision (see Chapter 2) is the amount of light needed to make the transition from the world of darkness to the world of low luminance levels. It is, however, one thing to detect that light is present in an otherwise dark environment and another to distinguish that two or more luminous stimuli differ in intensity. The ability to detect intensity differences is an essential part of identifying the location of the boundaries of objects and, hence, the shape of objects. This is of fundamental importance for spatial vision.

Difference thresholds and increment thresholds are two measures of intensity discrimination*

As mentioned in Chapter 1, in an increment threshold measurement, a test stimulus of luminance L_T is compared to an adjacent reference stimulus of luminance L (see Figure 1.1 in Chapter 1). The task is to determine how different L_T must be from L for it to be seen as different, (i.e., to determine the threshold ΔL that must be added to L or subtracted from L for L_T to be seen as different 50% of the time).

In a difference threshold test on the other hand, there are two separate stimuli, such as two luminous patches, that are often presented on a black background (see Chapter 1, Figure 1.1D). One of the stimuli is designated as a constant reference stimulus with a luminance, L. The other is designated as the variable test stimulus with a luminance, L_T. Again, the task is to determine the threshold ΔL by which L_T must differ from L to be seen as different. Under similar conditions, increment thresholds generally are smaller than difference thresholds.

In both situations, psychophysical methods are used to determine the threshold ΔL. At threshold, the test stimulus has a luminance that can be represented as $L_T = L + \Delta L$, if it is more intense than L, and $L_T = L - \Delta L$, if it is less intense than L (see Chapter 1, Figure 1.2). These measurements are relatively simple to make, and psychophysicists have determined the threshold ΔL under many conditions. They have found that the threshold ΔL usually has an orderly relationship to the reference luminance, L. When the threshold ΔL is plotted as a function of the reference luminance, the result is often described as a *threshold versus intensity function*.

Quantum fluctuations provide a theoretical lower limit for intensity discrimination by an ideal observer

In an intensity discrimination task, the smallest difference an observer could theoretically detect is when L and L_T are briefly presented and L_T differs from L by one quantum because one cannot divide a quantum into smaller units. Even if the visual system could discriminate a difference of one quantum, quantal fluctuations in the amount of light emitted from a stimulus set a theoretical limit. Recall from Chapter 2 that the number of quanta contained in a flashed stimulus is variable. If L_T, on average, was one quantum more intense than L, then, because of quantum fluctuations, there are many times in a series of stimulus presentations when L_T would actually contain fewer quanta than L. This is because a stimulus that contains, for example, a mean number of nine quanta when presented many times often actually contains seven or fewer quanta. Likewise, a stimulus with a mean number of eight quanta often con-

*This text uses the phrase "intensity discrimination." Many older texts and research papers use the phrase "brightness discrimination" to describe the same measurement of threshold ΔL. It also would be correct to use the phrase "luminance discrimination."

tains 10 or more (see Chapter 2, Figure 2.7). This variability means that it is physically impossible for an observer to always detect an intensity difference between two flashed stimuli that, on average, differ in intensity by only a small number of quanta.

Furthermore, as also shown in Figure 2.7 of Chapter 2, quantum fluctuation increases with the number of quanta in the stimulus. In a Poisson distribution, the variance is equal to the mean, and, therefore, the standard deviation is equal to the square root of the mean. Thus, the standard deviation of the quantum fluctuations increases as the square root of the mean number of quanta increases. Based on signal detection theory (see Chapter 1), it can be determined that, in a two alternative forced-choice task, for two luminances to be distinguished at a level of 75% correct responses (e.g., a 50% threshold), the luminance of the two stimuli must differ by 0.95 of a standard deviation (Laming 1991). This is the theoretical lower limit based on quantal fluctuations. In addition, as the stimulus luminance increases, the minimum discriminable threshold increases in proportion to the square root of the intensity level. This is mathematically expressed in the deVries-Rose law (deVries 1943; Rose 1948) as

$$\frac{\Delta L}{\sqrt{L}} = K \qquad\qquad \text{Eq. 3.1}$$

where ΔL is the threshold luminance difference, L is the reference luminance, and K is a constant.

Human observers follow the deVries-Rose law and behave as ideal detectors at low reference luminance levels

As shown in Figure 3.1, at low reference luminance levels, human increment thresholds approximately follow the deVries-Rose law for brief stimulus presentation times (approximately 10 milliseconds) and small test spots (approximately 10' in diameter) (Hess 1990). In these studies, the reference stimulus was a large background with luminance, L, on which the least spot of luminance L_T was presented. Decrement thresholds (L_T less intense than L) also follow the deVries-Rose law. At low levels of background luminance, decrement thresholds are slightly, but significantly, smaller than increment thresholds, however (Hess 1990). This is expected, based on the smaller standard deviation for a Poisson distribution of lower intensity. Thus, at low background luminance levels, human intensity discrimination thresholds are close to the theoretical limit.

At higher background luminance levels, Weber's law holds and the intensity discrimination threshold is higher than expected from an ideal detector

For more intense background luminance levels, in the range where L equals 1–1,000 **millilamberts**, the threshold ΔL is larger than predicted by quantum fluctuations. This means that the visual system is not an ideal detector over much of the range of intensities that are normally experienced in everyday life. As

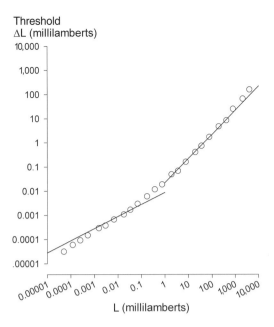

Threshold
ΔL (millilamberts)

L (millilamberts)

FIGURE 3.1 *Threshold ΔL versus the luminance, L, of the background. The threshold ΔL approximately follows the deVries-Rose law (solid line with slope of 0.5) for background luminance values up to approximately 1.0 millilambert in this example. At higher values of L, the threshold ΔL increases more rapidly, approximately following Weber's law (slope of 1.0). (Modified from S Hecht. 1934. Vision II. The nature of the photoreceptor process. In C Murchison [ed], Handbook of General Experimental Psychology. Worcester, MA: Clark University Press, 1934;704–828. Original data from A König, E Brodhun. Experimentelle Untersuchungen über die psychophysische Fundamentalformel in Bezug auf den Gesichtssinn. Sitzungsber. Berlin: Preuss Akad. Wiss., 1889;27:641–644.)*

shown in Figure 3.1, as L increases above approximately 1 millilambert, the threshold ΔL increases more rapidly (with a slope of 1.0 on the log-log plot indicated by the straight line).

Figure 3.2 replots the same data as Figure 3.1, except that the ordinate is the fraction threshold ΔL/L. This ratio is called the *Weber fraction*, after the early psychophysicist E. H. Weber. The x-axis of this graph still plots the background intensity level. In the region where the deVries-Rose law holds, the value of the Weber fraction decreases as L increases. In the region where L is greater than 1 millilambert, the Weber fraction approximately follows a horizontal line. In this region, if the background intensity is increased by a factor of 100 from 10 to 1,000, the threshold ΔL also increases by a factor of 100 from approximately 0.1 to 10; the ΔL/L thus remains constant at a value of approximately 0.01. The constant proportional relationship between the increment threshold ΔL and the background luminance is called *Weber's law*, which is mathematically expressed as

$$\frac{\Delta L}{L} = K$$ Eq. 3.2

where ΔL is the threshold luminance difference, *L* is the background (or reference), luminance, and *K* is a constant. Weber's law is useful for its predictive

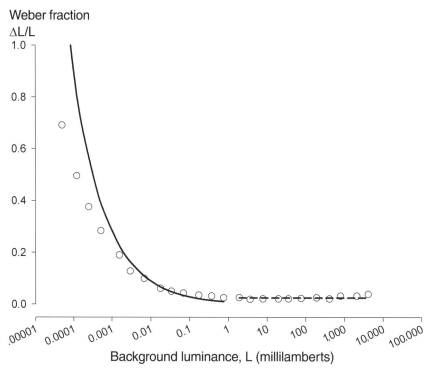

FIGURE 3.2   *The Weber fraction as a function of background luminance using the same data a shown in Figure 3.1. When the background luminance level is low, the Weber fraction decreases as the background luminance is increased, approximately following the prediction of the deVries-Rose law (curved solid line). When the background luminance is higher, the Weber fraction remains nearly constant with further increases in background luminance approximately following the horizontal solid line. (L = luminance of the background [reference] field; ΔL = threshold change in luminance needed to detect that the luminance of the test stimulus [L_T] differs from L.) (Modified from S Hecht. 1934. Vision II. The nature of the photoreceptor process. In C Murchison [ed], Handbook of General Experimental Psychology. Worcester, MA: Clark University Press, 1934;704–828. Original data from A König, E Brodhun. Experimentelle Untersuchungen über die psychophysische Fundamentalformel in Bezug auf den Gesichtssinn. Sitzungsber. Berlin: Preuss Akad. Wiss., 1889;27:641–644.)*

value. In the range where it holds, if one measures the threshold ΔL at a given background luminance, one can then calculate and predict the threshold ΔL at other background luminance values.

The proportional change in threshold ΔL with L means that the visual system is not detecting luminance differences at the theoretical limit. One possible explanation might be that the deVries-Rose law holds for rod-mediated vision and Weber's law holds for cone-mediated vision. This is not the case, however. As shown in Figure 3.3, the increment thresholds of a person whose retina contains only rods follows the deVries-Rose law at low values of L and Weber's law at higher luminance levels. Rather, the constancy of the Weber fraction in the region where Weber's law holds is evidence for a limitation on intensity discrimination based on neural processing in the retina or elsewhere in the visual system, as is discussed later in this chapter.

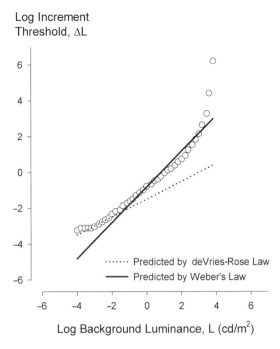

Log Increment Threshold, ΔL

Log Background Luminance, L (cd/m²)

······ Predicted by deVries-Rose Law
—— Predicted by Weber's Law

FIGURE 3.3   *Increment threshold data of a rod monochromat (circles) plotted along with the theoretical lower limit (deVries-Rose law, dotted line) and the predictions of Weber's law (solid line). (Modified from RF Hess, LT Sharpe, K Nordby. Night Vision: Basic, Clinical and Applied Aspects. Cambridge, UK: Cambridge University Press, 1990.)*

deVries-Rose and Weber's laws fail to account for thresholds at high light intensities

At high stimulus intensity levels, the Weber fraction becomes large. In other words, the threshold ΔL increases faster than L. This is because the response of the visual system is *saturating*, meaning that it is becoming unresponsive even to large values of ΔL. Figure 3.3 shows increment threshold data for a rod monochromat, a person who has only rods in the retina (Hess et al. 1990). At low light levels, the increment threshold data are consistent with the deVries-Rose law over a small range. At intermediate background intensities, the threshold ΔL increases at a slightly lower rate than would be predicted by Weber's law. As the background luminance reaches approximately 1,000 candelas per square meter (cd/m²), the threshold ΔL becomes extremely large. At the highest levels, the increment threshold increases by 4 log units (or 10,000 fold) for just a 1 log unit (10 fold) increase in background light level. As described in the Appendix, this luminance level can occur in brightly lit rooms and is easily exceeded outdoors. Rod monochromats must live with the effects of rod saturation at photopic light levels because they are not able to rely on cones to modulate visual function, as most observers do. They describe themselves as being blinded by high-intensity light, and tend to avoid it. They are blind, in a way; although they see a bright light, little detail can be discerned because their intensity discrimination threshold is high. Because normal observers do have cones, the effects of rod photoreceptor saturation are not seen, except under special testing conditions (Hess et al. 1990). The mechanisms that underlie rod saturation are discussed in Chapter 4.

The Weber fraction is affected by stimulus size, duration, wavelength, and retinal location

Just as the absolute threshold for detecting light is affected by a wide range of stimulus dimensions, so are intensity discrimination thresholds. Stimulus size, duration, wavelength, and retinal location, as well as the intensity of the background stimulus all can affect the threshold ΔL and, therefore, the value of the Weber fraction. This has practical consequences in visual assessment. For example, if increment thresholds are to be tested in a patient who is suspected of having ocular disease, it is important to use a background light with a luminance in the range where the Weber fraction does not vary greatly in normal observers so that the threshold measures will not be altered by ocular changes that reduce retinal illuminance.

Figure 3.4 shows the data from an increment threshold study (Blackwell 1946) that measured the Weber fraction as a function of background luminance for five test stimulus sizes. At low background intensities, where the deVries-Rose law holds, the Weber fraction decreases at a constant rate as the background intensity increases. Notice that Weber's law holds only over a small range of the background luminances that were examined in this study. For the 121' stimulus, the threshold $\Delta L/L$ is constant from a little less than 1 cd/m^2 to approximately 100 cd/m^2. For the 4' target, it is constant from approximately 100 to 1,000 cd/m^2.

Bear in mind that the smaller the value of the Weber fraction, the more sensitive the visual system is to differences in light intensity. A larger Weber fraction means that it is less sensitive. For a given background luminance, the Weber fraction increases as target size decreases. For instance, in Figure 3.4, the Weber fraction for the 121' test stimulus at a background luminance of 10.0 cd/m^2 is approximately 0.01. This means that the observers in this study were just able to detect a change in luminance of 0.1 cd/m^2 under these conditions. L_T must be approximately 1% greater than L to reach threshold. For the smallest (4') test stimulus, the Weber fraction was approximately 0.1, meaning that the threshold ΔL was 1.0 cd/m^2 or approximately a 10% change in luminance.

As an example of the predictive use of this type of data, consider the curve in Figure 3.4 for the 121' diameter stimulus. This is roughly the size of a dinner plate seen at 8 m. Suppose the plate has a luminance of 0.0102 cd/m^2 in a dimly lit room, and it is positioned against a tablecloth with a luminance of 0.01 cd/m^2. The difference between the plate and the background tablecloth, ΔL, is 0.0002 cd/m^2 and $\Delta L/L = 0.02$. This means that the luminance of the plate is 2% greater than that of the background. From the data in Figure 3.1, one can predict that the plate would not be visible under these conditions. The Weber fraction for this background luminance is the antilog of -1.5 or approximately 0.03 (3%). Because there is only a contrast of 2% between the plate and the tablecloth, one could not see the plate. There would have to be a 3% contrast to detect it.

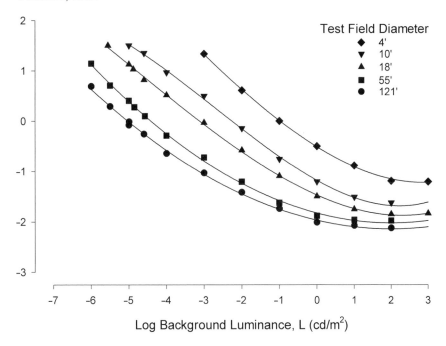

Log Weber
Fraction, ΔL/L

FIGURE 3.4 *Weber fraction versus background luminance at five different stimulus sizes. Stimuli were presented for 6 seconds. (cd = candela; L = luminance of the background; ΔL = threshold change in luminance to detect that L_T differs from L.) (Modified from HR Blackwell. Contrast thresholds of the human eye. J Opt Soc Am 1946;36:624–643.)*

In addition to the effect of test stimulus size, other stimulus parameters influence the increment threshold. For example, short duration flashes are less discriminable (e.g., the threshold ΔL is larger) than are longer duration flashes, as was shown in Chapter 2 (Bloch's law, see Figure 2.5) for flashed stimuli shorter than the critical duration.

The wavelength of the target and the background can affect the Weber fraction and can be of use in clinical vision testing. In short wavelength automated perimetry (SWAP) (Johnson et al. 1993), an intense yellow background is used to raise the increment threshold for cones sensitive to middle- and long-wavelength light. However, because the cones sensitive to short-wavelength light are relatively unaffected by this background luminance, their threshold ΔL for blue test stimuli remains low. SWAP can thus selectively measure the increment threshold of the short-wavelength–sensitive cone system (see Chapter 8). This is important clinically because recent studies (Quigley et al. 1989) have suggested that changes in these cones precede other changes during the development of glaucoma. Similar logic can be applied to determine combinations of background and increment wavelengths to selectively measure middle- and long-wavelength cone sensitivity.

Figure 3.5 shows the increment threshold as a function of retinal eccentricity for several levels of background luminance. Eight levels of background are illus-

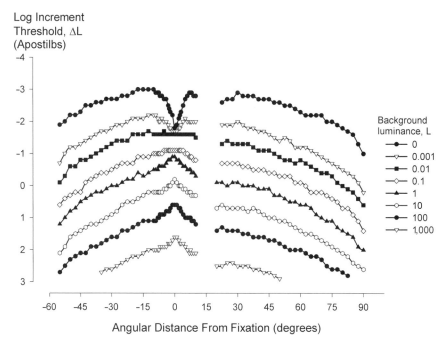

FIGURE 3.5   *Increment threshold as a function of eccentricity from the fovea for several luminance levels. The top line shows the threshold when the background reference luminance (L) is low (0 apostilbs). The bottom line shows the threshold for a background L of 1,000 apostilbs. Note that, on the y-axis, lower thresholds (higher sensitivities) are upwards on the graph. (Modified from JR Lynn, RL Felman, RJ Starita. Principles of Perimetry. In R Ritch, MB Shields, T Krupin [eds], The Glaucomas. St. Louis: Mosby, 1996;491–521.)*

trated, from complete darkness (L equals zero) to L equals 1,000 apostilbs (asb).* At high background levels (e.g., 1,000 asb; see bottom line of Figure 3.5) there is a noticeable increase in sensitivity (decrease in threshold) at the point of fixation corresponding to the high cone density in the fovea. Thus, the Weber fraction is lowest at the fovea. At the lowest background level (0 asb) where rods are used to detect the flashed spots, there is a noticeable decrease in sensitivity (increase in threshold, increase in the Weber fraction) at the fovea. This occurs because, at lower background levels, the cones are not sensitive enough to detect the flashed spot, so the more sensitive rods are used. Because there are no rods at the center of the fovea, there is a lower sensitivity (higher threshold) in compari-

---

*The apostilb (asb) is not a common unit of light measurement but is often used in specifying the stimuli used in perimetry. In terms of units more commonly used in the United States, 1,000 asb is the equivalent of 100 millilamberts, 318.3 cd/m^2, or 92.9 footlamberts. For comparison, the background luminance level on a computer monitor is the equivalent of approximately 250 asb. See the Appendix for further information on luminance.

son with the rod-rich peripheral retina. When thresholds are measured at these very low background luminances, people essentially have a blind spot at the fovea as well as at the optic disc. Knowledge of the influence of these stimulus parameters on the intensity discrimination threshold is important in choosing stimulus parameters in clinical visual perimetry tests.

Intensity discrimination can be limited at many places within the visual system

The variability of stimulus intensity at the level of quantum fluctuations places a basic limit on increment threshold as described by the deVries-Rose law. However, as described by Weber's law, the ability to discriminate the intensities of visual stimuli is often worse than can be predicted by quantum fluctuations. This reduction in increment threshold, relative to the theoretically possible value, must be due to limiting neural processing in the visual pathway.

The success of Weber's law in describing increment thresholds in the middle range of luminance values implies that the visual system loses information about the absolute number of quanta caught at the level of the photoreceptors when operating in this luminance range. Instead, it seems to process and transmit the ratios (or at least the relative luminance levels) of visual stimulus intensities. As is described in more detail in Chapter 6, this is appropriate for a visual system that analyzes the visual scene more in terms of the relative luminance content necessary to detect boundaries of objects than in terms of the actual stimulus intensity. Because, as described in the Appendix, surfaces always reflect a constant proportion of light at a given wavelength, it is important for the visual system to distinguish intensity differences and, sometimes, to de-emphasize absolute luminance values.

Information about stimulus luminance may be lost at the level of the photoreceptors or at subsequent steps of neural processing, or both. For instance, the intensity discrimination is affected by the type and density of photoreceptors at a given position within the retina. Rods and cones react differently to light intensity changes within the intensity range that they are active. This is due to the biochemical responses that occur after quantum absorption by the photopigment (Baylor 1996). There is a tremendous amplification of the response to quantum absorptions, and this amplification is affected by the background luminance, as is shown in Chapter 4. These effects can differ quantitatively in the rods and the cones.

Other locations in the visual pathway also modify a person's ability to discriminate intensity differences. The retinal bipolar cells, horizontal cells, amacrine cells, and ganglion cells have their own operating ranges and can affect the visual signal. In addition, there are many different classes of retinal ganglion cells, each responding a little differently to the signal from the photoreceptors and each affected a little differently by the conditions under which psychophysical testing is conducted. Thus, postreceptor neural factors significantly affect increment thresholds. These neural factors can be altered by changes in the size of the test target, the adaptation level, or the timing of the stimulus presentation (Harwerth et al. 1993).

Fechner attempted to relate magnitude of sensation to increment threshold

As described in Chapter 1, threshold measurements provide no information about the subjective sensory magnitude of a suprathreshold stimulus. Knowing that a 0.1 log unit flash is, under some circumstances, a threshold ΔL does not determine how bright the flash appears. Nor does knowing that a stimulus is above absolute threshold by a specific luminance value determine how bright that stimulus is. Many years before Stevens (see Chapter 1) derived his power law, Gustav Theodor Fechner (1801–1887) tried to use Weber's law to relate increment thresholds to sensory magnitude. Fechner assumed that Weber's law held over the entire range of stimulus intensities and suggested that each increment threshold, called a *just noticeable difference* (jnd), might be a basic unit of sensation. At a background luminance of 10, if the increment threshold were 0.1, then a stimulus of 10.1 would be 1 jnd larger than a stimulus with a luminance of 10. For a background luminance of 10.1, if the increment were 0.15, then a stimulus with luminance of 10.25 (10.1 plus 0.15) would be a second jnd brighter than the original stimulus with a luminance of 10. Based on Weber's law, each jnd is slightly larger than the one at the previous, lower stimulus intensity level. Fechner believed, however, that each jnd is equal in sensory magnitude. He devised a scale (Fechner's law) where Ψ is sensory magnitude, *k* is an arbitrary constant determining the scale unit, and Φ is the stimulus magnitude, such that

$$\Psi = k\log(\Phi) \hspace{4cm} \text{Eq. 3.3}$$

In Figure 3.6, stimulus magnitude is plotted on the abscissa. On the ordinate (y-axis), sensory magnitude is plotted using Fechner's law and Stevens' Power Law. The plot of Fechner's law is a curve that, at first glance, is not significantly different from a plot of Stevens' Power Law where the exponent is less than one. It now is believed that the Stevens' Power Law is generally a more accurate expression of the relationship between stimulus intensity and sensory magnitude. However, because Fechner's law was believed to be correct for many years, one finds many references to the visual system making a "logarithmic transform" of the stimulus intensity. Also, Fechner's law is the basis for the auditory decibel scale of loudness.

Fechner was in error when he assumed that Weber's law was correct for the whole range of stimulus intensities and when he assumed that all jnds were equal to each other in sensory magnitude. The latter is clearly not the case. As William James put it in 1899, "The many pounds which form the just perceptible addition to a hundred weight feel bigger when added than the few ounces which form the just noticeable addition to a pound."

Increment threshold measures are important in clinical vision testing

A goal of psychophysical measurement of visual function is to determine how the visual system functions under normal conditions, which, most of the time, involve

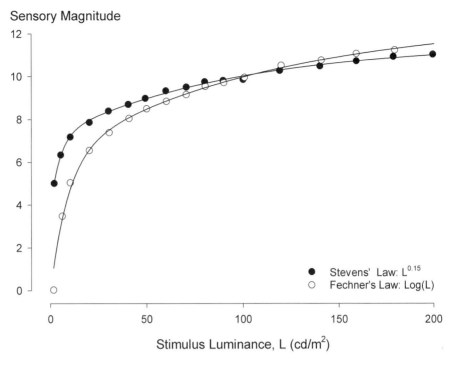

Sensory Magnitude

Stimulus Luminance, L (cd/m²)

● Stevens' Law: L^{0.15}
○ Fechner's Law: Log(L)

FIGURE 3.6   *Comparison plots of Fechner's law and the Stevens' Power Law. (cd = candela; L = luminance of the background.)*

relatively high luminance levels. For example, in visual acuity testing (see Chapter 5), the threshold for discriminating that gratings or letters are present is measured. In contrast sensitivity testing (see Chapter 6), the threshold for detecting a nonuniform distribution of light is measured. Several other types of increment thresholds are used in vision testing, including stereoacuity tests, which measure the thresholds for the detection of stimuli at different distances (depth) from the subject, and many types of color vision tests in which it is determined whether the difference threshold for color is normal (see Chapter 8). Establishing the range of normal values allows clinicians to determine whether a specific patient has a loss of visual function.

Measuring increment thresholds in patients is best done under conditions in which the Weber fraction is constant

To determine whether a patient's visual function is normal, it is important to choose stimulus conditions where slight changes in test parameters, such as the background L, do not produce large changes in the threshold. In other words, it is important to use background luminance values where Weber's law holds. For example, older observers differ from younger observers in the optical density of their lenses (Savage et al. 1993). Even with identical light sources, many older observers have a lower retinal illuminance than younger observers. If one measures increment thresholds in the older observers in a range of background luminance levels in which the Weber fraction changes with luminance level (see Figure 3.4), these patients might appear to have a loss of visual function (larger threshold

ΔL) because their thresholds are affected by the reduced background luminance. If tested at a comparable L, their thresholds might not actually differ from that of the younger observers. By paying careful heed to the manner in which stimulus conditions influence the increment threshold, one can avoid this source of error.

Visual field testing represents a major clinical application for use of the increment threshold

In concept, the simplest use of a threshold measurement to evaluate vision function is visual field testing. In this test, the increment threshold is determined for the position of a spot of light presented in the visual field against a constant background luminance. This is an important measure for detecting changes in vision that can be caused by eye disease or pathology of the visual pathways. Although the traditional visual acuity test is excellent for quantifying foveal vision, it tells the clinician nothing about the health of the peripheral retina. In measuring peripheral vision, rather than asking the patient to identify letters, the patient is asked just to respond to the presence or absence of a circular spot of light.

To measure the limits of the visual field of the eye, a stimulus is gradually moved from a peripheral position where it is not seen to a position where it is seen. Measured in this way, the visual field of a normal eye extends 60° superiorly from the point of fixation, 75° inferiorly, 100° temporally, and 60° nasally (Anderson 1987). Within these limits, the visual field is not uniform in its thresholds, however. As shown in Figure 3.5, at high background luminance levels, a target must be relatively intense to be detected in the periphery, whereas less intense targets can be detected when presented at the fovea. This nonuniformity for detecting small targets has been described by Traquair (1946) as being analogous to an "island" or "hill of vision" surrounded by a sea of blindness. It is hard to improve on his description of Figure 3.7:

> The coastline is somewhat ovoid in shape, and rises steeply so that the island is surrounded by cliffs vertical at one side, sharply sloping at the other. Above the cliffs is a sloping plateau which rises more rapidly again towards the somewhat eccentrically situated summit. This is crowned by a sharp pinnacle whose sides curve steeply upwards from a narrow base. To one side of this point is a pit (the blind spot) with sides almost vertical at first, but soon becoming perpendicular, which extends down to the level of the surrounding sea. To an observer situated in the air above the pinnacle a panoramic view of the whole island is presented. On the shore only large objects can be seen and colors cannot be distinguished. Immediately within the coastline along the top of the cliffs smaller objects are visible and colors can be recognized if in large enough patches, and as the neighborhood of the summit is approached smaller and smaller objects become apparent until at the apex of the pinnacle the most minute details can be detected. . . . The problem of perimetry is the survey of this surface.

In terms of Traquair's poetic vision, visual loss is an erosion of this hill of vision that, under extreme circumstances, leads to its sinking into a sea of blindness. A clinician can gain a rough estimate of the extent of visual field loss by using methods such as the *confrontation field*. This method tests the patient's

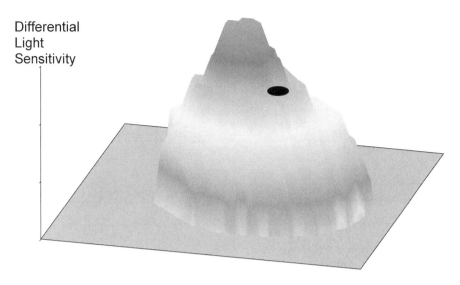

Differential Light Sensitivity

FIGURE 3.7   *Illustration of the "hill of vision." The fovea corresponds to the region of greatest sensitivity (smallest increment threshold). Small and dim spots may be seen at this point, but larger or more intense, or both, spots are needed to reach threshold, as the spot is presented further from the fovea. The black oval marks the optic disc where sensitivity is zero. In the usual plots of visual fields, this "hill" is represented on a two-dimensional plot as isopters (see Figure 3.8) or as a gray scale. (Modified from DR Anderson. Perimetry with and without Automation. St. Louis: Mosby, 1987.)*

ability to recognize, in the periphery of the visual field, a large target, such as a hand with a number of fingers extended. However, more detailed methods are needed to detect the often subtle erosions in visual sensitivity that can precede large losses in vision due to diseases, such as glaucoma.

In Figure 3.7, the height of the Traquair's hill of vision indicates the relative sensitivity of the observer to detect a target intensity as different from the background luminance at different retinal locations. At higher luminance levels, sensitivity is greatest at the point of fixation, which corresponds to stimulation of the fovea (see Figure 3.5). Under photopic conditions, the cones are more sensitive than the rods and the greatest density of cones is found in the fovea.

Isopters define points in the visual field with similar increment thresholds

If a dim small target is viewed against a photopic background, the visual field, defined by one's ability to detect that target, is quite small and centered around the point of fixation (fovea) in the normal observer. If one plots the limit (or perimeter) of the area of the visual field that can be seen with this target, this defines an *isopter*, a line connecting retinal regions with similar threshold. If a slightly larger target is used or if the luminance of the small target is increased, the visual field is larger. By using progressively larger or slightly more luminous targets, or both, a series of isopters is defined that demonstrates that one can see with larger portions of the retina. Within an isopter (i.e., closer to the fovea), the stimulus is suprathreshold and is seen by the patient (Haley 1986). Outside of the isopter, the stimulus is below threshold (subthreshold) and is not seen.

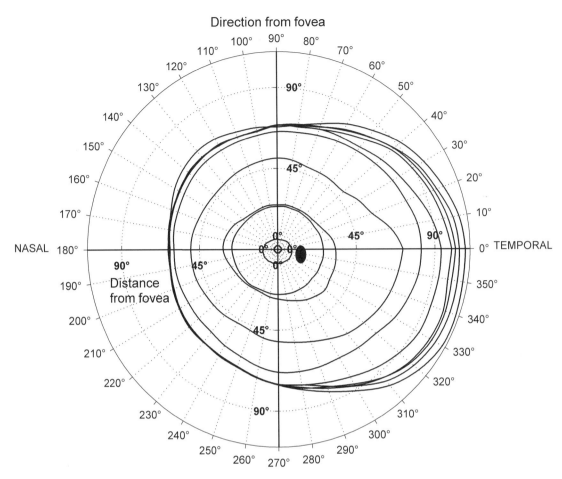

FIGURE 3.8   *Visual field plot using isopters that connect regions of similar threshold, similar to a topo-graphic map. (Modified from J Glaser, J Goodwin. Neuro-ophthalmologic Examination: The Visual System. In J Glaser [ed], Neuro-ophthalmology [2nd ed]. Philadelphia: Lippincott, 1990;9–36.)*

The location of an isopter depends jointly on the size and the intensity of the incremental test spot. The lower contour lines of Figure 3.7 (the "shore-line") on the hill of vision indicate the isopters for large or intense, or both, test targets. In clinical use, a two-dimensional plot of these isopters is drawn, as shown in Figure 3.8. The same data can be shown as a gray scale. In the gray-scale method of presentation, lighter areas represent high sensitivity, whereas darker areas represent lower sensitivity (and therefore are the result of mea-surement with a larger or more intense target).

Results of static and kinetic perimetry may differ

Increment thresholds in visual perimetry are measured in two main ways. In kinetic perimetry, an increment of constant size and intensity is moved across the patient's view, until the patient can notice it, thus defining a point on an isopter. A set of such points determined for a number of directions of target movement around the fixation point defines the isopter for the target used. Generally, the target is moved from "not-seeing" to "seeing," because more repeatable results are found this way. The tangent screen and the Goldmann perimeter are typical pieces of equipment for kinetic perimetry.

In static perimetry, increment thresholds are measured at many specific points in the visual field is measured. Computer-automated devices, such as the Humphrey Field Analyzer, are typically used for static perimetry. One does not always find equivalent results using the two techniques. Particularly large discrepancies may be due to the Riddoch phenomenon (Anderson 1987): In an abnormal part of the visual field, patients may have a much greater sensitivity to the moving target that is used in kinetic perimetry than to the target that is used in static perimetry.

If a patient has a loss of visual function, he or she may not be able to see any visual stimulus at a certain point within his or her visual field. This patient has an **absolute scotoma**. If the patient requires a larger or more intense stimulus than normal at threshold, the patient has a **relative scotoma**. Figure 3.8 shows the normal blind spot at the optic disc as an absolute scotoma in the temporal visual field (nasal retina). At this retinal position, there are no photoreceptors, only the bundle of individual optic nerve fibers exiting the eye through the optic nerve head.

The three main dimensions that are varied in visual perimetry are stimulus size, intensity, and retinal locus

Because Goldmann perimetry has served as the standard in kinetic perimetry, the Goldmann perimeter stimulus terminology has been retained with the modern development of automated perimetry. Target size progresses from Goldmann I (which subtends 0.11°) to Goldmann V (which subtends 1.72°). Each larger target size subtends twice the visual angle of the target that precedes it.

Target intensity in visual perimetry is usually defined in terms of the attenuation of the maximum target intensity possible for a given brand of perimeter. The amount of this attenuation is given in decibels (dB). Ten dB represents a decrease in intensity of 1.0 log unit or a factor of 10. A 3 dB decrease represents a –0.3 log unit change or a decrease in light intensity by a factor of 2.

The criterion for the detection of a change from normal is often that a patient needs 4 dB more light at a given point within the visual field. However, results using different manufacturers' products are not always comparable. Because different perimeters have different maximum intensities possible for their targets, results with one type of perimeter may differ from results with another.

More efficient perimetric tests are being developed by refining standard psychophysical methods

Much of visual field testing is performed using computerized visual field equipment to perform static perimetry using a staircase variation of the Method of Limits. A test flash is increased in 4 dB steps, until the patient detects it. It is then dimmed in 2 dB steps to obtain a finer estimate of the threshold. A complete visual field examination requires a repeat of this sequence at many points; this can be tiring for patients and is not always an efficient use of time.

Because stimuli that are much more intense or less intense than threshold are not informative, some faster strategies have been developed that attempt to present only near-threshold stimuli. One such strategy is to use the results of a patient's previous exam to suggest the starting point for threshold estimation. A second strategy refers to data from a control group of normal observers. Third, a screening test might use only a single value at which a point in the visual field would be measured. For example, in one strategy, patients are tested with targets that are 6 dB above threshold for normal observers. If the patient detects all the targets, the examiner can conclude that the patient does not have any absolute scotomas, and any relative scotoma is less than 6 dB. The test may be made even more efficient by evaluating only points suggested by a preliminary diagnosis of pathology for a given patient. Some such test procedures can screen a monocular visual field in less than 5 minutes. For example, using frequency doubling technology a visual field can be screened in approximately 40 seconds (see Chapter 7).

There may be substantial anatomical loss before visual field deficits are detected

It has been surprisingly difficult to determine how much retinal damage is associated with a particular threshold elevation. This is because threshold changes do not seem to be directly related to neural losses. If the loss of neurons were proportional to the increase in threshold, a 6 dB loss (which is a sensitivity that is 25% of normal) would correspond to a loss of 75% of the neurons at that target location, assuming the remaining neurons have normal sensitivity. However, recent research suggests that, in glaucoma, there is a substantial loss of retinal ganglion cells before any detectable increase occurs in threshold, such that some patients have lost as much as 50% of their optic nerve fibers when visual field testing first reveals an erosion of the "hill of vision" (Quigley et al. 1989). This leads to some interesting questions: Can more sensitive psychophysical tests be devised to detect changes when fewer optic nerve fibers have been lost? What should be the criterion for loss, neural loss, or functional loss? Does visual field testing as presently performed give us an adequate measure of a patient's functional loss? These questions remain unanswered as of yet, but many researchers are trying to develop more sensitive and efficient methods of examining visual fields and measuring visual field loss. New microscopic techniques to measure the thickness of the nerve fiber layer are also being developed as a direct way to assess neural loss.

Glare is ambient light that interferes with increment or difference threshold detections

Older patients often mention that they have trouble driving at night when they are confronted with glare from oncoming headlights. Some contact lens wearers and some patients who have had refractive surgery have similar complaints. The effect of car headlights on visual performance is called *disability glare* and is due to the effects of scattered light on visual acuity. Glare can also produce another, poorly understood effect called *discomfort glare* (Pitts & Kleinstein 1993). Patients can experience discomfort from glare but still have no loss of visual acuity; they can also have a decrease in visual acuity without sensing any discomfort. The two phenomena appear to have different mechanisms.

Any clouding of the normally clear optical media of the eye can scatter light, resulting in changes in vision. If the particles causing the scatter are small compared to a wavelength of light, the light scatter (called *Rayleigh scattering*) is inversely proportional to λ^4. Small particles scatter 400 nm light 16 times more than 800 nm light. If the particles are large, light scatter is independent of wavelength and called *Mie scattering*. It is the difference between these two kinds of scattering that causes the thick scleral fibers of a healthy patient to appear white (Mie scattering) and the thin scleral fibers of osteogenesis imperfecta to appear blue (Rayleigh scattering) (Miller 1991).

Scattered light causes a veiling luminance over the retinal image that is proportional to the square of the angle of displacement of a glare source from a directly viewed light. This is described by the Stiles-Holladay formula, which, for a young eye, is

$$L_v = K\left(\frac{E_0}{\theta_0^2}\right) \qquad \text{Eq. 3.4}$$

where L_v is the veiling luminance, K is a constant, E_0 is the illuminance of the glare source, and θ_0 is the angle between the glare source and the fixated target.

This veiling luminance adds together with the background luminance with the result that the increment necessary for threshold detection must be increased. Suppose, for instance, that the Weber fraction for a given test configuration is 0.1. The threshold increment for detection against a 100 cd/m^2 background is 10 cd/m^2. If a glare source is placed in the area adjacent to the test stimulus, such that it casts a veiling luminance of 20 cd/m^2 at the point of the retina being examined, the Weber fraction for a 10 cd/m^2 increment will drop to 10 divided by 120, or 0.083. This would be below threshold for the observer; the increment would need to be increased to 12 cd/m^2 to be seen.

Study Guide

1. Distinguish between a difference threshold and an increment threshold.
2. Define the deVries-Rose law.
3. Define the Weber fraction.
4. Define Weber's law.
5. Over (approximately) what range of luminance values does the deVries-Rose law hold?
6. Over (approximately) what range of luminance values does Weber's law hold?
7. Draw a graph showing a typical relationship of threshold ΔL to the L.
8. Draw a graph showing a typical relationship of the Weber fraction to L.

9. Be able to use Figure 3.4 to determine whether a target (L_T) with a particular luminance and size could be seen against any specified background luminance.
10. Define Fechner's law.
11. Compare and contrast Fechner's law with Stevens' Power Law.
12. What stimulus parameters affect the Weber fraction?
13. Define the "hill of vision."
14. Describe a typical psychophysical procedure for testing visual fields.
15. What is the influence of angular distance from the fovea on threshold ΔL?
16. Approximately what fraction of optic nerve fibers are lost in glaucoma before a visual field test detects a loss in sensitivity?
17. What is the relationship between wavelength and light scatter caused by small particles?
18. Define the Stiles-Holladay formula.
19. Distinguish between Rayleigh scattering and Mie scattering.

Glossary

Absolute scotoma: a complete loss of function at a point in the visual field.
Millilambert: a unit of measure of luminance. 1 millilambert = 0.31416 candelas per square meter (cd/m^2).
Relative scotoma: a partial loss of function at a point in the visual field that results in a higher-than-normal threshold for detecting visual stimuli.

4   Adaptation to Light and Dark

Thomas T. Norton and David A. Corliss

Overview

The material presented in this chapter exemplifies how extraordinarily sensitive measurements of visual function can be to small changes in stimulus dimensions. The visual system operates over a range of retinal illuminance levels of more than 10 orders of magnitude. This means that the sensitivity of the visual system can range from detecting a few quanta of light in complete darkness to seeing a polar bear on a background of snow on a bright, sunny day. Four mechanisms are used to allow vision to occur over this very wide range: (1) two different photoreceptor sub-systems, the rods and the cones; (2) change in the pupil size; (3) change in the concentrations of bleached and unbleached photopigment; (4) and changes in neural responsiveness.

Light adaptation refers to the process that decreases the visual system's light sensitivity (increases threshold) in response to an adapting light. Dark adaptation is the increase in sensitivity (decrease in threshold) that occurs as a function of time in darkness. A dark adaptation curve potentially consists of a cone branch and a rod branch with a rod-cone break at the transition between the two. However, the dark adaptation curves one obtains have rather different shapes and time courses depending on whether rods or cones, or both, are affected by the adapting light and by the test flash. Dark adaptation can be affected by ocular abnormalities and eye disease.

Although neural ("network") changes can produce rapid adaptation without photopigment changes, and neural adaptation can occur before photoreceptor adaptation, the level of bleached photopigment accounts for much of the retinal sensitivity change that occurs during light and dark adaptation. The equivalent background theory demonstrates that the threshold during dark adaptation is equivalent to the threshold that would be measured in the presence of an adapting light that bleaches the same amount of pigment. The level of light adaptation controls the magnitude of the photoreceptor responses to test flashes.

The visual system uses four mechanisms to adapt to a wide range of light levels

The visual system is able to operate as the level of retinal illuminance changes over more than 10 orders of magnitude, ranging from starlight to bright sunlight. The main question addressed in this chapter is how the visual system can be so sensitive at absolute threshold and still mediate vision without being saturated by an overpowering amount of light on a bright sunny day at the beach. The visual system actually uses four basic mechanisms to allow vision to occur over this very wide range of illuminance.

First, there are two different photoreceptor subsystems, the rods and the cones. Rods are used in low-luminance (**scotopic**) conditions and cones are used in high luminance (**photopic**) conditions. This was originally called the **duplicity theory** when it was proposed by Schultz (1866). It is now an established fact, rather than a theory. As described in Chapter 2, rods can be sensitive to very small amounts of light. Cones are not activated by these low luminance levels. At higher luminance levels, the rods saturate, that is, they are not able to respond to luminance changes above a certain level, and the cones are used instead. There is a middle (**mesopic**) range of luminances where rods and cones are used. The rod system in humans sacrifices color information and has low spatial acuity and temporal acuity to gain sensitivity by summating over a larger retinal area and over a longer time than does the cone system. The cone system sacrifices sensitivity to gain color vision (critically important for primates, such as humans) along with better spatial and temporal acuity. The range of light levels to which the rods are sensitive, when added to the range over which the cones are sensitive, nearly doubles the range of light intensities to which the visual system can respond. The eye is often compared to a camera; in the case of the duplicity theory, the analogy would be to changing film—at low light intensities, one uses sensitive film, which is usually grainy and, to get the most sensitivity, black and white. At higher light intensities, one uses a less sensitive, high-resolution color film.

A second mechanism used to adapt the visual system to different luminance levels is to change the pupil size, which takes less than 1 second. If the smallest pupil size is approximately 2 mm and the largest approximately 8 mm, a change in pupil size can only alter the retinal illuminance by approximately 1.2 log units (a factor of 16×). Thus, if the eye is exposed to a 2 log unit increase in luminance, pupillary constriction cannot fully compensate to keep the retinal illuminance constant. In addition, the pupil itself shows adaptation to a given light level: After initially constricting to an increase in luminance, there is a slight, gradual dilation.

A third, and very important, mechanism is a change in the concentration of photopigment. In fact, the level of bleached photopigment explains much of visual adaptation. A fourth mechanism, and one that can change the sensitivity of the visual system 1–2 log units within a second without changes in photopigment concentration, is a change in neural responsiveness (also called *network* responsiveness). The last two are discussed in detail later in this chapter.

The classic dark adaptation curve has a cone and a rod portion

Visual adaptation is the process whereby the visual system adjusts its operating level to the prevailing light level. **Light adaptation** is the process that increases threshold luminance (decreases sensitivity) in response to an increased prevailing level of illumination. **Dark adaptation** is defined as the decrease in threshold luminance (increased sensitivity) as a function of time in darkness. Everyone with a normal visual system has experienced the basic phenomenon of dark adaptation after walking into a darkened room from a lighted one—it takes time before the features of the room become discernible and dim lights, not initially perceived, become visible. Dark adaptation is easily measured in the laboratory or the clinic by using standard psychophysical threshold techniques. First, the eyes are exposed for a period of time to a suprathreshold **adapting light** of fairly large spatial extent and desired wavelength composition. After this adapting light is turned off, at an instant called *time zero*, a test flash of designated wavelengths and spatial extent is presented at intervals to designated retinal locations. The Method of Limits (ascending only, or tracking) or the Method of Adjustment is usually used to determine the threshold luminance (L_T) required to detect the test flash. The test flash must be presented for a short enough duration (less than 1 second) and infrequently enough to prevent the test flash itself from light adapting the eye.

Figure 4.1 shows the classic curve observed in a dark adaptation study. The time scale begins, the instant that the high luminance white adapting light is turned off. The measurements of the threshold over a period of 40 minutes when the subject remained in the dark were made using a short-wavelength violet test flash that stimulates rods and cones. At time zero, both the rods and

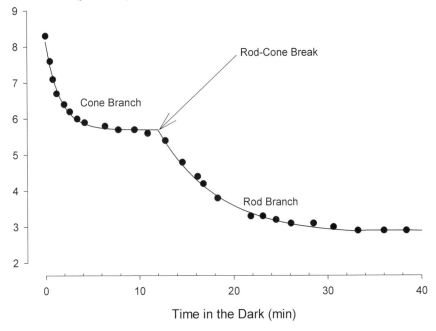

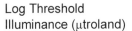

Log Threshold
Illuminance (μtroland)

FIGURE 4.1 *Typical dark adaptation curve after exposure to an intense adapting light that light adapted rods and cones. The test flash subtended 5°, was located on the nasal retina 30° from the fovea, and consisted of wavelengths that could stimulate rods or cones. (Modified from S Hecht, C Haig, AM Chase. The influence of light adaptation on subsequent dark adaptation of the eye. J Gen Physiol 1937;20:831–850.)*

the cones begin to dark adapt. The first thing to note is that there are two branches to the adaptation curve. For the first 10 minutes or so after time zero, there is an upper cone branch during which the test flash is detected by the cones. The rods are slower to dark adapt and have a threshold that is higher than the threshold of the cones during this period. The subject can identify the color of the stimulus at threshold during this part of the dark adaptation curve.

During approximately the first 3 minutes after the adapting light goes off, the cone branch shows a rapid decrease in threshold luminance. This is followed by a period that lasts until approximately 11 or 12 minutes, during which there is little decrease in the threshold and the cones approach their lowest threshold level because they are fully dark adapted. At threshold, the test flash appears either white or colored depending on its wavelength composition. After approximately 12 minutes, the subject's threshold begins to drop again as the rods become more sensitive than the cones. At threshold, the stimulus appears gray or colorless. The rod branch of the curve shows the dark adaptation of the rods, but only after the point in time at which they became more sensitive than the cones. The point during dark adaptation at which rods become more sensitive than cones is defined as the **rod-cone break**. This divides the portion of the dark adaptation curve where the subject detected the test flash with cones from the portion where rods were used to detect the test flash. After approximately 30 minutes, the rod portion of the curve reaches a plateau region where there is little further decrease in threshold because the rods are fully dark adapted. If one measures a dark adaptation curve of a rod monochromat (see Figure 4.11), a person who lacks cones, the dark adaptation curve does not have a break in it and shows only the rod branch of the curve.

The explanation of the dark adaptation curve in the previous paragraph is based on several principles that have been discovered through many psychophysical and neurophysiological investigations over the past 100 years: (1) Rods and cones both start dark adapting at time zero, (2) the more sensitive system determines the threshold at any time, (3) cones adapt faster than rods, and (4) the lowest threshold obtained with cones is much higher than the lowest threshold obtained using rods because the rods are ultimately more sensitive than the cones. It is important to remember that the rods begin to dark adapt at the same time as the cones, but they are initially less sensitive than the cones and they are slower to dark adapt.

The shape of the dark adaptation curve is extremely sensitive to changes in many stimulus dimensions because of the duplex nature of the retina

The shape and time course of a dark adaptation curve is dictated primarily by whether rods or cones, or both, are affected by the adapting light and by the test flash. Substantial variations occur with small changes in the stimulus dimensions first described in Chapter 1. These include (1) the retinal location that is stimulated by the test flash, (2) the size of the test flash, (3) the wavelength of the adapting light, (4) the wavelength of the test flash, (5) the intensity and (6) duration of the adapting light, and (7) the task that the subject is asked to perform.

The rod portion of the dark adaptation curve is more prominent if the test flash stimulates a retinal region with high rod density

Figure 4.2 shows the dark adaptation curves obtained by Hecht et al. (1935) when a 2° test spot was used to test the threshold at different locations on the retina. Before dark adaptation began, the subject was exposed to a 300 milli-lambert (approximately 10^3 candelas per square meter [cd/m^2]) broad-spectrum adapting field for 2 minutes. When the adapting light went off the 2° test spot was flashed for 1 second every 2 seconds. The subject adjusted the intensity to find the threshold luminance as a function of time. When this spot was centered on the fovea, there was only a slight decrease in threshold over time as the cones reached their minimum threshold, and there was no rod-cone break. This was because the central 2° of the visual field contain almost only cones that can never become very sensitive. Even though there were many rods elsewhere in the retina that became very sensitive, the test flash did not measure the threshold of those rods because of its position.

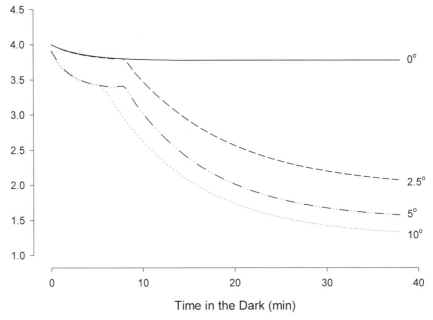

FIGURE 4.2 *Dark adaptation measured with a 2° test flash placed at various angular distances (0°, 2.5°, 5°, and 10°) from the fovea. (Modified from S Hecht, C Haig, G Wald. Dark adaptation of retinal fields of different size and location. J Gen Physiol 1935;19:321–337.)*

When Hecht et al. (1935) placed the test spot 2.5° from the fovea, a distinct rod-cone break was detected, and the final, rod-mediated threshold was much lower than when the spot had been centered on the fovea. Placement of the test spot 5° from the fovea and then 10° from the fovea also produced a rod-cone break and an even lower final threshold, presumably because (1) the rod density was greater at 10° than at 5° or 2.5°, and (2) the receptive fields of the ganglion cells were progressively larger, so that there was a greater likelihood that enough of the quanta in the flash would be absorbed within the receptive fields of enough cells to produce the preception of light in the subject.

A larger test flash generally yields a more prominent rod branch of the dark adaptation curve

Figure 4.3 shows that the size of a foveally fixated test flash dramatically alters the shape of the dark adaptation curve. The light-adaptation procedure, the testing conditions, and the subject were the same as in Figure 4.2. As in Figure 4.2, the 2° diameter test flash, which stimulated almost only cones, produced a small rapid decrease in cone threshold. The final threshold after 30 minutes of dark adaptation was high because essentially no rods were stimulated by the test flash.

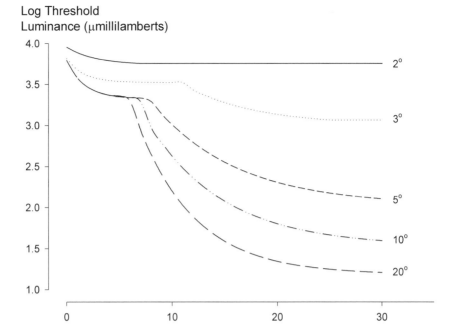

Log Threshold
Luminance (μmillilamberts)

FIGURE 4.3   *Dark adaptation measured with centrally fixated test flashes of different diameters, indicated to the right of each curve. (Modified from S Hecht, C Haig, G Wald. Dark adaptation of retinal fields of different size and location. J Gen Physiol 1935;19:321–337.)*

When larger test flashes were used, the rod branch of the curve became much more prominent. The final threshold after 30 minutes became much lower because the larger test flashes covered larger and larger regions of the retina where they could stimulate more and more rods. Given that the threshold is always set by the most sensitive retinal mechanism available, the odds of detecting a large test flash are greater than the odds of detecting a smaller test flash of the same intensity, even after the flash is large enough (5° or more) that it always stimulates some rods.

Different rod and cone sensitivities to the wavelength of the test flash affect the shape of the dark adaptation curve

Figure 4.4 shows how the wavelength of the test flash affects the shape of the measured dark adaptation curve. The main factor is that the peak sensitivity of the rods is approximately 510 nm in an intact eye. If the test flash contains 510 nm, then the rod branch of the curve is more prominent and the final threshold is relatively low. If the test flash contains only long wavelengths, which primarily stimulate cones but not rods, the cone branch of the curve predominates; when the test flash contained only wavelengths longer than 680 nm, it was detectable only by the cones. The dark adaptation curve shows no rod branch,

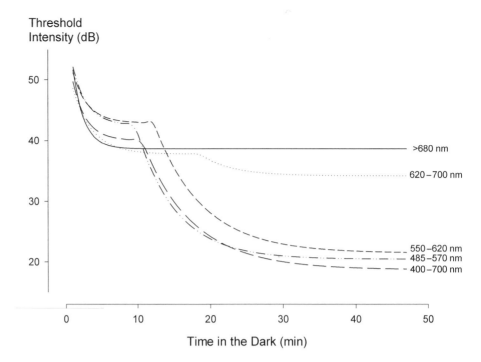

FIGURE 4.4   *Effect of test flash wavelength on dark adaptation curves. The adapting light (35° diameter, 2,000 millilamberts for 5 minutes, centered 7° temporal to the fovea) contained a broad spectrum of wavelengths so that it light adapted rods and all three cone types. The shape of the curve depended on whether the test flash stimulated cones only or rods and cones. On the ordinate, dB is decibels, a log scale in which zero equals absolute threshold and 10 dB equals 1 log unit. Values do not reach absolute threshold because the stimulus conditions are not as well controlled as in the Hecht et al. study described in Chapter 2. (Modified from A Chapanis. The dark adaptation of the color anomalous measured with lights of different hues. J Gen Physiol 1947;30:423–437.)*

even though the rods in the subject's eye must have had a low threshold after 40 minutes.

Rods can be dark adapted in relatively high-luminance conditions if the adapting-light wavelength primarily affects cones

Figure 4.5 shows a combination of two effects: the use of (1) a relatively dim white adapting light and (2) a red adapting light that does not effectively adapt rods. When a white (broad-spectrum) adapting light was used, its intensity was so low (36.9 millilamberts) that it did not produce much light adaptation (as is the case in Figure 4.6 for the 263 troland curve). Thus, the rods were quite sensitive as soon as the adapting light was turned off and there was no cone branch to the curve.

The red adapting light used in this experiment is similar to that used in ready rooms on military installations when pilots must be ready to rush out into the night and take off. It stimulates the cones almost exclusively, so that a person in this situation can still read and find his or her way around. This light

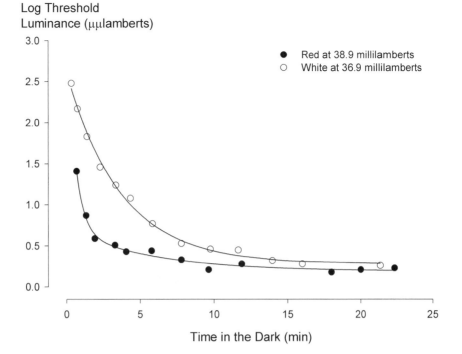

Log Threshold
Luminance (μμlamberts)

FIGURE 4.5   *Average dark adaptation curves after light adaptation to a red or white adapting light of approximately the same luminance for 5 minutes. The test flash was short wavelength (blue), 3° in diameter, and 200 milliseconds in duration and was presented 7° nasal to the fovea. (Modified from S Hecht, Y Hsia. Dark adaptation after light adaptation to red and white lights. J Opt Soc Am 1945;35:261–267.)*

does not effectively stimulate rods because rods are not as sensitive to long wavelengths as are cones. Thus, a situation is created in which the rods are, effectively, in the dark while the person is using the red-sensitive cones to see. Figure 4.5 clearly shows that when the red adapting light was turned off, the rods were almost fully dark adapted (filled circles) as evidenced by the fact that dark adaptation occurs faster and a lower threshold is reached than when the white adapting light was used. A person emerging from this situation into darkness could use the rods to navigate in a a darkened world better than a person who had been exposed to white light of similar luminance.

A more intense or longer-duration adapting light makes the cone branch of the dark adaptation curve more prominent and prolongs dark adaptation

A more intense adapting light produces greater light adaptation as shown in Figure 4.6. This is evidenced by the facts that, as the retinal illuminance of the adapting light was decreased, the threshold test flash luminance was lower immediately after the adapting light went off, the rod-cone break occurred sooner after time zero, and rod adaptation was complete in a shorter time after time zero. For the lowest two adapting light values, the rods were more sensi-

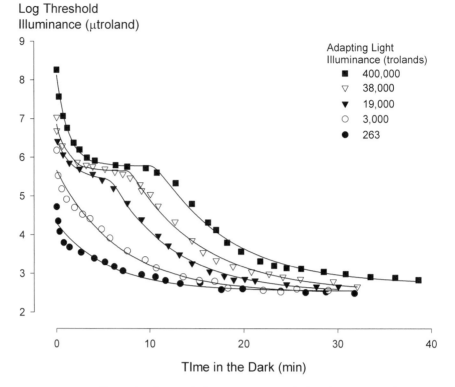

Log Threshold
Illuminance (µtroland)

FIGURE 4.6   *Effect of adapting-light intensity on dark adaptation. Adapting-light intensities ranged from 263 to 400,000 trolands of white light. The test flash was a short-wavelength violet light. (Modified from S Hecht, C Haig, AM Chase. The influence of light adaptation on subsequent dark adaptation of the eye. J Gen Physiol 1937;20:831–850.)*

tive than the cones as soon as the adapting light went off, so there was no cone branch to the dark adaptation curve.

Figure 4.7 shows an effect similar to that in Figure 4.6. In this case, the investigators altered the length of the time that the adapting light was on before dark adaptation began. The longer an intense adapting light was presented, the more light adapted the subject became. From Figure 4.6 and Figure 4.7, it is evident that being more light adapted causes (1) a higher initial threshold, (2) a more prominent cone branch, (3) a rod-cone break that (4) occurs later, and (5) a longer time until complete rod dark adaptation occurs.

If the threshold task requires the subject to have good acuity, cones must be used

Figure 4.8 shows that the type of task that the subject must perform also influences the shape of the dark adaptation curve. The curve in the graph measured without a grating is a typical dark adaptation curve in which the subject detects the presence of a test flash. It shows both a rod branch and a cone branch. When the investigators required that the orientation of a

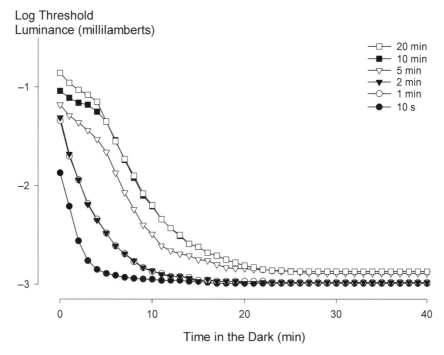

FIGURE 4.7 *Effect of adapting-light duration on dark adaptation. The adapting light had a luminance of 333 millilamberts. (Modified from G Wald, AB Clark. Visual adaptation and the chemistry of the rods. J Gen Physiol 1937;21:93–105.)*

grating be detected, rather than just the presence of the test flash, the shape of the curve changed, and more light was needed in the test flash to reach the threshold. As the grating became finer, the subject needed better acuity and even more light to reach threshold. In Figure 4.8, the curves in which visual acuity equals 1.04 and 0.62 occurred when gratings with the narrowest lines were used. This task could only be mediated by the cone system (see Chapter 5). Thus, the test flash intensity had to be high enough to stimulate only the cones. This is why there was no rod branch in the dark adaptation curve.

Early dark adaptation is a small but very rapid decrease in threshold mediated by neural changes

In Figures 4.1–4.8, dark adaptation was measured on a time scale of minutes. Baker (1953) examined the threshold for detecting the test flash within 2 seconds after time zero and found that there is a rapid decrease in threshold within 0.3 seconds after the adapting flash was turned off (Figure 4.9). Baker used adapting lights of 57, 1,800, and 57,000 trolands. The test flash was 1° in diameter, 20 milliseconds in duration, and was centered on the fovea. Over the course of many trials, he light adapted the subject and then presented the test flash at varying times before, at the same time as, and after the adapting

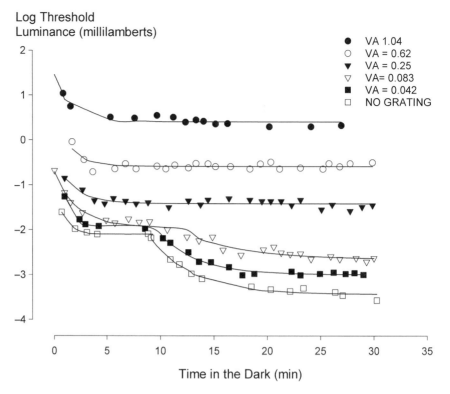

FIGURE 4.8 *Luminance thresholds needed for a subject to detect the orientation of a grating. The visual acuity (VA) is the reciprocal of the visual angle subtended by each grating bar that the subject was required to detect. In the bottom curve, a flashed spot was used instead of a grating. (Modified from JL Brown, CH Graham, H Leibowitz, HB Ranken. Luminance thresholds for the resolution of visual detail during dark adaptation. J Opt Soc Am 1953;43:197–202.)*

light was extinguished. The main finding was that the threshold for detecting the test flash drops very rapidly after the offset of the adapting light. Indeed, when the most intense adapting light was used, the threshold dropped more than 1 log unit within the first 0.3 second. Thus, **early dark adaptation** begins very rapidly after the offset of the adapting light. This is due to neural (network), rather than photopigment, changes.

The rise in threshold before the adapting light goes off is due to the duration of the neural response to the test flash

An even more interesting result of Baker's study is that the elevation in threshold for detecting the test flash begins shortly before the adapting light goes off. This is because the response to the test flash has a duration of several milliseconds. As shown in Figure 4.10A and B, the same on-center retinal neurons that respond to the test flash with an increase in action potentials also respond to the offset of the adapting light with a decrease in action potentials. When these two response patterns overlap in time, the response to the test flash is cut off

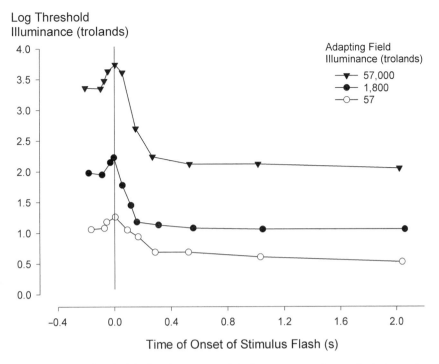

Log Threshold
Illuminance (trolands)

FIGURE 4.9   *Thresholds for detecting a brief (0.02 second) test flash immediately before and after the adapting light was turned off. The time that the adapting light was turned off is indicated as zero. Retinal illuminance of the adapting light, in trolands, is as labeled. Note that the time scale in this figure is in seconds, rather than the minutes shown in the previous figures. (Modified from HD Baker. The instantaneous threshold and early dark adaptation. J Opt Soc Am 1953;43:798–803.)*

(see Figure 4.10D), making it difficult to detect. If the test flash intensity is raised, the firing rate of the cell becomes higher so that enough of the response to the test flash can occur before the response to the adapting light is offset so that the test flash can be detected.

Detecting the test flash at the same time the adapting light is turned off is a signal detection task

When test flashes are presented well before the adapting light goes off (see Figure 4.10C) or well after the adapting light goes off (see Figure 4.10F), the thresholds are at their lowest. Note in Figure 4.9, however, that the threshold for detecting the test flash is at its highest when it is presented precisely at the time that the adapting light is turned off. As shown in Figure 4.10E, this increase in threshold can be due to the difficulty in detecting the neural activity produced by the test flash (the signal) against the reduction of activity in the on-center neurons that is produced by turning off the adapting light. In other words, the net number of action potentials that occur in response to the test flash is reduced to the point that the response is below threshold for flash intensities that would have been detected before or after the adapting light offset.

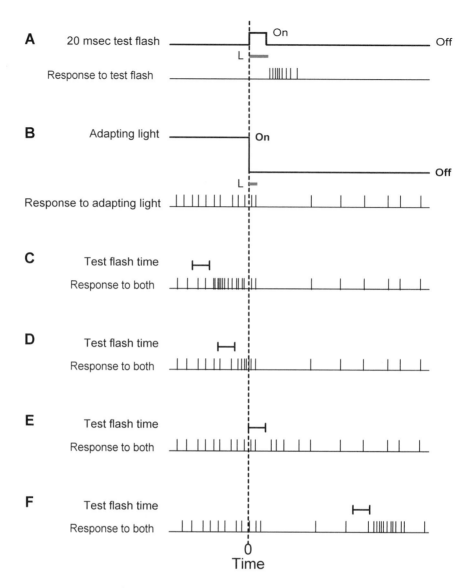

FIGURE 4.10   **A.** The hypothetical response of an on-center retinal ganglion cell to a 20 millisecond test flash. The cell responds to the threshold flash after a latency (L) shown by the short horizontal line. To be detected, all of the action potentials in the response need to occur. If fewer occur, the spot will not be seen. **B.** The response of the same cell to the offset of an adapting light. In this case, the cell responds by ceasing to produce action potentials. The latency is shown as being shorter than that of the test flash because the adapting light was more intense. **C–F.** Responses of the cell to presentation of the test flash when the test flash precedes **(C–D)**, is coincident with **(E)**, and follows **(F)** the adapting light offset at time zero. In **C–F**, the bracket indicates when the test flash is presented.

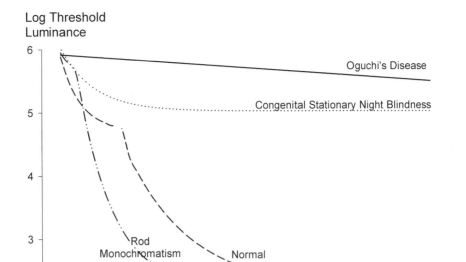

FIGURE 4.11   *Normal dark adaptation contrasted with types of abnormal dark adaptation. (Modified from JWM Hart. Visual Adaptation. In RA Moses, JWM Hart [eds], Adler's Physiology of the Eye [8th ed]. St. Louis: Mosby, 1987;389–414.)*

Dark adaptation can be affected by ocular abnormalities and eye disease

Measurement of dark adaptation curves can be of use in clinical practice. An example mentioned earlier in this chapter is the dark adaptation curve of rod monochromats, who have no cones. As shown by the lowest dashed line in Figure 4.11, when tested under conditions that would produce a rod-cone break in a normal patient, a rod monochromat shows only a rod dark adaptation curve. Conversely, patients with congenital, stationary (i.e., nonprogressive) night blindness, in which there is abnormal rod functioning, show only cone adaptation. Patients with Oguchi's disease (a congenital, nonprogressive inherited condition with unusual discoloration of the fundus and normal acuity) complain of night blindness and show minimal dark adaptation right after an adapting light is turned off. After prolonged dark adaptation (it can take up to a day), rod thresholds decrease to normal levels. Abnormal dark adaptation also occurs in degenerative retinal diseases (e.g., retinitis pigmentosa) and hereditary cone degeneration. Vitamin A deficiency increases the thresholds in the rod portion of the curve but does not affect the rate of dark adaptation. Drugs, such as quinine and thioridazine (a tranquilizer), can increase rod thresholds, as can alcohol intoxication (Hart 1987).

The level of bleached photopigment explains much of visual adaptation

Earlier in this chapter, four basic mechanisms for controlling the sensitivity of the visual system were listed: duplicity theory (changing between rods and cones), pupil size, the amount of unbleached retinal photopigment, and neural changes. Previous sections have primarily described how changing between using cones and rods dramatically affects the sensitivity of the visual system. Pupil size is not considered further, as it can contribute only a little more than a 1 log unit change in sensitivity. The next section discusses changes in sensitivity that are related to the amount of photopigment. These are generally measured in the rods because they have only one photopigment, rhodopsin. Photopigment-related changes during dark adaptation tend to be relatively slow, occurring over several minutes. Changes in sensitivity that are related to neural adaptation, rather than photopigment concentration, occur more quickly, as already discussed (see Figure 4.9).

The time course of dark adaptation matches the time course of photopigment regeneration

If one observes a retina that has been dark adapted and then exposed to light, its color changes from pink to white—it bleaches. This is caused by changes in the light-capturing photopigment molecules, primarily rhodopsin. As has been shown in animals and humans, if there are no unbleached photopigment molecules in the photoreceptors, they can not capture any quanta of light and respond, thus rendering the visual system completely insensitive to light. Regeneration of photopigment after it has been bleached takes place over several minutes as shown in Figure 4.12.

The amount of bleached rhodopsin declines exponentially as a function of time in the dark

Figure 4.12 is a plot of the time course of the regeneration of rhodopsin after a complete bleach, as determined by **retinal densitometry**. At time zero, 100% of the rhodopsin was in the bleached state (i.e., the proportion of bleached rhodopsin was 1.0). Examination of the figure shows that, after approximately 5 minutes, only 50% of the pigment was still bleached (0.5 on the y-axis). After approximately 10 minutes, only 25% remained bleached. By approximately 15 minutes, 12.5% was bleached, and so on. This curve is an exponential decay curve similar to that used to calculate radioactive decay. It can also be used in the more general situation in which some unknown amount of pigment has been bleached from exposure to light. This general equation is

$$B = B_0 \times (0.5)^{(t/\tau)} \qquad \text{Eq. 4.1}$$

where B is the fraction of pigment remaining bleached, B_0 is the initial fraction of bleached pigment, t is the time after the adapting light has been turned

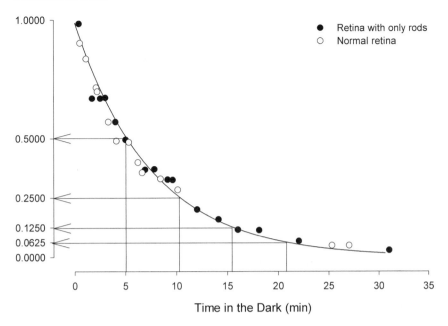

Proportion of Pigment
in Bleached State

- ● Retina with only rods
- ○ Normal retina

FIGURE 4.12   *Time course of regeneration of rhodopsin in a normal eye (open circles)
and the eye of a rod monochromat (closed circles). (Modified from WAH Rushton. The
Ferrier lecture. Visual adaptation. Proc R Soc Lond B Biol Sci 1965;162:20–46.)*

off, and τ is the half time* for the process. τ is 5.2 minutes for rhodopsin, as
shown in Figure 4.12. Thus, whatever fraction of the rhodopsin was bleached
at a given time, half of that amount is still bleached after 5.2 minutes in the
dark. For cone pigment regeneration (not shown), the half time is approximately 1.7 minutes because cone photopigments regenerate more rapidly
than does rhodopsin.

The log of the threshold elevation is related to the fraction of bleached rhodopsin

It should not be surprising that sensitivity to light is related to the amount of
bleached photopigment. It would be logical to predict that there would be a
linear relationship between the two, so that maximum sensitivity would occur
with 0% bleached photopigment (e.g., after 45 minutes of dark adaptation)
and that there would be a 50% reduction in sensitivity if 50% of the rhodopsin

*One also can use a *time constant* in a slightly different equation. The time constant is the amount of time for B_0 to decrease to $1/e$ of the original value, where e is
the base of the natural logarithm. The time constant in this example is approximately 7.5 minutes, which is where the amount of bleached photopigment is
approximately 37% of its original value.

were bleached. This was proposed by Hecht (1942) but was subsequently found not to be the case. Careful measures revealed that the threshold was increased by approximately 8 log units (a factor of approximately 100 million) when 50% of the rhodopsin was bleached.

From the work of William Rushton and his students and colleagues (Rushton 1965) in humans and John Dowling and his students and colleagues (Dowling 1987) in animals, an equation was derived that approximately relates the amount of bleached pigment to visual sensitivity:

$$\log\left(\frac{\Delta I_t}{\Delta I_0}\right) = 10HB \qquad \text{Eq. 4.2}$$

where I_t is the threshold for detecting the test stimulus, I_0 is the absolute threshold, H is a constant, specific for the test conditions and with a value of approximately 2, and B is the fraction of pigment that is still bleached. Thus, if 10% of the pigment were bleached, 10 HB would be $10.0 \times 2.0 \times 0.1 = 2$. This means that the threshold (I_t) would be 100 times higher than absolute threshold when only 10% of the pigment is bleached.

This equation is only an approximation because the threshold is lower for large stimuli than for small ones (see Figure 4.3), even though the amount of bleached rhodopsin is the same at any given time after time zero. Figure 4.13

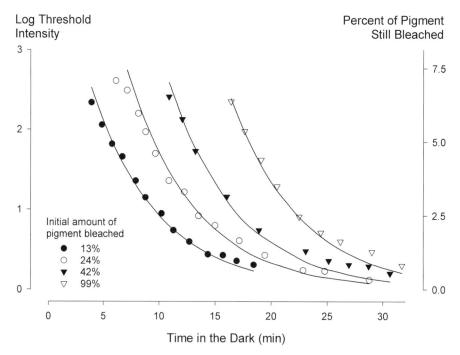

FIGURE 4.13   *Relationship of bleached rhodopsin to visual threshold. The circles and triangles are thresholds, 3° test spot centered 10° temporal to the fovea, measured during dark adaptation after an adapting light bleached varying amounts of rhodopsin. The solid lines show simultaneous measurements by retinal densitometry of the amount of bleached rhodopsin still present in the retina. (Modified from WAH Rushton & DS Powell. The rhodopsin content and the visual threshold of human rods. Vision Res 1972;12:1073–1081.)*

shows a direct comparison between the amount of bleached rhodopsin and the visual threshold. It appears that, under these specific test conditions, Equation 4.2 slightly underestimates the amount of the increase in threshold as a function of the fraction of bleached rhodopsin (i.e., H actually has a value larger than 2). In any case, the threshold was always closely related to the amount of bleached rhodopsin. Whenever a particular percent of rhodopsin was still bleached, say 5%, the threshold was the same (approximately 1.8 log threshold intensity) no matter what the initial amount of bleached rhodopsin was or how long it had been since time zero.

The equivalent background theory relates threshold during dark adaptation to threshold during light adaptation

As noted earlier (see Figure 4.3), the shape of a dark adaptation curve depends on the size of the test target used to measure the threshold. One would like to be able to find a common physical variable that is independent of such variations in the stimulus but is related to dark adaptation in a systematic way. If such a variable relates to dark adaptation in a consistent manner, then it should also relate to the amount of bleached photopigment in a systematic way. The **equivalent background theory** (EBT) (Crawford 1947) provides just such a common variable. The EBT states that, during dark adaptation, the threshold for detecting a spot is equivalent to the threshold for detecting the same spot against a background that bleaches the same fraction of rhodopsin as remains bleached at that point in dark adaptation.

The EBT is based on the observation that, during recovery from an adapting light that bleaches rhodopsin, it is almost as if there were a veiling background intensity against which a test target must be detected. This is similar to the veiling luminance in glare described in Chapter 3. It is as though the subject were looking at a background luminance instead of a dark field. Unlike a real background, however, the veiling luminance fades because it is stabilized on the retina.* The issue then is to learn whether there are real background luminances that are equivalent to the veiling luminance at various times during dark adaptation.

Based on the earlier work of Crawford (1947), Blakemore and Rushton (1965) examined dark and light adaptation for test flashes of various sizes. They studied this in a rod monochromat so that they could work with the rod system without interference from the cones. Figure 4.14 shows the results. The left side of the figure is the familiar dark adaptation curve of threshold luminance versus time in the dark for two different stimulus diameters (5' and 6°). One can clearly see that the shapes of the curves are different: They are not simply displaced vertically or horizontally from each other. The right side of the figure shows the threshold luminance for detecting the same two target sizes against a real background. Again, notice that the curve for the 5' spot is not parallel to the curve for the 6° flashed spot.

---

*A real image fades in exactly the same way if it too is stabilized on the retina; this is known as the **Troxler effect**.

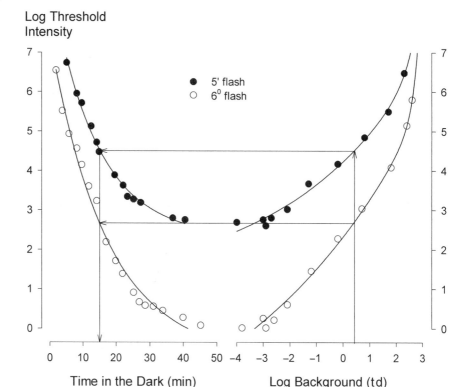

FIGURE 4.14   *Illustration of the equivalent background theory of dark adaptation. On the left are dark adaptation curves for two stimulus sizes after a 2 minute exposure to a 4.9 log troland adapting light. On the right are the threshold luminances for detecting the same size stimuli against a background with a variety of luminance levels. (td = troland.) (Modified from C Blakemore, WAH Rushton. The rod increment threshold during dark adaptation in normal and rod monochromat. J Physiol [Lond] 1965;181:629–640.)*

Blakemore and Rushton (1965) found that the threshold luminance for detecting a flashed spot when there is a real background predicts the threshold for detecting the same spot during dark adaptation. The key is that a real background luminance bleaches a certain fraction of the rhodopsin. During dark adaptation when the fraction of bleached rhodopsin crosses that same point on the way from having a lot of bleached rhodopsin to having little bleached rhodopsin, the threshold for detecting the spot is the same as it would be if there were a real background present. It is equivalent to a real background.

To see how this works, begin on the right side of the figure at a background luminance of 0.4 log trolands. Follow the vertical line from that point until it intersects the threshold curve for the 6° spot. Note (on the right vertical axis) that the threshold for detecting the spot against this background was approximately 2.8 log units above the minimum threshold. Following the horizontal line to the left, one reaches the curve for the 6° spot that was tested against no background in the dark adaptation study. Following the vertical solid line down to the x-axis, it can be seen that this threshold occurred after approximately 14 minutes of dark adaptation. The thought here is that a background of 0.4 log trolands bleaches as much rhodopsin as was present after 14 minutes of dark adaptation. If this is the case, then the threshold for detecting the smaller 5' diameter spot should be the same after 14 minutes of dark adaptation as it is when tested against the real background luminance of 0.4 log trolands. By starting on the right side of the figure again, going up to the 5' curve, over to the left to the dark adaptation curve for the 5' spot, and then back down vertically to the x-axis, one can see that there is a match.

The net result of going through this exercise for the entire range of background luminances and dark adaptation times is shown in Figure 4.15. Notice that the points related to the 6° flash (open circles) fall on the same curve as do the points related to the 5' flash (filled circles). Thus, in this plot, the effect of target size has been eliminated from the dark adaptation curve revealing a more general relationship: the equivalent background value as a function of time. The threshold to detect a spot of light at any particular time after the start of dark adaptation (the x-axis) can be related to an equivalent background luminance (the y-axis).

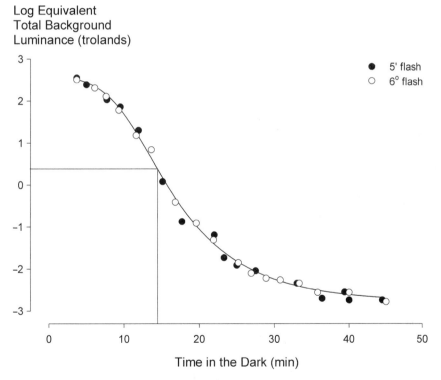

FIGURE 4.15   *Equivalent background versus time in the dark generated from the data in Figure 4.14. The intersection of the vertical line with the horizontal line indicates that approximately 14 minutes in the dark was equivalent to detecting a target against a background luminance of 0.4 log trolands regardless of target size. (Modified from C Blakemore, WAH Rushton. The rod increment threshold during dark adaptation in normal and rod monochromat. J Physiol [Lond] 1965;181:629–640.)*

The level of light adaptation controls the magnitude of responses of photoreceptors to flashes of light

Previous sections have shown that a great deal of light adaptation and dark adaptation can be explained by the amount of bleached photopigment in the photoreceptors. This section describes how the photoreceptors actually respond during adaptation. These responses, in turn, determine the responses of the bipolar cells, ganglion cells, and, ultimately, the cortical cells that produce the perception of light.

The obvious approach to looking for the neurophysiological basis of the psychophysical phenomena of light adaptation is to record the responses from photoreceptors during light and dark adaptation. Figure 4.16 represents the

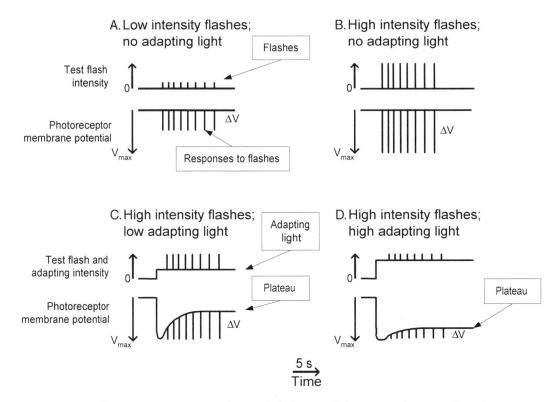

FIGURE 4.16   Schematic representation of intracellularly recorded responses from a gecko rod. **A.** Hyperpolarizations (change in voltage [ΔV]) of the rod membrane potential in response to a series of low-intensity 100 millisecond test flashes. **B.** Hyperpolarization (ΔV) of the rod membrane potential in response to a series of higher-intensity 100 millisecond flashes. At this intensity, the hyperpolarizations reach the maximum voltage (V_{max}), the greatest hyperpolarization that the photoreceptor can produce. **C.** Membrane potential changes to the onset of a low-intensity adapting light. Test flashes were presented in addition to the adapting light such that the total intensity was the same as that in **B.** **D.** Membrane potential changes to the onset of an adapting light of higher intensity. In **C** and **D**, the membrane potential in the plateau region did not return to the initial depolarized value. The more intense adapting light in **D** caused the membrane potential in the plateau region to be closer to V_{max}. Thus, the largest ΔV that could occur to the test flashes was smaller than in **C**. (Modified from JE Dowling. The Retina: An Approachable Part of the Brain. Cambridge, MA: Belknap Press of Harvard University Press, 1987.)

response of the membrane potential of a rod in a reptile (a gecko) to two events: (1) a background adapting light that was turned on and remained on and (2) the presentation of short-duration test flashes. Before the adapting light was turned on (see Figure 4.16A), the photoreceptor was dark adapted and was, therefore, in its expected depolarized state. When the low-intensity adapting light was turned on (see Figure 4.16C), a rapid hyperpolarization occurred, as indicated by the vertical drop in the membrane potential toward the maximum voltage (V_{max}). After approximately 1 second, the membrane potential then rose, returning most of the way back to the depolarized resting level.

Thus, after initially responding to the onset of the adapting light, the rod settled down at a membrane potential (the plateau) that was somewhat hyperpolarized. Turning to the second event shown in Figure 4.16C, the series of vertical lines shows the change in voltage (ΔV) of the membrane potential in response to brief test flashes that were presented while the adapting light remained on. In Figure 4.16C, in the first 2–3 seconds after the adapting light was turned on, the ΔV in response to the test flash was small because the rod could not hyperpolarize any farther than V_{max}. As the membrane potential recovered from its response to the onset of the adapting light, the ΔV increased, even though the test flash intensity did not change. Note that the ΔV of the rod in the plateau region was smaller than in Figure 4.16B. This is important because the change in release of neurotransmitter from the rod is related to the size of ΔV. Thus, a small ΔV produces a small effect on the bipolar cells to which the rod connects, and a larger ΔV has a larger effect. This, in turn, is passed along to the ganglion cells.

Figure 4.16D shows how the rod membrane potential responded when a more intense adapting light was used. As in Figure 4.16C, the membrane potential moved to V_{max} when the adapting light came on and then depolarized somewhat. Because the adapting light (which remained on) was more intense than in Figure 4.16D, the membrane potential in the plateau region was closer to V_{max} than in Figure 4.16C. Because the response (ΔV) of the photoreceptor to the test flash cannot exceed V_{max}, the ΔV was smaller when a test flash of the same intensity was presented.

Figure 4.17 summarizes the results of presenting flashes at a variety of intensities when the photoreceptor was dark adapted and exposed to two different background intensities. Each data point shows the response (ΔV) produced by a particular test flash intensity at one of the three background intensities. This figure shows three important points about the responses of photoreceptors. First, the same flash intensity produces a smaller response (ΔV) when the amount of light adaptation increases. Second, at each adaptation level, there is a linear region of intensities where equal increases in flash intensity produce equal increases in ΔV. This is called **gain control**. Third, at each adaptation level, there is a maximum response (ΔV) that the photoreceptor can produce, and this maximum response decreases as the adapting light becomes more intense. With an intense adapting light, the plateau would be at V_{max}, and ΔV would be zero for even the most intense flash. At this point, the photoreceptor would be *saturated*.

The first point was previously described for Figure 4.16C and D but can also be seen in this figure: The size of the response of the rod to any given flash

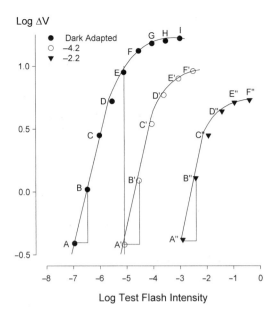

Log ΔV

- Dark Adapted
○ −4.2
▼ −2.2

Log Test Flash Intensity

FIGURE 4.17   *Responses of gecko rods to light flashes presented when the photoreceptor was in the plateau region (see Figure 4.16) at three levels of adaptation. The ordinate plots the log of the change in V (ΔV) in mV, the transient voltage change produced by the test flash. (Modified from JE Dowling. The Retina: An Approachable Part of the Brain. Cambridge, MA: Belknap Press of Harvard University Press, 1987.)*

intensity decreases as the intensity of the adapting light is increased. For instance, in Figure 4.17, the point labeled E and the data point labeled A' were produced by test flashes with the same intensity. The response (ΔV) of the photoreceptor, however, was smaller at A' because the adapting light had caused the photoreceptor membrane potential to remain somewhat hyperpolarized.

This has implications for detecting the flash. Starting at the photoreceptor level, the response of the visual system to a light flash of a given intensity is decreased when the retina is more light adapted. If a certain level of response (some criterion increase in spikes per second) has to be produced for the owner of the visual system to detect the light, then it follows that the threshold for detecting light increases as light adaptation increases. This was shown on the right in Figure 4.14 and also in Chapter 3 (see Figure 3.1). Thus, the responses of photoreceptors help to explain why the psychophysical threshold for detecting a light flash increases in a human subject as the retina becomes more light adapted.

A second important point that is shown in Figure 4.17 is that, within the response region of the photoreceptor in which the line connecting the data points is straight, a presentation of a flashed stimulus that is more intense than another stimulus causes a nearly identical increase in response, regardless of the adaptation level. For instance, when the background luminance was zero (dark adapted conditions), the point B shows that a particular ΔV was produced by a flash with an intensity of approximately −6.6. The flash that produced the response at B was approximately 0.3 log units more intense than was the flash that produced the ΔV at point A, and, hence, the ΔV in the rod was greater for the flash of intensity B than for the flash of intensity A. The triangle shows that a particular change in ΔV was produced when the flash intensity increased from A to B. A similar increase in ΔV was produced when the intensity changed from A' to B'. As indicated by the similar slopes of the three lines that connect the points, this increase in membrane potential for a particular change in luminance also holds for A'' and B''. The bipolar and horizontal cells leading to the ganglion cells receive their signals from the photoreceptors and base their responses on the change in the photoreceptor membrane potential. Thus, once the visual system is adapted to a particular luminance level, the same increase in physical luminance produces the same change in response from the visual system. This process has been referred to as gain control, and it probably contributes to the phenomenon of brightness constancy in which objects appear to have the same brightness whether they are out in the sunshine or under the shade of a tree (see Chapter 6).

Finally, it can be seen that, as the intensity of the adapting light increases, the maximum ΔV that the photoreceptor can produce becomes less (the regions connecting points G, H, and I; E' and F'; and D'', E'', and F''). This is the same phenomenon that was shown in Figure 4.16 in which the membrane potential in the plateau region moves closer to V_{max} as the intensity of the adapting light is raised. For even higher adapting light levels, no response can be produced from the photoreceptor, even to extremely intense light flashes. In this condition, the rod is saturated, and vision must be mediated by the cones, which, in turn, can also saturate at high background intensity levels. Rod saturation can occur without complete bleaching of the rhodopsin, possibly because all of the sodium ion (Na^+) channels in the photoreceptor membrane are closed (Dowling 1987).

Neural (nonphotopigment) changes also produce light and dark adaptation

Although the amount of bleached photopigment clearly has a strong effect on threshold, photopigment concentration is not the complete story. The fourth mechanism that helps to produce light and dark adaptation is changes in the responses of the photoreceptors and the retinal cells that receive input from the photoreceptors. These changes work to alter the sensitivity of the visual system more rapidly than can occur with photopigment changes and can cause light and dark adaptation without photopigment changes. For instance, Dowling (1987) found that as background luminance is increased from zero, light adaptation occurs in photoreceptors without detectable changes in rhodopsin concentration until the background luminance is 2–3 log units above the totally dark adapted level. The neural basis for this change is not yet known. When the adapting light is turned off, rapid dark adaptation occurs, as was seen in Baker's study of early dark adaptation (see Figure 4.9).

Even when the photoreceptors are not light adapted, neural adaptation has been found to occur in ganglion cells. Figure 4.18 shows the results of a study in the retina of the skate (a type of fish) that illustrate this point. In this experiment, the adapting light was dim, so that it did not bleach a significant fraction

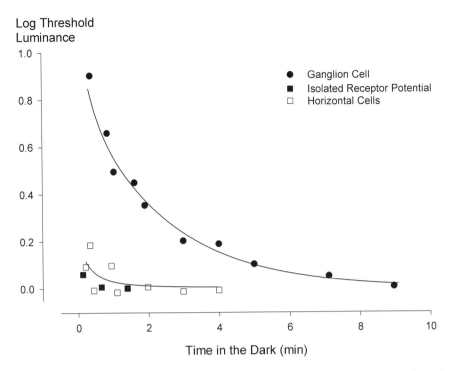

Log Threshold
Luminance

FIGURE 4.18   *Threshold light intensity needed to evoke a criterion response from the various retinal cell types in the skate retina after exposure to a dim adapting light. The "isolated receptor potentials" show the photoreceptor thresholds. Horizontal and ganglion cell responses were measured with a microelectrode. The ganglion cells had a higher threshold than the photoreceptors and horizontal cells when the adapting light was turned off. This difference in threshold, which disappears after approximately 10 minutes, must be due to neural, not photoreceptor, adaptation. (Modified from DG Green, JE Dowling, IM Siegal, H Ripps. Retinal mechanisms of visual adaptation in the skate. J Gen Physiol 1975;65:483–502.)*

of the rhodopsin. Based on the data of the previous section, the rods should not have had an elevated threshold immediately after the adapting light went off. Indeed, the rod threshold was only slightly elevated and readapted to its minimum threshold within 1 minute after the adapting light was turned off. The horizontal cell showed a similar pattern to the photoreceptors. In contrast, the threshold intensity needed to elicit a particular criterion response from the ganglion cell was initially approximately 1 log unit higher than the threshold for the rods or the horizontal cell. Furthermore, it took approximately 10 minutes for the ganglion cell threshold to reach the same level as the photoreceptors. Because the amount of photopigment bleached was negligible, the threshold elevation and longer adaptation time must have been due to a postphotoreceptor neural adaptation mechanism.

The mechanisms by which neural adaptation is accomplished are still being determined. Several facts are known regarding ganglion cells. One is that changes in the release of the neurotransmitter dopamine are involved in receptive-field changes of some ganglion cell classes. Second, in a completely

Log Threshold
Luminance

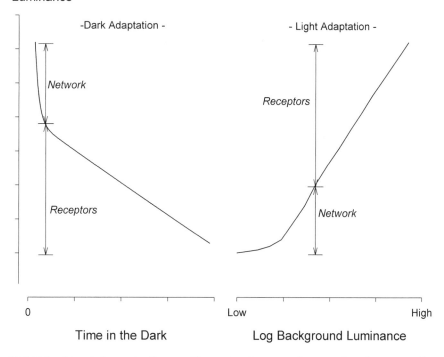

-Dark Adaptation -   - Light Adaptation -

Network

Receptors

Receptors

Network

0   Low   High

Time in the Dark   Log Background Luminance

FIGURE 4.19   *Schematic diagram illustrating that neural (network) adaptation affects the sensitivity of the visual system more quickly than does pigment bleaching (receptors); both play a role in adaptation. Note the similarity to Figure 4.14. (Modified from JE Dowling. The Retina: An Approachable Part of the Brain. Cambridge, MA: Belknap Press of Harvard University Press, 1987.)*

dark adapted retina, the antagonistic receptive-field surround disappears. The receptive-field surround makes a ganglion cell less responsive to large spots of light, because light falling on the surround reduces the response that would occur if only the center were stimulated. When the surround is functionally removed, the ganglion cells become more sensitive to light spots of any size. This is a benefit in conditions in which the detection of any light present in the environment is needed by the retina's owner. A third fact (which really is a side effect of inactivating the receptive-field surround) is that the effective size of the receptive-field center is increased. This also helps to increase the sensitivity of the visual system, but it has a cost: The acuity of the visual system is decreased, as is discussed in the next two chapters.

Figure 4.19 illustrates that neural adaptation occurs before photoreceptor adaptation. On the left side of the figure, during dark adaptation, the neural changes occur temporally before there is significant pigment regeneration, so that sensitivity increases fairly rapidly after the adapting light is turned off (as shown in Baker's study [see Figure 4.9]). The neural adaptation can provide a 1 to 2 log unit head start for the visual system to become more sensitive than would be possible if it had to wait for photopigment regeneration to occur. On the right side of the figure (which is similar to the right side of Figure 4.14), if one starts with a dark adapted visual system and gradually increases the background luminance, the light intensity needed to reach threshold also increases. At low background levels where there is minimal pigment bleaching, this light adaptation is mediated by neural retinal mechanisms. As the background luminance is increased further, the neural adaptation reaches its limit (approximately 1–2 log units), and photopigment bleaching becomes the mechanism that changes the threshold.

Study Guide

1. Define dark adaptation and light adaptation.
2. What are the four mechanisms that the visual system uses to adapt to varying light conditions, in order of decreasing importance?
3. Be able to draw a typical dark adaptation curve, showing and labeling the cone branch, the rod branch, and the rod-cone break. Be sure to know the labels and scales that go on the x- and y-axes.
4. Explain what is happening in the retina when the rod-cone break occurs (i.e., why the subject didn't see with the rods at an earlier point in time and doesn't see with the cones after the rod-cone break).
5. Explain how and why the dark adaptation curve is affected by the
    a) part of the retina that is stimulated by the test flash
    b) size of the test flash
    c) wavelength of the adapting light
    d) wavelength of the test flash
    e) intensity of the adapting light
    f) duration of the adapting light
    g) task required of the subject
6. Know what happens to the threshold luminance a few milliseconds before and after the adapting light is turned off.
7. Why is there an elevation in threshold around the time that the adapting light goes off?
8. What is the duplicity theory?
9. Why is the Method of Constant Stimuli rarely used to measure dark adaptation?
10. In Figure 4.9, how can one be sure that Baker was measuring the early light adaptation of cones?
11. Use Equation 4.1 to calculate the fraction of rhodopsin that remains bleached 10 minutes after the start of dark adaptation if 44% was bleached when the adapting light went off.
12. Write the equation that gives the approximate threshold elevation as a function of the fraction of bleached photopigment.
13. Explain why the line labeled "99%" in Figure 4.13 is to the right of the line labeled "13%."
14. Explain why the correspondence of the data points with the lines in Figure 4.13 shows that the percent of bleached rhodopsin has an important effect on visual threshold.

15. Explain, for Figure 4.14, how the percent of bleached rhodopsin accounts for the dark adaptation data (left side of the figure) and the increment threshold data (right side of the figure).
16. Explain how the plateau value of the rod membrane voltage accounts for the reduced response of the photoreceptor during light adaptation.

Glossary

Adapting light: any source of retinal illuminance that decreases sensitivity to light.

Dark adaptation: the increase in sensitivity (decrease in threshold luminance) as a function of time in darkness.

Duplicity theory: the proposal (Schultz 1866) that two different photoreceptors are used in low luminance conditions (rods) and high luminance conditions (cones).

Early dark adaptation: the small (approximately 1 log unit) decrease in threshold that occurs within 400 milliseconds after time zero.

Equivalent background theory (EBT): during dark adaptation, the threshold for detecting a spot is equivalent to the threshold for detecting the same spot against a background that bleaches the same fraction of rhodopsin as remains bleached at that point in dark adaptation.

Gain control: the presence, at each adaptation level, of a linear region in which a given increase in flash intensity produces a given increase in ΔV.

Light adaptation: the process that decreases sensitivity (increases threshold luminance) in response to an adapting light.

Mesopic: luminance conditions in which vision occurs through the use of rods and cones (approximately 10^{-2} to 10^{2} cd/m^2).

Photopic: luminance conditions (greater than approximately 10^{2} cd/m^2) in which vision occurs through the use of only cones.

Retinal densitometry: A technique for measuring changes in photopigment concentration in an intact, living eye by measuring the amount of light that is reflected back out of the eye.

Rod-cone break: the point during dark adaptation at which rods become more sensitive than cones.

Scotopic: luminance conditions in which vision occurs through the use of only rods (approximately 10^{-6} to 10^{-2} cd/m^2).

Troxler effect: the fading of a stabilized image or a large image with fuzzy edges presented in the peripheral visual field.

5   Spatial Acuity

Harold E. Bedell

Overview

Measurement of spatial visual acuity is one of the most important and most common psychophysical measures of the functioning of the eye and visual system. This chapter provides a foundation for understanding why visual acuity measurements are performed in particular ways in the clinic.

Spatial visual acuity is the smallest spatial detail that can be detected, discriminated, or identified. The major types of spatial visual acuity are detection, localization, and resolution acuity. Detection acuity is the angular size of the smallest visible target and, fundamentally, a threshold intensity discrimination task. Localization acuity is the smallest spatial offset or difference in location between targets that can be discriminated. Resolution acuity is the smallest spatial separation between two nearby points or lines that can be discriminated—that is, the minimum angle of resolution.

In part because grating acuity is relatively insensitive to optical defocus, identification acuity is the measure that is most often used clinically and is considered by many to be a fourth acuity type. It is a measure of the details in the smallest letter or other complex target that can be recognized and thus is a form of resolution acuity. Although the standard resolution acuity is defined to be 1 minute of arc (1'), most people have better than the standard acuity. Clinical charts are now designed to use letters with standard shapes with approximately equal legibility, constructed with consistent spacing between neighboring letters and lines.

Although various scales are used to represent acuity results, the logMAR scale provides estimates of acuity that are probably the easiest to interpret and compare across individuals and conditions. Letter acuity becomes worse with optical defocus, reduced target luminance or contrast, and distance from the fovea. Visual acuity also is degraded for moving and for briefly presented targets. Another limitation of visual acuity can be neural defocus, which results from the convergence of spatial information onto neurons with large receptive-field centers.

Spatial visual acuity is one of the most common psychophysical measurements made by eye-care professionals

Spatial visual acuity measures provide absolute and relative benchmarks about a person's visual condition. For instance, if a person's resolution acuity meets or exceeds that of a *standard observer* (able to resolve details of 1'), it implies that a clear image is formed on the retina and that the central retinal structures and subsequent neural pathways involved in visual processing are probably healthy. When acuity measurements are compared over time for the same person, they provide information about stability or change in that person's refractive state, ocular media, and visual-processing structures. This chapter considers some of the choices that are made when an acuity test is designed and used. These choices highlight many of the factors that influence visual acuity in normal vision and in conditions where the visual system is not normal.

Spatial acuity is defined as the finest spatial detail that can be detected, discriminated, or resolved

Most people associate the measurement of visual acuity with the letter chart found in doctors' offices. However, spatial visual acuity can be and has been assessed using a variety of targets in addition to letters. Although each of the spatial targets provides a measure of spatial acuity, these measures do not all produce equivalent results.

Three types of spatial acuity are described in this chapter: **detection acuity** (also called *minimum visible acuity* or *minimum distinguishable acuity*), **localization acuity** (also called *minimum discriminable acuity* or *hyperacuity*), and **resolution acuity** (sometimes called *minimum separable acuity*). Many researchers and clinicians consider that **identification acuity** (also called *minimum recognizable acuity*) constitutes a fourth type of spatial acuity. In identification acuity, the task is to identify letters by resolving their details. Although its purpose is to determine the resolution threshold, letter acuity testing does not give identical results to other measures of resolution acuity. Table 5.1 lists the typical stimuli that are used to measure each type of acuity with the minimum thresholds obtained in healthy, normal people.

As described later in this chapter, measuring acuity is a threshold determination. Although any of the three psychophysical methods (see Chapter 1) can be used, the descending Method of Limits is most commonly used.

Detection acuity is the angular size of the smallest visible target

The diameter of the smallest spot or the width of the smallest line that can just be seen provides a measure of detection acuity. However, detection acuity depends primarily on the luminance or contrast of the retinal image of the spot or line, not on the angular size of the stimulus. When objects are very small, the size of the image they create on the retina is limited by the eye's optics. Consequently, the illuminance of the image on the retina, and not the size, decreases as the object becomes smaller. For example, consider the star, Aldebaran—the bright eye of the bull in the constellation Taurus. Aldebaran is approximately 35 million miles in diameter and approximately 4×10^{14} miles away from earth. The angular subtense of this star at the eye is, therefore, 0.018". As illustrated in Figure 5.1, the image of this star or any point of light on the foveal region of the retina is much broader than 0.018" in diameter. Depending on the size of the pupil, the

Table 5.1 Comparison of spatial acuity tasks and thresholds

Acuity task	Typical stimulus	Minimum Threshold (")
Detection	Single black spot	15–20
	Single black line	0.5–1.0
Localization	Spatial interval	2–4
	Vernier lines	3–6
Resolution	Two black lines/spots	30–40
	Grating	30–40
Identification	Letters or numerals	30–40

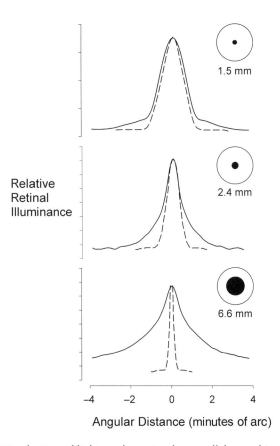

Relative Retinal Illuminance

Angular Distance (minutes of arc)

FIGURE 5.1   *Distribution of light on the retina for a well-focused image of a point of light, such as a star, for three pupil diameters. The image is measured across the line, and not along the line. The distribution for a spot would be similar. The solid lines show the distribution of retinal illuminance, and the dashed lines show the theoretical illuminance distributions based on the size of the pupil alone. The sharpest image is achieved with an intermediate (2.4 mm) pupil size. (Modified from F Campbell, R Gubish. Optical quality of the human eye. J Physiol 1966;186:558–578.)*

image is spread over a region several minutes of arc across, mostly because of the limitations that are inherent in the optics of the human eye. Nevertheless, at night, this star is readily visible because sufficiently more quanta reach the retina from the star than from the immediately surrounding region of the sky. If the sky around the star had extremely low luminance, and the star's image was centered on the fovea, whether or not the star is visible would depend on the absolute threshold for dark-adapted cones (see Chapter 2). Thus, extremely small lights may be detected if they are sufficiently intense. During the day, the same luminance of the star (L_T) is not detectable against the more intense background of the sky (L) because the star's luminance is below the increment detection threshold (ΔL) of light-adapted cones at that luminance level (see Chapters 3 and 4).

The narrowest black line that can just be detected against a field of high luminance is approximately 0.5" (Hecht et al. 1947). Similar to the situation with the star, the visibility of a line depends on the ability of the visual system

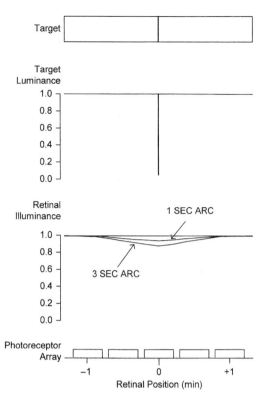

FIGURE 5.2   *A high-contrast black line subtending 1" or 3" (**top**) produces a retinal image of similar width (**bottom**) because of the optical properties of the eye. The depth of the luminance decrement in the image depends on the thickness of the line. The line can be detected when the luminance decrement is of sufficient contrast. (Modified from G Westheimer. The spatial sense of the eye. Proctor lecture. Invest Ophthalmol Vis Sci 1979b;18:893–912.)*

to detect a slightly different (but lower, in this case) luminance region ($L_T = L - \Delta L$) against a homogeneously illuminated (higher, in this case) luminance field (L): a decrement threshold task (see Chapter 3). As illustrated in Figure 5.2, the optics of the eye spread a 1" low-luminance region into an image that spans approximately ± 1'. The minimum retinal illuminance is approximately 2% less than the background. The shadow produced by a line 0.5" wide would be half as dark, which corresponds well to the threshold ability of the visual system to detect a 1% luminance decrement with a small stimulus (see Chapter 3, Figure 3.5).

A black spot viewed against a high-luminance background is just detectable when its diameter is approximately 15" (Hecht et al. 1947). One reason that the just-detectable spot is wider than the just-detectable line is because the visual system has less opportunity to spatially summate contrast information for a spot, as it can along the length of the line (see Chapter 2). A second reason is that the maximum contrast in the retinal image of the spot is lower because its contrast is spread out across two dimensions of the image instead of only one. A test that uses a spot as the detection target occasionally is used to estimate the resolution acuity of young children (Kirschen et al. 1983).

However, using the finest black line that can just be detected as a clinical test in adults is impractical owing to printing limitations. A line that subtends 0.5″ would be only 15 μm wide at a distance of 6 m and less than 1 μm wide at a distance of 40 cm.

Localization acuity is the smallest spatial offset or difference in location between targets that can be discriminated

Two examples of localization acuity tasks are **spatial-interval acuity** and **Vernier acuity**, as illustrated in Figure 5.3. Other targets can be used, such as judging the alignment of two spots or whether one line is tilted relative to another. Under optimal conditions, high-contrast targets with spatial offsets on the order of 2–6″ can be discriminated. This is much finer than the spacing between the foveal photoreceptors. This characteristic of localization acuity tasks has led to their designation as *hyperacuities* (Westheimer 1979b) and to the conclusion that the neural mechanisms for localization acuity occur in the visual cortex, rather than in the retina. As with detection acuity, the implementation of these tasks on an eye chart for use in a clinical situation is difficult. A spatial offset of 6″ corresponds to approximately 0.17 mm at a distance of 6 m and only approximately 0.01 mm (10 μm) at 40 cm.

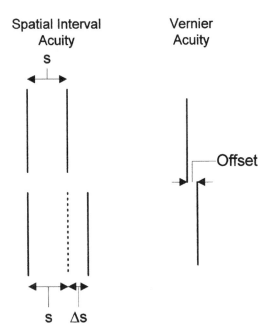

FIGURE 5.3   *Spatial-interval acuity (**left**) is specified by the smallest change in the separation (ΔS) between two targets that can be discriminated as larger or smaller than a standard separation (S). Vernier acuity (**right**) is specified by the smallest offset between two targets that can be discriminated as a deviation of one target rightward or leftward from perfect alignment.*

Performance on localization (hyperacuity) tasks is degraded by optical defocus if the targets are close

The effect of optical defocus on localization acuity tasks varies systematically with the separation between the targets. When the targets to be compared are very close together (less than 10–15' vertical separation between the ends of the lines in Figure 5.3), localization thresholds increase with defocus. When the localization targets are farther apart (approximately 1°), the thresholds for focused images are higher than when the targets are close together. Under these conditions, defocus has much less of an effect (Williams et al. 1984). These and other effects of target separation on localization acuity have led to the suggestion that the visual system uses different information to determine the relative locations of targets that are close together versus targets that are more widely separated (Waugh & Levi 1993).

Resolution acuity is the smallest spatial separation between two nearby points or lines that can be discriminated

In an optical system, the smallest angular separation at which a pair of points just can be resolved as two instead of one depends on how sharp the image of each point is and the "grain" of the imaging surface. In a photographic camera, for example, resolution depends on the quality of the camera optics and the size or "grain" of the silver particles in the film. In the human eye, resolution in the central retina depends on the quality of the eye's optics and the spacing between the adjacent photoreceptors (Figure 5.4).

When two thin high-luminance lines are viewed, the optics of the eye produce a distribution of retinal illuminance for each line, shown by the dashed lines in Figure 5.4. If the lines are close together, as in the figure, the images overlap, and the net illuminance profile is shown by the solid line. If the lines are sufficiently separated, there is a region with reduced luminance in between the peaks that are related to each line. If the region with reduced luminance is sufficiently wide and sufficiently deep, it is possible that at least one foveal cone will be significantly less hyperpolarized than the cones on either side. For a region of reduced retinal illuminance to be detected, there must be a small enough spacing between the foveal cones, so that, as in Figure 5.4, one cone is centered under the region of decreased luminance, while adjacent cones are under the regions with higher luminance.

Under optimal imaging conditions, the eye's optics and the spacing of the foveal cones (center-to-center spacing of 20–40" in the fovea [Curcio et al. 1990]) allow some subjects to resolve two points or two lines that are approximately 30–40" (0.5') apart (Geisler 1989; Wilcox 1932). This is called the **minimum angle of resolution (MAR)**. Not all eyes are able to achieve a MAR of 0.5' even when they are using an optimal correction for any refractive error. Figure 5.5 shows the cone array at the fovea in eyes from two different people and demonstrates that some people have small cones in the foveal center, whereas others have larger cones. If the optics of the eye provide sharp enough images, a fovea with smaller cones would be expected to resolve smaller separations between images than a fovea with larger cones.

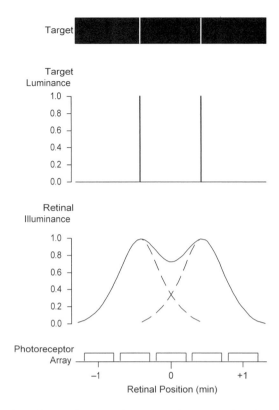

FIGURE 5.4   At best focus, the retinal images of two nearby, thin high-luminance lines overlap because of the optical properties of the eye. Theoretically, an observer can resolve that there are two lines instead of one when a centrally located photoreceptor is illuminated sufficiently less than its neighbors. (Modified from G Westheimer. The spatial sense of the eye. Proctor lecture. Invest Ophthalmol Vis Sci 1979b;18:893–912.)

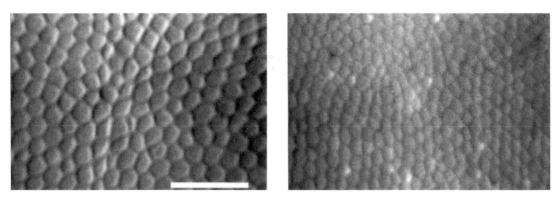

FIGURE 5.5   Optical sections of the human foveal cone mosaic that show variability between individuals. Both photos are from the foveal center and contain only cones. The smaller cones in the retina on the right produce a much higher density of cones that, presumably, could mediate higher resolution acuity than could the fovea on the left. The scale bar is 10 μm, which is approximately 2' on the retina. (Reprinted with permission from CA Curcio, KR Sloan, RE Kalina, AE Hendrickson. Human photoreceptor topography. J Comp Neurol 1990;292:497–523.)

Resolution acuity for two spots or lines is difficult to implement as a clinical test

There are many reasons for using letters instead of spots to measure resolution acuity clinically. The most important reason is that, as the gap between a pair of spots or lines is increased, they appear as a slightly fatter single spot or line before they can actually be resolved as two. Unless special precautions are taken (e.g., using spots or lines of different thickness), individuals may be able to correctly answer whether two spots or lines are present before they can actually resolve the gap between them. A second reason, which applies to the resolution of high luminance spots or lines, is that the two retinal images spread into each other at high luminance levels, so that, unlike other forms of acuity (see following sections), resolution actually worsens as the luminance of the targets increases (Wilcox 1932). Finally, over one-half of the clinical population has at least 0.25 diopters (D) of **astigmatism** that produces different amounts of image defocus for targets in different orientations. Spot or line targets would have to be presented in multiple orientations to reliably detect an acuity loss that results from astigmatism.

Resolution acuity can be measured using multiple lines (gratings)

Several of the difficulties associated with measuring resolution acuity are alleviated if resolution threshold is measured for a target consisting of many lines instead of just two. Targets consisting of multiple, evenly spaced black-and-white lines (Figure 5.6) are called *square wave gratings*. The sensitivity of the visual system to gratings is considered in detail in Chapter 6. An estimate of resolution acuity is determined by finding the thinnest grating lines that a person can just detect. With normal room illumination, the threshold line width (i.e., the MAR) that is required for a normal adult to distinguish a square-wave grating from a gray target is approximately 0.75' (45") (Virsu et al. 1981).

Grating targets are used routinely in clinical settings to evaluate the resolution acuity of infants (see Chapter 9). They are also used with patients who do not read letters, particularly in countries with low literacy rates. Gratings are sometimes used to estimate resolution acuity in patients who have cataracts or other opacities of the media (Goldmann 1972). This is possible because gratings can be formed on the retina by the interference between two coherent beams of light that enter the eye at different pupillary locations. These interference gratings are affected minimally by imperfections of the ocular media of the eye, so they can provide an estimate of what a patient's resolution acuity would be if the opacities were removed.

Grating acuity measures are relatively insensitive to optical defocus

People who normally wear a spectacle or contact lens correction are well aware that resolution acuity for letter targets is markedly degraded by optical

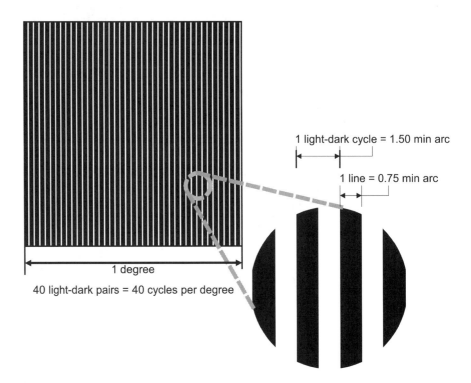

FIGURE 5.6   *A square-wave grating contains black-white pairs of lines. Each pair of black and white lines is called a* cycle. *Each black, or white, line of the grating shown subtends 0.75', and each black-white pair is 1.5' wide, so the grating contains 40 cycles per degree (cycles/deg) of visual angle.*

defocus, as illustrated in Figure 5.7. For instance, 2 D of myopic defocus, which represents a relatively mild refractive error, reduces the MAR on a letter chart from approximately 1' (0 **logMAR**) to worse than 5' (0.7 logMAR). On the other hand, more than 10 D of myopic defocus is required to reduce resolution acuity for a grating target from approximately 1' to 5'. This insensitivity to defocus makes gratings less than optimal for testing resolution acuity in adults.

The cause of the insensitivity of grating targets to optical defocus is a phenomenon called *spurious resolution*. The defocused images of the adjacent elements in a repetitive spatial pattern overlap to produce regions of greater and lower intensity well outside of the image plane (Smith 1982). These are not really images (neither are they interference patterns), because they are formed from multiple, rather than individual, components in the original object. Nevertheless, because regions are visible as lighter or darker, this phenomenon can lead to a false estimate of resolution acuity.

Letter charts are most commonly used clinically to measure the minimum angle of resolution

As described in the previous sections of this chapter, there are a variety of tests for the smallest spatial detail that the visual system can detect or dis-

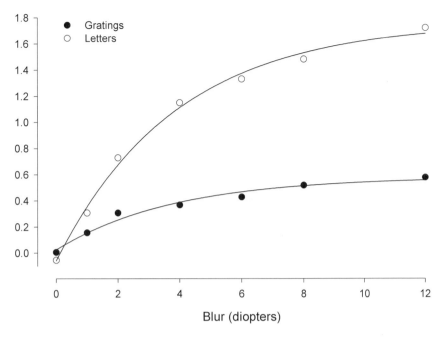

LogMAR

FIGURE 5.7   *Acuity for letters, measured by the logMAR, worsens dramatically as the amount of imposed optic defocus increases (open circles). Resolution acuity for square wave gratings (filled circles) is influenced much less by optical defocus. Data are the average of seven normal observers. (Modified from F Thorn, F Schwartz. Effects of dioptric blur on Snellen and grating acuity. Optom Vis Sci 1990;67:3–7.)*

criminate. Various visual acuity tasks are used in specialized testing situations, but different acuity tasks do not necessarily respond to changes in the stimulus or the observer in the same way. In addition, different acuity tasks probably do not all measure the same characteristics of the visual system. For example, although resolution represents an important component of identification acuity, the recognition of complex targets, such as letters, apparently involves other spatial processing as well (Herse & Bedell 1989; Levi & Klein 1982; see also Chapter 6). This, along with the differences seen in Figure 5.7, provides the basis for considering identification acuity as a distinct type of acuity, even though its aim is to measure resolution. The use of letter charts is widely preferred for the clinical evaluation of visual acuity in adults and in children who are old enough to name the letters consistently. The following sections examine some considerations involved in constructing and administering a letter acuity test. In this context, some further advantages of using letters over other **optotypes** to measure resolution acuity become apparent.

Some reasons for using letter charts in an identification task are (1) letters comprise a highly familiar and easily identified set of stimuli for many people, permitting quick and reliable testing; (2) letter acuity is sensitive to the effect on vision of common clinical entities, such as refractive errors, media abnormalities such as corneal swelling, cataract, and diseases that affect the macular region of the retina; and (3) letter identification includes an *indicator response* (i.e., naming the letter) and is therefore much less influenced by guessing than tasks based on simple detection (see Chapter 1). Because most of the people in the world do not read English letters, charts using letters in other languages or Chinese or Japanese characters have been devised. The same principles apply to the design of those charts. Because the identification of letters or characters on charts is the most commonly used way to assess resolution acuity, in the remainder of this chapter, the phrase "visual acuity" is used instead of "resolution acuity" or "identification acuity." Visual acuity in this context is often abbreviated as VA.

The stroke width is the key element in each chart letter

To identify a letter, a person must resolve the details of the letter. The spatial detail that must be resolved corresponds to the width of the strokes that make up the letter. In the United States, the uppercase letters on acuity charts usually conform to a standard configuration in which each letter is as tall as it is wide and each stroke width corresponds to one-fifth of the total letter size (Committee on Vision 1980). A different convention holds in the United Kingdom, in which acuity letters conform to a matrix that is 5 units high by 4 units wide; each stroke width is one-fifth of the height (Ophthalmic Standards Committee 1968) (Figure 5.8). The main strokes of acuity letters may have small secondary projections called *serifs* (e.g., Snellen letters) or not (e.g., Sloan letters).

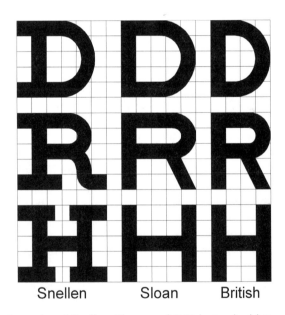

Snellen   Sloan   British

FIGURE 5.8   *Examples of Snellen, Sloan, and British standard letters. Each square in the background grid is 1 unit × 1 unit.*

A standard observer is defined as having a visual acuity that allows him or her to just identify letters with a stroke width of 1'

Regardless of whether the letters include serifs, *visual acuity* is defined in terms of the visual angle subtended by the stroke width of the smallest letters that the person can reliably identify. Consider a group of letters presented at 6 m, each comprised of strokes with a width equal to 1.75 mm. Each letter is 8.75 mm tall, because the height of each letter is five times the stroke width. At 6 m, each 1.75 mm stroke width corresponds to a visual angle of 1'—that is,

$$\tan^{-1}\left(\frac{1.75 \text{ mm}}{6,000 \text{ mm}}\right) = 1''$$

Eq. 5.1

Suppose one examines a person whose acuity is poorer than the standard observer: To identify a group of letters at 6 m, the stroke widths have to be larger than 1'. Assume that this person can identify letters at 6 m only if the stroke width is four times larger than required by the standard observer (4', equal to 7 mm). Because the stroke width and letter height are now four times larger, the standard observer would just be able to identify these letters at a four times greater distance (24 m), where each stroke width once again subtends an angle of 1' (Figure 5.9). This hypothetical calculation

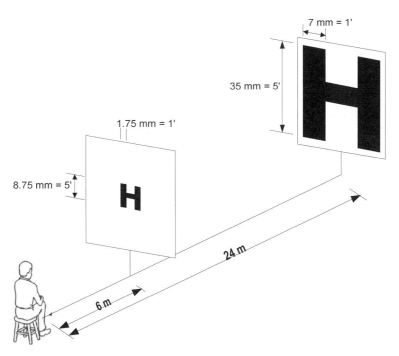

FIGURE 5.9   *A standard observer can just identify letters with a stroke width corresponding to 1'. At 6 m (approximately 20 ft), these letters are 8.75 mm tall. At 24 m (approximately 80 ft), letters with a stroke width that is four times larger (35 mm tall) subtend the same visual angle and, therefore, can still just be identified by a standard observer.*

defines the **Snellen fraction**. A person who, like the standard observer, can just identify letters with a stroke width of 1' at 6 m has a visual acuity of 6/6. The person with poorer acuity, who can just identify letters that are four times larger at 6 m has an acuity of 6/24. This fraction is the ratio of the distance at which the tested person can just identify letters of a certain size (the numerator) to the distance at which the hypothetical standard observer can identify letters of the same physical size (the denominator).

Another way to view the Snellen fraction is that the numerator is 1' times the test distance and the denominator is the tested observer's MAR times the test distance. Six meters is a standard test distance internationally because the stimulus is far enough away to not stimulate accommodation. However, acuity measures can be made at other distances. Six meters is very nearly 20 feet, so, in the United States, the visual acuity of the standard observer is expressed in Snellen notation as 20/20. The person whose threshold was 4' would have a Snellen acuity of 20/80.

Many people have better than the standard (1') visual acuity

Although 1' visual acuity is designated as standard normal acuity, as shown in Figure 5.10, it is common for people to resolve smaller separations when tested with gratings of letters. The average visual acuity is somewhat poorer in older normal individuals (see Chapter 10) and starts out substantially worse than 1' in infants (see Chapter 9).

Relative legibility and confusions influence the selection of the letters on a visual acuity chart

Even when letters are constructed to a standard format and are all the same size, some are easier to identify and some are more difficult. For example, the upper case letters L and T are highly legible, and the upper case letters S and B are more difficult to identify (Bennett 1965). One way to define the relative legibility of letters is to specify the differences in size that are required for each letter to reach its identification threshold—that is, the size at which each letter is identified correctly 50% or more of the time. For uppercase letters, relative legibility spans a range of approximately ± 30%, which means that the most difficult letters are identified correctly at threshold when they are approximately twice the size of the easiest letters (Bennett 1965; Hedin & Olsson 1984).

When observers are examined with the descending Method of Limits, they read down an acuity chart to a level at which they do not identify all of the letters correctly. The mistakes they make are not random, however (Banister 1927; Gervais et al. 1984). Rather, they are much more likely to misidentify an uppercase C as an O or G, but not as an R or M). Letters that observers often mistake for one another are called **confusion letters**. In addition, the letters that an observer identifies incorrectly vary to some extent with his or her uncorrected refractive error, particularly if it includes astigmatism. An observer with myopic astigmatism at axis 180 experiences

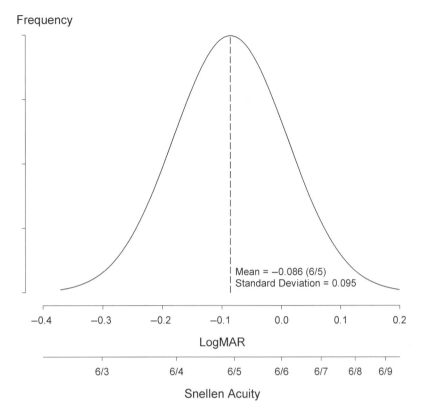

FIGURE 5.10   *Distribution of visual acuities based on results from 400 normal adults who were 40–49 years of age, measured with a letter chart while they wore the proper refractive correction if needed. The upper x-axis scale is the logMAR. On this scale, the standard acuity of 1' is at 0. The equivalent metric Snellen notation is presented on the lower x-axis scale. Notice that the mean of the acuity distribution is less than 1', such that 82% of adults in this sample have acuities of 1' or better. (Data from FW Weymouth. Effect of Age on Visual Acuity. In MJ Hirsch, RE Wick [eds], Vision of the Aging Patient. Philadelphia: Chilton Co., 1960;37–62.)*

defocus of vertical contours, making letters like V and Y difficult to distinguish. The same error has much less effect on other letters like E and F. Because of these factors, the set of letters used on each line of an acuity chart should have similar average legibility and should include a similar number of confusion pairs. Several sets of acuity letters have been suggested based on these criteria (Bailey & Lovie 1976; Bennett 1965; Sloan 1959).

One way to ensure equal legibility is to use charts that contain just a single letter

Charts have been designed that use only either an E or a C in different orientations. Typically the C (called a *Landolt C*) has a gap that is the same width as the stroke of the letter. Although it presents a less straightforward task to the patient (and to the examiner) than identifying different letters, charts consisting of the letter C in four orientations have been adopted as a standard method for measuring visual acuity (Committee on Vision 1980). The presentation of letters at other than horizontal and vertical orientations is discouraged because even observers without any astigmatism have poorer acuity for obliquely oriented stimuli than for horizontally or vertically oriented stimuli (Appelle 1972).

Various scales are used to represent visual acuity results

The outcome of a visual acuity test is expressed numerically. The three scales that have been introduced in this chapter are the MAR, the **logMAR scale**, and the Snellen fraction. Additional scales have been devised and used, including the **decimal visual acuity scale** and the Snell-Sterling visual efficiency scale. Different scales are defined and compared for several acuity performance criteria in Table 5.2. When evaluating the appropriateness of

TABLE 5.2 Comparison of acuity values and inverse slopes for several scales

	Visual acuity scale					
	MAR (min of arc)	*Denominator of Snellen fraction (metric)*	*Denominator of Snellen fraction (English)*	*Decimal (min of arc)$^{-1}$*	*Snell-Sterling visual efficiency (percent)*	*LogMAR log (min of arc)*
Scale definition		6 × MAR	20 × MAR	1/MAR	0.836$^{(MAR-1)}$	log(MAR)
Performance criterion						
Normal adult	0.82	4.9	16.4	1.22	103.3	−0.09
Estimated inverse slope	0.25	1.5	5	0.37	4.6	0.13
Standard	1.00	6	20	1	100	0
Estimated inverse slope	0.30	1.8	6.1	0.30	5.4	0.13
Unrestricted driving	2.00	12	40	0.50	83.6	0.30
Estimated inverse slope	0.61	3.7	12.2	0.15	9	0.13
Moderate visual impairment	3.50	21	70	0.29	64	0.54
Estimated inverse slope	1.06	6.4	21.3	0.09	11.9	0.13
Legal blindness	10	60	200	0.10	20	1
Estimated inverse slope	3.04	18.2	60.8	0.03	10.5	0.13
Profound visual impairment	25	150	500	0.04	1.4	1.40
Estimated inverse slope	7.60	45.6	151.9	0.01	2	0.13

LogMAR = log (minimum angle of resolution); MAR = minimum angle of resolution.

these scales, it is important to remember that the scale that is used sets the change of the stroke width, the letter height, and even the spacing between lines of letters, from line to line in the chart. This affects (1) the utility of the chart for making comparisons between acuity values at different positions on the scale, and (2) the accuracy with which one may make a judgment about whether the acuity has changed.

When using a letter chart, visual acuity is measured in terms of the angular size of the spatial detail (the stroke width) of the smallest letters that can be correctly identified. However, patients typically do not progress from identifying all of the letters correctly on one line to none of the letters correctly on the next smaller line. Instead, the percentage of correct responses usually decreases systematically from 100% to chance performance as the letter size becomes smaller. This is depicted in Figure 5.11, which illustrates hypothetical psychometric functions (see Chapter 1) for visual acuity. When using a descending Method of Limits procedure, most clinicians define acuity as the last line on which the patient correctly identifies at least four out of five (or five out of six) letters. This corresponds to 80% correct or higher on the psychometric function. Even though the point on the psychometric function that can be estimated most reliably is half way between 100% correct and 0% correct (e.g., 50% in Figure 5.11), where the slope of the function is steepest, many clinicians are hesitant to define threshold as a letter size that the patient can identify only half the time. However, in most serious clinical research studies, the subject is required to continue reading lines with smaller and smaller stroke widths, until chance performance is reached (Bailey et al. 1991). This allows comparisons to be made between the various scales, as shown in Figure 5.11.

An important parameter of the psychometric function is the **inverse slope**, defined as the change in stroke width (Δx) required for a criterion change in the percentage of correct responses (Δy), say, from 84% correct to 50% correct (see Figure 5.11). A change from 84% to 50% correct has been selected because it corresponds to one standard deviation of a cumulative normal probability distribution, which is assumed to form the basis of the psychometric function.* It has been found that the inverse slope generally corresponds to approximately a 30% change in the size of the letter for a decrease in the percent correct from 84% to 50% (Horner et al. 1985; Prince & Fry 1956). Under some conditions, such as uncorrected astigmatism, fluctuating accommodation, and unsteady eye movements, the psychometric function can be considerably flatter. This means that the inverse slope is commensurately larger. It should be apparent that the flatter the slope of the psychometric acuity function, the more error there can be in the estimate of acuity (see Figure 5.11). The larger the error of estimate, the less certainty a clinician can have about classifying a patient's acuity as normal versus abnormal or deciding whether the patient's acuity has changed as the result of disease or treatment. Clinicians can obtain, and increasingly are obtaining, information about the inverse slope of the psy-

---

*As mentioned in Chapter 1, if the values of a normal distribution are summed cumulatively from left to right (small letter sizes to large), a psychometric function results. If one assumes that the mean of the distribution is 50% correct, one standard deviation above the mean occurs at 84% correct.

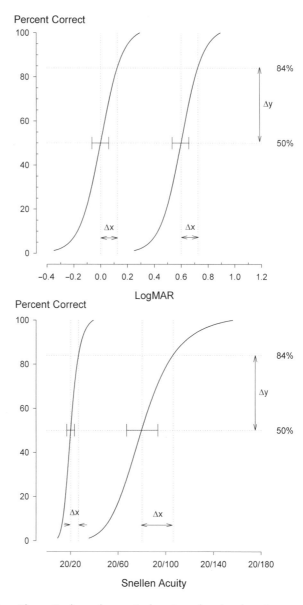

FIGURE 5.11 *Theoretical psychometric functions for visual acuity are plotted on the logMAR and Snellen scales, assuming that testing was with acuity charts containing 10 letters per line. Note that better acuity (smaller minimum angle of resolution) is to the left on the x-axis. If the descending Method of Limits were used, the patient's percent correct would be assessed first on rows with large letters, yielding 100% correct, and then on rows with smaller and smaller letters yielding fewer correct identifications. On each plot, the 50% correct acuity threshold for the left-hand function corresponds to 0 logMAR (6/6 Snellen) and the threshold for the right-hand function corresponds to 0.6 logMAR (6/24 Snellen). The inverse slope of the psychometric function (Δx/Δy) does not vary with the value of acuity on the logMAR scale but increases as acuity becomes worse on the Snellen scale. The size of the confidence interval (horizontal error bars) remains constant on the logMAR scale, but varies with the value of acuity on the Snellen scale, because the confidence interval depends on the inverse slope of the psychometric function. (Δx = change in stroke width; Δy = change in percentage of correct responses.)*

chometric acuity function and an estimate of the likely measurement error by recording the number of correct responses that a patient makes on each line of the chart, from 100% down to 50% or fewer correct (Committee on Vision 1980; Flom 1966).

The log of the minimum angle of resolution (logMAR) is the preferred scale for representing visual acuity

Based on the two factors considered in the previous section, it has been found that a logMAR scale provides the most reasonable estimates of acuity change, especially when the acuity is better than 1" or much worse (see Table 5.2). Many researchers and clinicians now prefer the logMAR visual acuity scale and have begun using it routinely. The major advantage of this scale is that the inverse slope of the psychometric acuity function remains more or less independent of the acuity value (Horner et al. 1985; Westheimer 1979a). Thus, when acuity is expressed using the logMAR scale, and an equal number of letters is presented on each line, the associated measurement error remains approximately constant (see Figure 5.11 and Table 5.2). Consequently, an acuity change of 0.10 logMAR is equally significant whether the initial acuity is 6/6 (0 logMAR) or 6/60 (1.0 logMAR).

On acuity charts designed according to the logMAR scale, the letters on each line are approximately 26% (0.1 log unit) larger or smaller than those on the line just below or above (Figure 5.12)—a size change that corresponds roughly to the inverse slope of the psychometric function. These charts can be viewed from different distances with no change in the relative sizes or the spacing of the letters. Moreover, because there are five letters on a row, each letter can be assigned a value of 0.02 log units. If a person correctly identified all the letters on the 0.3 logMAR line and then two more of the letters on the 0.2 logMAR line, he or she would be given an acuity score of 0.26. This provides a scale that is five times finer than would result from a row-by-row scoring (Bailey et al. 1991).

Letter acuity is affected by the spacing between adjacent targets

The ability to identify a letter depends not only on its size, but also on how near it is to other letters or other high-contrast contours, such as the edge of the chart. This *contour interaction* phenomenon does not result from interference between or overlap of the retinal images of neighboring letters or contours, because the effect remains if the test letter is shown to one eye and the neighboring targets are presented to the other eye (Flom et al. 1963). In addition, the maximum degradation of legibility is usually produced when a letter and neighboring contour are separated by approximately half a letter width; larger or smaller separations produce less interference (Figure 5.13). Contour interaction is greater and extends over a larger region of the retina when the letters are viewed with nonfoveal vision (Jacobs 1979).

Besides interference from nearby contours, other factors, such as inaccurate eye movements, can contribute to reduced visual acuity on charts that present

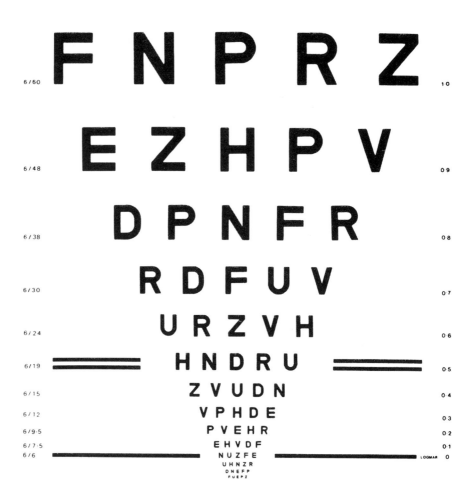

FIGURE 5.12 *An example of an acuity chart constructed using the logMAR scale. The spacing between the letters on each line is proportional to the letter size, and letter size progression is in equal steps of 0.1 log unit. Because each line contains five letters, one letter corresponds to an increment of acuity equal to 0.02 logMAR. Notice also that the spacing between the rows of letters is proportional to the letter size. (Reprinted with permission from I Bailey, J Lovie. New design principles for visual acuity letter charts. Am J Optom Physiol Opt 1976;53:740–745.)*

several different letters in each line (Flom 1991). The aggregate of all of these influences is labeled the **crowding effect**. Visual acuity can be evaluated independently of the crowding effect by presenting letters to the patient one at a time on a background with no other nearby contours. The effect of inaccurate eye movements can be selectively eliminated by presenting a series of charts, each consisting of multiple representations of the same letter in the same orientation, so that where the patient looks on the chart is not an issue (Harris et al. 1985). Typically, modern letter charts do not eliminate contour interaction and related effects but, instead, standardize them by ensuring that the separa-

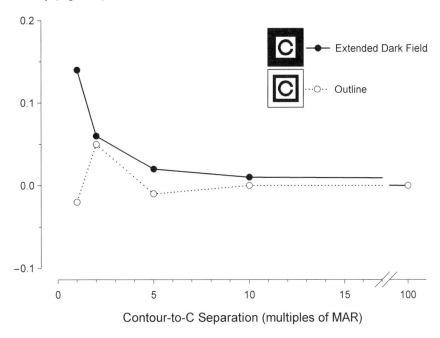

Normalized Visual Acuity (logMAR)

Contour-to-C Separation (multiples of MAR)

FIGURE 5.13   *Spatial interactions between an acuity target and nearby contours impair visual acuity. Contour interaction was produced by the inside edge of an extended low-luminance field* (filled symbols) *or the edge of an outline square with the same stroke width as the Landolt C acuity target* (unfilled symbols). *The x-axis indicates the spatial separation between the acuity target and the nearby contour, expressed in multiples of the acuity target's stroke width. Data are the average of six normal observers, normalized to 0 logMAR in the absence of any nearby contours (infinity on the x-axis). (MAR = minimum angle of resolution.) (Modified from ST Chung, HE Bedell. Effect of retinal image motion on visual acuity and contour interaction in congenital nystagmus. Vision Res 1995;35:3071–3082.)*

tion of the letters on each line and between lines is proportional to their size (Bailey & Lovie 1976; Ferris et al. 1982; Flom 1966).

Retinal illuminance affects visual acuity

Everyone has had the experience that visual tasks, such as reading, become more difficult under conditions of low luminance. Recall from Chapter 4 that vision at high levels of luminance is mediated primarily by cone photoreceptors and at low levels of luminance by rod photoreceptors. In Figure 5.14, the shift from cone (filled circles) to rod (open circles) vision is demarcated by a transition in the acuity versus retinal illuminance function. Starting at luminance levels just above the cone threshold, as retinal illuminance is increased,

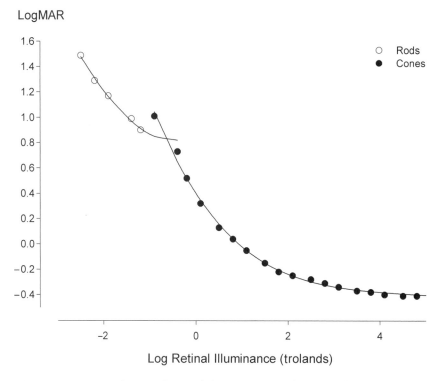

LogMAR

FIGURE 5.14   *Visual acuity for Landolt C targets as a function of retinal illuminance. Separate lines are drawn through results obtained for rod- and cone-mediated vision. On the x-axis, 3 log trolands correspond to a target luminance of approximately 100 candelas per square meter (cd/m²), assuming a pupil diameter of 3.5 mm. (Modified from S Shlaer. The relation between visual acuity and illumination. J Gen Physiol 1938;21:165–188.)*

visual acuity first improves fairly rapidly and then much more gradually. Clinically, acuity is measured on the section of the curve at which luminance has relatively little effect (approximately 100 candelas per square meter [cd/m²]), so that small fluctuations in room illumination or differences from observer to observer in pupil size or intraocular scattering and absorption (which influence the amount of light that reaches the retina) do not substantially influence the result.

At low illuminance levels, visual acuity that is mediated through the rods also improves as the illuminance is increased (see Figure 5.14). The maximum visual acuity reached by normal observers under scotopic lighting conditions is 5'–10' (0.7–1.0 logMAR), which corresponds reasonably closely to the visual acuity achieved by rod monochromats (individuals who lack cones) (Haegerstrom-Portnoy et al. 1996). Because the foveal region normally lacks rod photoreceptors, optimal scotopic acuity is achieved when the observer aims his or her fovea to one side of the acuity target. However, best scotopic acuity occurs at a much smaller retinal eccentricity than 20°, the location at which the density of the rod photoreceptors is highest (see Chapter 2). As is discussed later in this chapter (see the section Visual acuity is determined largely by optical and "neural" defocus), this clearly points out that scotopic acuity depends strongly on neural processing that occurs beyond the level of the photoreceptors (i.e., the convergence of rods onto bipolar cells to form receptive-field centers).

Visual acuity is better for targets of high contrast than of low contrast

As described in the Appendix, if black letters are presented against a white screen, their contrast is negative. When high-luminance letters are presented on a lower-luminance screen, contrast is positive. Fortunately, over a reasonably wide range, the response of the visual system is approximately the same to targets of negative and positive contrast (Alexander et al. 1993; Newacheck et al. 1990).

For well-focused targets that are presented on the fovea, the letter acuity becomes worse (i.e., the MAR increases) as contrast is reduced. In Figure 5.15, note that acuity initially remains good as contrast is reduced and is strongly

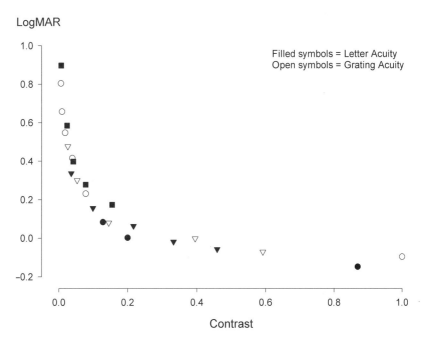

FIGURE 5.15   *Visual acuity for letter targets (filled symbols) and grating targets (open symbols), compared for several studies. Acuity for both types of target is affected in the same way by changes in contrast. Acuity changes little for a wide range of high levels of contrast (expressed here as $[L_{max} - L_{min}]/(L_{max} + L_{min}]$, where L_{max} is the maximum luminance level and L_{min} is the minimum luminance level, as described in the Appendix). Consequently, small changes in the contrast of standard letter targets do not strongly influence measured acuity. (Modified from PR Herse, HE Bedell. Contrast sensitivity for letter and grating targets under various stimulus conditions. Optom Vis Sci 1989;66: 774–781.)*

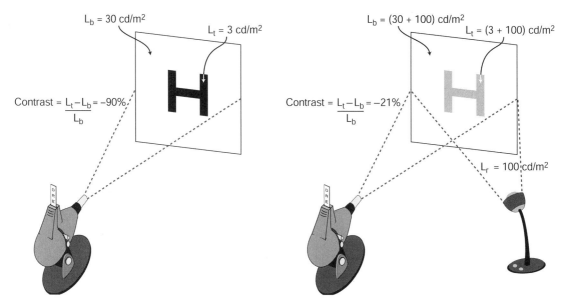

FIGURE 5.16   *Ambient room illumination can reduce the contrast of projected acuity targets. Contrast is defined here as $(L_t - L_b)/L_b$; see the Appendix. Contrast is reduced because the room illumination (L_r) adds equally to the luminance of the target (L_t) and its background luminance (L_b).*

affected only when contrast falls below approximately 0.2. With continued decrease in contrast, the MAR increases greatly. Because standard clinical acuity tests use high-contrast letters, small changes in the contrast (e.g., from low ancillary room luminance when using a projected chart) do not substantially affect the measured acuity. However, the contrast of projected letter charts can be significantly decreased if lights in the room, other than projector, are allowed to illuminate the screen, providing a veiling luminance, as shown in Figure 5.16 (see also Chapter 3).

Some researchers and clinicians have advocated using low- as well as high-contrast acuity charts (Pelli et al. 1988; Regan & Neima 1983). An example of a low-contrast acuity chart is shown in Figure 5.17. The rationale for using low-contrast charts is that some ocular or neurologic conditions may selectively degrade the visual mechanisms responsible for detecting large objects, although leaving acuity for small targets relatively normal. Defects of this kind would not be detected with high-contrast letters but should appear when acuity is tested with large, low-contrast letters.

Resolution and localization acuity become worse with eccentricity from the fovea

In daylight or at normal indoor luminance levels, visual acuity is best when the targets are imaged on the center of the fovea because of the small, tightly

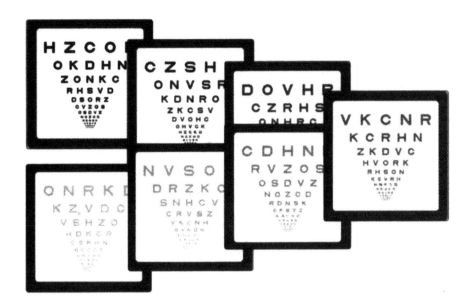

FIGURE 5.17   A representation of low-contrast Bailey-Lovie type logMAR charts produced by Precision Vision. All of the letters on each chart are the same contrast, but the contrast of each chart decreases from 100% (**top left**) to 1.25% (**center**). (Courtesy of Precision Vision, La Salle, Illinois.)

packed cones in this region. Acuity is systematically poorer for targets presented to other retinal regions, even when the targets remain within the rod-free fovea (Weymouth et al. 1928). Weymouth (1958) showed that, to a first approximation, the change in photopic acuity is linear with retinal eccentricity when acuities are expressed as the MAR. However, the rate at which acuity worsens with distance from the fovea differs according to the acuity task. As shown in Figure 5.18, acuity worsens more rapidly for localization acuity and more slowly for grating resolution and letter identification (Levi et al. 1985). When expressed as MAR, letter and grating acuity worsen to twice the foveal value at eccentricities of approximately 2.0° and 2.5°, respectively. The rate at which resolution changes with eccentricity is not the same for different retinal meridians: Acuity worsens more slowly along the horizontal than along the vertical meridian of the field and is better in the temporal than in the nasal visual field (Wertheim 1980). The unequal rates of change for different visual acuity tasks have been interpreted to mean that different neural factors probably limit these kinds of acuity.

As described in a previous section, under scotopic lighting conditions, the rod-free fovea becomes "blind" (see also Chapter 3, Figure 3.14) and the best acuity is achieved at a peripheral retinal location. Scotopic acuity is limited primarily by the neural convergence that occurs onto bipolar cells from the rod photoreceptors, rather than by the increased spacing between adjacent rods (D'Zmura & Lennie 1986). As a result (see the filled squares in Figure 5.19), optimal scotopic acuity occurs at retinal eccentricities that are much

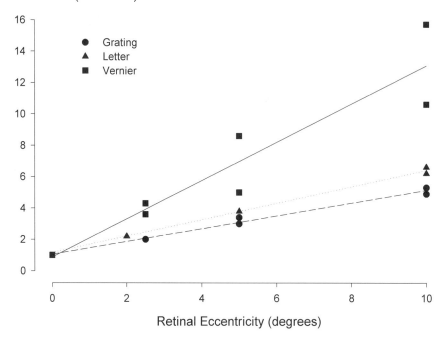

Relative Acuity
Threshold (min of arc)

- ● Grating
- ▲ Letter
- ■ Vernier

Retinal Eccentricity (degrees)

FIGURE 5.18 *Visual acuity worsens approximately linearly with retinal eccentricity when expressed in terms of the minimum angle of resolution. Vernier acuity worsens at a much more rapid rate than resolution or identification acuity. Note that foveal performance for each kind of acuity is accorded a value of 1 in this graph, even though Vernier acuity has a much lower threshold. The data are from several studies. (Modified from PR Herse, HE Bedell. Contrast sensitivity for letter and grating targets under various stimulus conditions. Optom Vis Sci 1989;66:774–781.)*

closer to the fovea than the retinal region with the maximum rod density (at approximately 5° from the foveal center instead of at approximately 20° of eccentricity) (Mandelbaum & Sloan 1947). At mesopic luminance levels (see the inverted triangles in Figure 5.19), when the cones and rods are active simultaneously, acuity varies little with eccentricity within the central 15–20° of the retina. It is noteworthy that despite the poor levels of visual acuity achieved at low levels of luminance, letter acuity is degraded still further by the introduction of optical defocus (Johnson & Casson 1995).

Visual acuity is degraded for moving and very brief-duration targets

Visual acuity for high-contrast targets is not impaired by low velocities of retinal image motion, such as occur when an observer sits or stands quietly and attempts to look at a stationary target (Steinman & Levinson 1990). On the other hand, visual acuity worsens progressively when the retinal image velocity increases beyond a few degrees per second (Figure 5.20). A necessary conse-

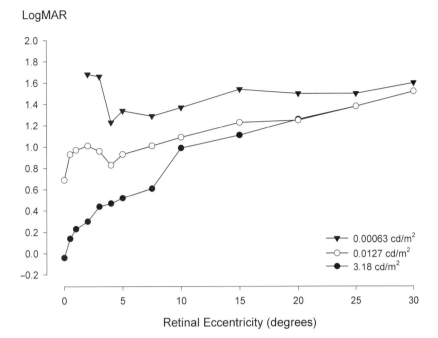

LogMAR

FIGURE 5.19   *Visual acuity that is measured using Landolt C targets varies differently with retinal eccentricity for targets of photopic* (circles), *mesopic* (inverted triangles), *and scotopic luminance* (squares). *Scotopic acuity cannot be measured in the rod-free fovea. (Modified from J Mandelbaum, LL Sloan. Peripheral visual acuity. Am J Ophthalmol 1947;30:581–588.)*

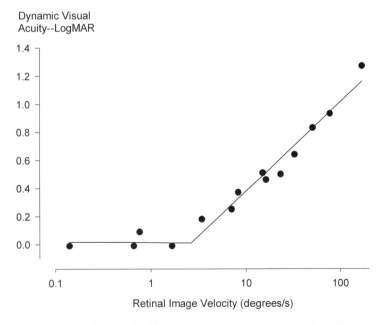

FIGURE 5.20   *Visual acuity for high-contrast Sloan letters is unaffected by retinal image velocity up to approximately 2° per second. At higher image velocities, acuity worsens systematically. (Modified from JL Demer, F Amjadi. Dynamic visual acuity of normal subjects during vertical optotype and head motion. Invest Ophthalmol Vis Sci 1993;34:1894–1906.)*

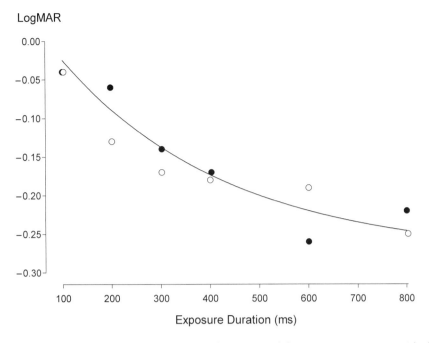

LogMAR

FIGURE 5.21   *Visual acuity as measured using Landolt C targets improves with the exposure duration of the target. Data are for two observers. (Modified from W Baron, G Westheimer. Visual acuity as a function of exposure duration. J Opt Soc Am 1973;63: 212–219.)*

quence of retinal image motion is that the target's image shifts from the fovea to nonfoveal retina. However, the falloff of acuity away from the fovea accounts for only a fraction of the amount that acuity is degraded during motion (Ludvigh 1949). Motion also limits the time that the target's image remains at each location on the retina. Because the visual system can summate information from the target over time, visual acuity for flashed targets improves up to a duration of approximately 500 milliseconds as shown in Figure 5.21.

Retinal image motion can result when either the target or the observer is in motion. Visual acuity that is measured when the target or the observer is in motion is called *dynamic visual acuity*. As expected, performance on a dynamic visual acuity test is determined by how well the observer's eye movements compensate for the imposed motion to maintain a fairly stable image of the target on the fovea (Brown 1972; Demer & Amjadi 1993). Retinal image motion occurs in certain patients because of abnormally large, uncontrolled eye movements. In patients who make abnormal eye movements, acuity is also determined largely by how long a low-velocity image of the target remains on or near the fovea (Abadi & Pascal 1991).

Visual acuity is determined largely by optical and neural defocus

This chapter has identified a number of parameters that influence visual acuity: defocus, luminance, contrast, retinal location, motion, and exposure duration. Conceptually, most or all of the parameters that influence visual acuity can be collapsed into two main categories. These two categories are defocus, which is considered in an expanded sense in the following discussion, and the detectability of the target.

The optics of the eye transmit the pattern of higher and lower luminance from an external object to the retinal photoreceptors. As illustrated earlier in this chapter, the optics of even a normal eye are imperfect, which results in a minimum, irreducible amount of defocus in the retinal image. The amount of retinal image defocus varies with the size of the pupil, reaching a minimum when the pupil is between 2 and 3 mm in diameter (see Figure 5.1). Larger pupils result in increased defocus because of the optical aberrations of the eye, and smaller pupils introduce defocus from the diffraction of light.

Regions of higher and lower illuminance in the retinal image are encoded into a spatial pattern of hyperpolarization in the retinal photoreceptors—that is, a neural image. Potentially, acuity can be lost during the photoreceptor encoding process if adjacent receptors are spaced further apart than the details in the retinal image. However, the spacing of the photoreceptors in the human fovea is well matched to the spacing of the finest details that the optics of the eye can produce in the retinal image. Consequently, little or no improvement of acuity would result if the foveal photoreceptors were packed even closer together. The correspondence between photoreceptor spacing and the optical properties of the eye does not hold outside the foveal region where the spacing between adjacent cone receptors is too coarse to accurately encode all of the details in the retinal image (Geisler 1989).

Just as the retinal image is transduced by the photoreceptors into a neural pattern of activity, subsequent levels of processing transform the neural image that is received from the photoreceptor layer. This process of successively transforming the neural image continues through the retina and into central visual structures, with each transformation providing an opportunity for the introduction of neural defocus, analogous to optical defocus, which blends together the details of an object in the retinal image. Neural defocus blends together gradations between the responses of neighboring photoreceptors at later processing stages. For example, if the different signals from many photoreceptors converge onto a single neuron at a subsequent level of processing, then the neural image at this more subsequent level is, effectively, defocused. In fact, the receptive fields of ganglion cells in the peripheral retina combine (via the bipolar cells) information from a large number of photoreceptors, thereby introducing neural defocus and degrading visual acuity (Banks et al. 1991). The convergence of photoreceptor signals at the ganglion cells is more extensive for peripheral rods than cones (D'Zmura & Lennie 1986), which accounts, in part, for the reason why peripheral visual acuity is worse under scotopic than photopic lighting conditions, even though the spacing is less between the peripheral rod receptors than the cones (see Figure 5.19).

Neural defocus can also impair visual acuity if the visual system is forced to rely on neurons with large receptive fields instead of small ones. For example, neural defocus apparently limits visual acuity when a target moves so quickly that small receptive fields become insensitive (Chung et al. 1996) or when the normal development of small receptive fields is disrupted by abnormal visual experience (Levi & Klein 1990).

The second main factor that influences visual acuity is the detectability of the target. As discussed previously, detectability determines the dimensions of the finest line and the smallest dot that a person can see. A substantial limitation on the detection and discrimination of targets arises because of fluctuations over time in the number of quanta that form the target's retinal image or different parts of the target's image. Increasing the luminance, the contrast, or (within the interval over which Bloch's law holds) the exposure duration of an acuity target provides the visual system with a larger number of quanta in the retinal image and a relatively smaller amount of quantal fluctuation (as discussed in Chapter 2). Two-point resolution, grating acuity, and spatial-interval acuity improve with photopic luminance and target contrast as expected from a statistical analysis of the quantal fluctuations in the image (Banks et al. 1987; Geisler 1989).

Visual acuity provides important information about the integrity of the visual system

As has been described in this chapter, a variety of targets and tasks can be used to estimate the several types of visual acuity. These tasks do not necessarily yield identical numerical values for acuity and probably reflect a number of different facets of visual processing. Visual acuity is influenced by a wide variety of stimulus parameters that help to establish its sensitivity as a psychophysical test (i.e., good acuity can occur only when the eye and visual system function well). The use of letter targets to assess visual acuity has a number of clinical advantages. When administered and interpreted appropriately, visual acuity is a robust psychophysical test that provides information about the optical properties of the eye, the central retina, and subsequent stages of neural processing.

Acknowledgments
I am pleased to acknowledge the assistance of Suzanne Ferimer, Curg Click, Douglas Ingram, Dennis Levi, Thanh Nguyen, Saumil Patel, Ming Qi, Lewis Reich, and Enita Torres, who contributed in important ways to the completion of this chapter. Preparation of the chapter was supported in part by research grant R01-EY05068.

Study Guide

1. Define visual acuity.
2. Know the three (or four) types of acuity, how each is tested, and the normal limits of each (see Table 5.1).
3. Explain how the minimum visible acuity for a single black line is a threshold $\Delta L/L$ task.
4. Explain how the minimum resolvable acuity is a threshold $\Delta L/L$ task involving the grain of the photoreceptors.
5. List two localization acuity tasks and how they are tested.

6. Define minimum angle of resolution (MAR).
7. Explain how the retinal image, photoreceptor grain, and neural convergence (neural defocus) each can limit the minimum resolvable acuity.
8. Define optotypes.
9. Define confusion letters.
10. Why is it preferable to use letter charts to measure acuity instead of spots or gratings?
11. Be able to design a Snellen letter and achieve a specified stroke width (in minutes of arc) at any specified distance.
12. If one was lost on a desert island and wanted to make a sign saying HELP that could be seen by a pilot flying at a height of 10,000 m (32,809 ft), and the pilot were corrected to resolve stroke widths of 2', how tall would the letters need to be? (Answer: 29.1 m [95.44 ft])
13. Define inverse slope.
14. Why is logMAR the preferred scale for representing visual acuity?
15. Be able to readily convert between Snellen notation, MAR, and logMAR.
16. What is contour interaction? Why is it a potential problem? How do clinicians deal with it?
17. Explain why acuity worsens with defocus.
18. Explain why acuity worsens at very low contrast.
19. Explain why acuity worsens with retinal eccentricity.
20. Explain why acuity declines with decreasing luminance.

Glossary

Astigmatism: a condition of refraction in which rays emanating from a single luminous point are not focused at a single point by the eye but rather are focused as two line images at different distances, generally at right angles to each other.

Confusion letters: chart letters that observers often mistake for one another.

Crowding effect: interference from nearby contours (contour interaction) and other factors, such as inaccurate eye movements, that can contribute to reduced visual acuity on letter charts compared to visual acuity for isolated letters.

Decimal visual acuity scale: the inverse of the MAR (i.e., 1 divided by MAR) in decimal notation.

Detection acuity (also called *minimum visible acuity* or *minimum distinguishable acuity*): the angular size of the smallest visible target.

Identification acuity (also called *minimum recognizable acuity* and commonly referred to as *visual acuity*, because letters are most frequently used clinically): an acuity measure in which the subject's MAR is determined by the ability of the subject to identify a letter, number, or character.

Inverse slope: the change in acuity (Δx) required for a criterion change in the percentage of correct responses (Δy), for example, from 84% to 50% correct.

Localization acuity (also called *minimum discriminable acuity* or *hyperacuity*): the smallest spatial offset or difference in location between targets that can be discriminated.

LogMAR: the log of the minimum angle of resolution.

LogMAR scale: a scale plotting the logarithm of the minimum angle of resolution. Also, an arrangement of letter sizes on an acuity chart such that the stroke width is smaller by 0.1 unit on lines arranged down the chart.

Minimum angle of resolution (MAR): the threshold angular separation that can be discriminated in a test of resolution acuity.

Optotypes: symbols used to determine resolution or identification acuity.

Resolution acuity (sometimes called *minimum separable acuity*): the smallest spatial separation between two nearby points of lines that can be discriminated.

Snellen fraction: the ratio of the distance at which the tested person can just identify letters of a certain size (the numerator) to the distance at which the hypothetical standard observer can identify letters of the same physical size (the denominator). Another way to view the Snellen fraction is that the numerator is 1 minute of arc times the test distance and the denominator is the tested observer's MAR times the test distance.

Spatial-interval acuity: a localization acuity that measures the smallest change in the separation (ΔS) between two targets that can be discriminated as larger or smaller than a standard separation (S).

Spatial visual acuity: the finest spatial detail that can be detected, discriminated, or resolved.

Vernier acuity: a localization acuity that measures the smallest offset between two targets that can be discriminated when one target is deviated rightward or leftward (or upward or downward) from perfect alignment.

6   **Spatial Vision**

Thomas T. Norton, Vasudevan Lakshminarayanan, and Carl J. Bassi

Overview

The visual system evolved to detect and recognize objects from patterns of light and dark on the retina. This chapter, therefore, concentrates on the psychophysical measurement of the mechanisms the visual system uses to consistently process complex patterns of light and dark under a variety of luminance conditions.

Absolute luminance is less important in spatial vision than relative luminance levels because luminance levels vary greatly in the environment, but relative luminances (contrast) for visual stimuli do not. The visual system responds to the luminance differences (contrast) at the boundaries between objects and their background, which is the basis for brightness constancy. The brightness of a surface is not always predicted by its luminance, as shown by simultaneous contrast and assimilation.

Seeing objects requires detecting their edges (boundaries). The visual system accentuates the differences at luminance boundaries as demonstrated by the existence of Mach bands. Retinal ganglion cells with center-surround receptive fields respond in a way that emphasizes contrast boundaries associated with the edges of objects and can account for Mach bands.

Spatial contrast sensitivity is a psychophysical measure used to assess the sensitivity of the visual system to spatial luminance changes of various spatial frequencies. The human spatial contrast sensitivity function (spatial CSF) is band-pass with a peak contrast sensitivity in the range of 3–10 cycles per degree. The cutoff high spatial frequency approximately matches spatial resolution acuity. Optical defocus mainly affects the cutoff high frequency of the spatial CSF.

The neural basis for the human spatial CSF is the receptive field of retinal and, eventually, cortical neurons. The receptive-field center size determines the optimal spatial frequency for any one neuron. Spatial frequency "channels" have been demonstrated psychophysically in humans using contrast adaptation at specific spatial frequencies. The brightness enhancement of Mach bands can be predicted by the spatial frequency content of visual stimuli, coupled with the human spatial CSF.

The detection of low-to-intermediate spatial frequencies is a critically important part of normal spatial vision. Patients with low vision often have losses in spatial contrast sensitivity and clinical contrast charts allow measurement of spatial CSF losses. No pattern of contrast sensitivity loss at specific spatial frequencies has been selectively associated with particular ocular pathologies.

The visual system recognizes objects from patterns of light and dark

Whereas previous chapters have dealt with measuring thresholds using targets, such as spots, lines, gratings, and letters, they have not considered that objects in the real world are represented to the eye as complex patterns of reflected light and that an object can be recognized when viewed under a variety of different luminance conditions. It is possible, for example, to recognize a face bathed in direct sunlight or lit by moonlight filtered through the leaves of a tree. This ability raises the question of what is being extracted from the image that remains constant enough from one lighting condition to another to enable the brain to recognize the two luminance patterns as the same object. An important part of the answer is that the visual system processes spatial luminance information in a manner that emphasizes the luminance differences that typically occur at the boundaries or edges of objects. Thus, the visual system, like other sensory systems, provides information about changes in the environment.

Absolute luminance is less important in spatial vision than relative luminance

The absolute luminance of an object is less important for detecting and recognizing objects than is the relative amount of light coming from one spatial location in comparison to another. Because the proportion of incident light reflected (reflectance) from real objects does not vary, objects with a higher reflectance always have a higher luminance than objects of lower reflectance when both are viewed at any given luminance level. If **contrast** is defined as $(L_T - L_B)/L_B$, where L_B is the luminance of the background and L_T is the luminance of the object, the contrast between an object and background is constant under different overall light levels and characterizes the object.

The visual system is a very poor light meter. In keeping with the fact that object contrast, rather than absolute luminance, remains constant in the environment, neurons in the visual system respond similarly to the relative luminance of objects across a wide range of luminance levels (see Chapter 4, Figure 4.17). As a result, the brightness of objects is judged to be relatively invariant, even though the absolute luminance varies widely. This is called **brightness constancy**. The fact that objects do not look much brighter or darker when the room lights are of high or low intensity is an example of brightness constancy. The neural basis for this was described in Chapter 4 (see Chapter 4, Figure 4.17).

A.

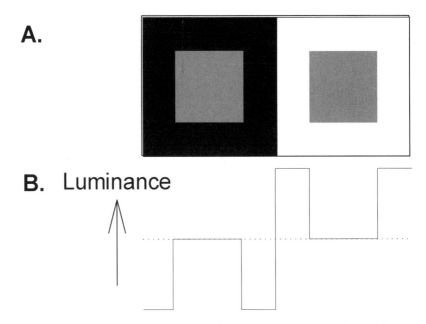

B. Luminance

FIGURE 6.1 **A.** *Simultaneous contrast. The two center squares of equal luminance appear to have different brightnesses induced by their backgrounds.* **B.** *Relative luminance profile of the stimulus, showing that the retinal illuminance produced by the central square is the same on the right and left sides of the figure.*

The brightness of an object is not always predicted by its luminance

Another example of how the brightness of an object depends on contrast more than on absolute luminance is **simultaneous contrast**. This effect occurs when a stimulus of a given luminance is viewed against backgrounds of lower and higher luminance. In Figure 6.1, the center squares are of equal reflectance and thus produce equal retinal illuminance. It is clear that the square surrounded by the background with the higher luminance appears darker than the square surrounded by the background with the lower luminance. Thus, the brightness of the center panel is affected by the local contrast at the boundary between the center panel and the surrounding background panels. Positive contrast (on the left side of the figure) increases the brightness, and negative contrast (on the right side of the figure) lowers the brightness.

Figure 6.2 shows the phenomenon of **assimilation**, a more complex version of simultaneous contrast. The center square and the intermediate square are identical on the left and right sides of the figure. The only difference is that the outermost panel is black on the left and white on the right. The intermediate squares show simultaneous contrast just as the center squares do in Figure 6.1. The small center squares also show a brightness difference, such that the left center square appears brighter than the one on the right. The brightness of the smallest center square has assimilated some of the apparent brightness of the surrounding intermediate panels. Because the contrast between the center

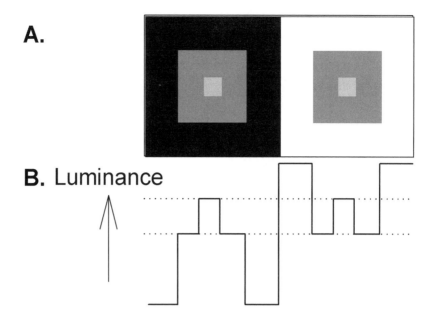

A.

B. Luminance

FIGURE 6.2   **A.** *Assimilation. The two center squares of equal luminance, located on gray backgrounds also having equal luminance, appear to have different brightnesses induced by other backgrounds. The central square on the left should appear slightly brighter than the central square on the right.* **B.** *Relative luminance profile of stimulus showing that the retinal illuminance produced by the central square and the dark grey background is the same on the right and left sides of the figure.*

panel is the same on the left and right sides of the figure, the brightness is additive with the brightness of the intermediate panel. The intermediate panel on the left appears brighter than the intermediate panel on the right, so the central panel on the left appears brighter than the central panel on the right. In assimilation, the brightness co-varies with the brightness of the immediately surrounding region (the intermediate panels), whereas in simultaneous contrast, the brightness is inversely related to the background.

Assimilation may originate in the visual cortex because it seems absent in the retina (Shapley 1991). It has been found that the amount of assimilation depends on the amount of simultaneous contrast and that the assimilation effect is approximately one-half as strong as simultaneous contrast (Shapley & Reid 1985). In all three instances (brightness constancy, simultaneous contrast, and assimilation), the visual system judges brightness based primarily on the local contrast at luminance boundaries.

Boundaries provide critical information for form perception

Given that the visual system essentially discards information about absolute luminance in favor of brightness constancy and, in turn, judges the brightness of a surface on the basis of what surrounds it, there must be some other characteristic of the image that provides information that remains stable over a range of lighting conditions. As the following sections show, the visual system

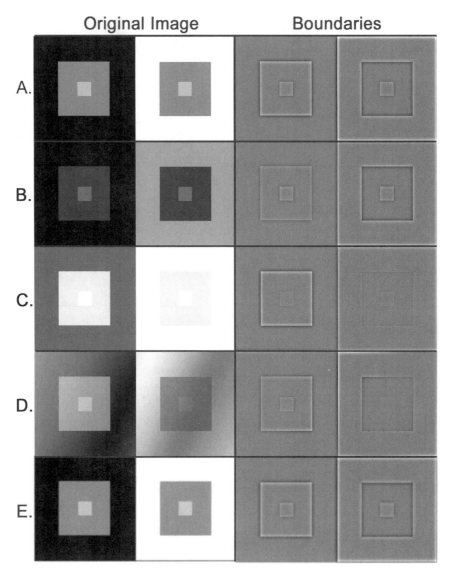

Original Image   Boundaries

A.

B.

C.

D.

E.

FIGURE 6.3 *An example of boundary information extracted from variations on the same original image. See text for details.*

is ideally suited to extracting information about contrast boundaries. To get an idea of how this works consider Figure 6.3.

The left-hand pair of columns in Figure 6.3 shows variations on the same image that was used to demonstrate assimilation in Figure 6.2. In Figure 6.3A, the image is unaltered. Images B–E have been darkened, lightened, overlaid with a gradient luminance, and blurred, respectively. The right-hand pair of columns shows the results of filtering the image in a manner that tends to equalize the luminance while accenting the contrast boundaries. Note the contrast at the boundaries in the filtered images: It tends to be lighter on the side in which the original area was light and darker in which the original area was darker. The visual system responds to the contrast boundaries on the left side of the figure in a similar way, creating the same kind of boundary as on the right side of the figure.

Mach bands are produced by a mechanism that accentuates luminance changes at surface boundaries

Perhaps because spatial luminance boundaries are so important for the detection of objects, the visual system responds to them in a way that emphasizes boundary information in comparison with spatial areas of unchanging or slowly changing luminance. This accentuation of luminance differences at boundaries affects the brightness near boundaries as is shown in Figure 6.4A. This figure consists of a series of panels, with each panel to the right having lower reflectance than the one to its left. Each individual panel does not appear uniformly bright, however. Each panel appears darker on its left and brighter on its right than it does in its center, particularly if the page is held close to the eye. These darker and brighter vertical regions are called **Mach bands** after Ernst Mach who first described them in 1865. The luminance profile of the bars is represented in Figure 6.4B. The brightness of the panels is illustrated in Figure 6.4C.

Mach bands are the visual system's way of accentuating luminance differences. The example shown in Figure 6.4 has sharp boundaries between the areas of constant luminance, but Mach bands also appear in instances in which the transition from one luminance to another are not as sharp.

The dependence of brightness on contrast and the brightness enhancement of Mach bands can be explained by retinal receptive-field center–surround interactions

As has been described in previous chapters, many retinal ganglion cells have a center-surround organization in which the center (either on-center or off-center) is produced by direct connections from photoreceptors to bipolar cells. The antagonistic surround (off-surround or on-surround) is produced by indirect connections from photoreceptors to horizontal cells to bipolar cells within the outer plexiform layer (Oyster 1999; Rodieck 1998). These indirect connections produce **lateral inhibition**, whereby the response of the bipolar cell is affected in an opposite, or antagonistic, way by luminance levels in the receptive-field surround than it is to luminance levels in the center. For instance, an on-center bipolar cell depolarizes in response to increased illuminance within its center. Increased illuminance in the surround causes the opposite effect: hyperpolarization. These effects cancel each other so that when illuminance is increased in both the center and the surround, the net effect is a slight depolarization. The center-surround organization is passed on to the ganglion cells, which produce action potentials that leave the retina via the optic nerve.

To see how the center-surround organization produces Mach bands, consider the luminance boundary between the evenly luminous light and dark

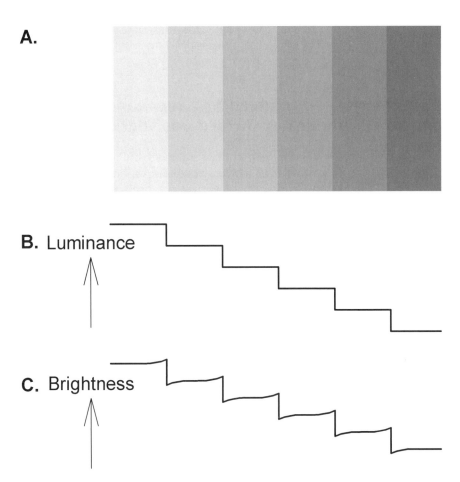

FIGURE 6.4 **A.** *Mach bands are visible at the borders between each of the panels. Each panel appears darker on its left and brighter on its right.* **B.** *Relative luminance profile of the five panels in* **A.** **C.** *The brightness profile of the panels, showing the Mach bands. (Modified from TN Cornsweet. Visual Perception. New York: Academic, 1970.)*

panels illustrated in Figure 6.5. Of the many ganglion cells that would actually be stimulated by such an arrangement, the receptive fields of four on-center, off-surround retinal ganglion cells are illustrated. Note that the receptive fields of these cells are shown in the figure, not the neurons themselves. The right side of Figure 6.5 shows that the amount of excitation that occurs in these on-center cells (measured as the number of action potentials produced per second) varies with their position relative to the light-dark boundary.

Receptive field 1 is located in a region in which the center and the entire surround are totally in the region of high luminance. Because this is a region of high luminance, the receptive-field center tends to cause the cell to respond with a high firing rate of action potentials. The antagonistic off-surround is also stimulated by the same high luminance, however. Because of lateral inhibition, it acts to reduce the cell's firing rate to a level that is lower than it would be if the center alone were stimulated by the light. Because the center is somewhat stronger than the surround, the net result is that the cell produces

Receptive field positions relative to
light and dark panels

Neural
responses

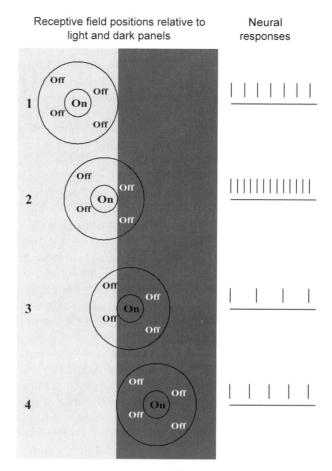

FIGURE 6.5.   *Illustration of how on-center off-surround retinal ganglion cells would respond to a sharp luminance boundary when located at different positions with respect to the boundary. The relative firing rates of the cells are indicated on the right of the figure.*

action potentials at a moderately high rate, as indicated by the neural responses on the right side of the figure.

Receptive field 4, on the other hand, is located entirely within the low-luminance region. Its on-center tends to cause the cell to fire at a moderate firing rate, and the antagonistic surround reduces this slightly, with the net result that the cell has a somewhat lower firing rate than the cell with receptive field 1.

The cell with receptive field 2 has the highest firing rate. This is because the on-center is entirely in the high-luminance region, which tends to produce a high firing rate by the cell, and the off-surround is partly in the low-luminance region. As a result, the off-surround has less of an antagonistic effect than in the case of the cell with receptive field 1, so the cell responds with a high firing rate.

The cell with receptive field 3 has the lowest firing rate. Its on-center is in the low-luminance region, which tends to produce a moderate firing rate, but part of its off-surround is in the high-luminance region, so it has a stronger antagonistic effect than in the case of the cell with receptive field 4. The net result is that this cell has a low firing rate.

The firing rates of the cells whose receptive fields are shown in Figure 6.5 are representative of other on-center cells near a sharp luminance boundary. Cells with their receptive field centers just on the higher-luminance side and part of their surround in the lower-luminance side all tend to respond with higher firing rates than any other on-center cells in the region. The on-center cells whose receptive-field centers are just on the low-luminance side of the boundary have the lowest firing rates. To the extent that the rate of production of action potentials is related to perceptual brightness, the region just to the right of the boundary in Figure 6.5 is seen as darker than the region farther away from the boundary, and the region just to the left of the boundary is seen as brighter than other regions of low luminance that are located farther away from the luminance boundary.

Off-center cells would respond with a symmetrically opposite pattern, such that a row of off-center cells whose receptive-field centers are located just to the right of the luminance boundary in Figure 6.5 would respond with the highest firing rates of any off-center cells in the region. Information from on-center and off-center cells tends to remain separate, at least until it reaches the primary visual cortex (V1) where a high firing rate of off-center cells could produce a perceptual response of darkness. Off-center cells located just to the right of the boundary would have high firing rates, which constitutes a strong darkness signal.

Taken together, the center-surround organization of on-center and off-center retinal ganglion cells generates responses that accentuate a boundary in which luminance changes abruptly in the visual scene. This response by the visual system acts to overemphasize or enhance the brightness difference at the boundary. In contrast, when the intensity changes gradually over a large distance, the responses of the neurons across that region of space are essentially identical. As a result, the visual system de-emphasizes or even ignores gradual changes in retinal illuminance.

The sensitivity of the visual system to spatial luminance changes is measured with sine-wave gratings of varying spatial frequency and contrast

Given that the visual system responds well to spatial changes in luminance across the retina, an obvious way to characterize the ability of the visual system to detect such changes is to measure the threshold contrast needed to see spatially varying stimuli. This is often accomplished with sine-wave gratings because they can be specified very precisely. On the right side of Figure 6.6 are examples of several vertically oriented gratings as they might appear on a computer monitor. At first glance, panels A and B may appear simply to be gratings composed of alternating black and white bars like those in panel D. The profiles on the left of the figure illustrate the luminance levels of the gratings as one might measure them with a tiny light meter moved across the grating. In panels A, B, and C, the luminance changes gradually, rather than suddenly, from low to high and back to low. The luminance changes can be described mathematically by a sine function, which is why these patterns are referred to as *sine-wave gratings*.

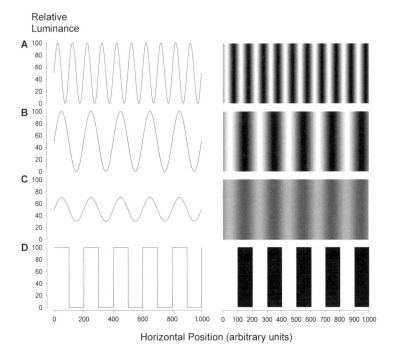

Relative Luminance

Horizontal Position (arbitrary units)

FIGURE 6.6   *Luminance profiles (**left**) and appearance (**right**) of three sine-wave gratings (**A–C**) and a square-wave grating (**D**). (Modified from TC Prager. Essential Factors in Testing for Glare. In MP Nadler, D Miller, DJ Nadler [eds], Glare and Contrast Sensitivity for Clinicians. New York: Springer-Verlag, 1990;33–44.)*

The grating in Figure 6.6D differs from the gratings in panels A, B, and C. Each white bar has a constant, high luminance, and there is a sudden shift to the constant, low luminance of the black bars. The profile of the luminance levels has sharp ("square") transitions, so this is referred to as a *square-wave grating*. Square-wave gratings were described in Chapter 5 as a tool to measure the minimum angle of resolution (MAR).

A sine-wave grating is more useful for studying the thresholds of the visual system than any other waveform because it is composed of a single spatial frequency. As is discussed later in this chapter, the square-wave grating is more complex because it is composed of many different spatial frequencies. Although the retinal images of visual scenes usually vary in spatial frequency in both the horizontal and vertical dimensions, for simplicity, this chapter considers only the responses of the visual system to sine-wave gratings in which the luminance variation occurs in only the horizontal dimension.

The spatial frequency of a sine-wave grating is specified in terms of the number of cycles per degree of visual angle

Figure 6.7 shows the luminance profiles of two sine-wave gratings. A *cycle* is illustrated as a smooth change from the mean luminance to a minimum, back to

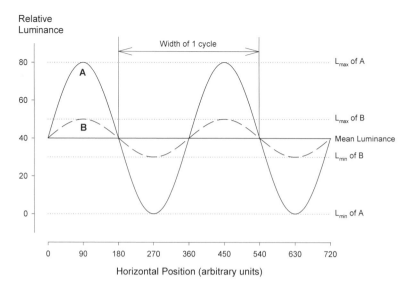

FIGURE 6.7 *Relative luminance profiles for high-contrast **(A)** and low-contrast **(B)** sine-wave gratings. (L$_{max}$ = maximum luminance; L$_{min}$ = minimum luminance.)*

the mean, then to a maximum, and finally back to the mean. This cycle, if it were to be viewed in isolation, would appear as a dark area on the left and a light area on the right. Had the length of the cycle been marked starting at 0 on the x-axis, the light bar would be on the left and the dark bar on the right. The figure shows two complete cycles extending from 0 to 720 units on the x-axis. If these two cycles were to extend across 1° of visual angle on the retina, the spatial frequencies of the sine waves in Figure 6.7 would be 2 cycles per degree.

As a further illustration of the concept of spatial frequency, look back at Figure 6.6A and Figure 6.6B. When viewed from a distance of 28.5 cm (approximately 11 in.), the width of these gratings subtend an angle of roughly 8° on the retina. The grating in A has 10 cycles in that 8°, and thus has a spatial frequency of 1.25 cycles per degree. The grating in B has only 5 cycles in the same 8°, and thus has a spatial frequency of 0.625 cycles per degree. It should be clear from this example that wider bars constitute a lower spatial-frequency grating, and that as the width of the bars is decreased, the gratings become higher in spatial frequency for a constant viewing distance.

Grating contrast is defined differently from the contrast of a target against a background

The sine-wave grating in Figure 6.6C has the same spatial frequency as the grating in Figure 6.6B but has lower contrast. The dark bars are not as low in luminance, and the light bars do not have as high a luminance. Because the luminance of a sine wave stimulus does not consist of a background or a target with constant luminance values, the **contrast** of a grating is defined in terms of two parameters that can be physically measured: the maximum (L$_{max}$) and minimum (L_{min}) luminance illustrated in Figure 6.7. Using these values, grating contrast (known as the *Michelson contrast*) is defined as

$$\text{Contrast} = \frac{(L_{max} - L_{min})}{(L_{max} + L_{min})} \qquad \text{Eq. 6.1}$$

Defined in this manner, contrast can vary between 0, when L_{max} equals L_{min}, and 1, when L_{min} equals 0. Contrast is often expressed as a percentage, that is, a contrast of 0.5 is referred to as 50% contrast. Although L_{max} and L_{min} are measured luminance values and have dimensions, such as candelas per square meter (cd/m^2), contrast is a dimensionless number.

Note that in Figure 6.7, L_{max} and L_{min} are symmetrically arranged around the **mean luminance (L_m)**, which is defined as

$$L_m = \frac{(L_{max} + L_{min})}{2} \qquad \text{Eq. 6.2}$$

L_m is 40 for both sine waves in Figure 6.7. The amplitude of the sine wave is $L_{max} - L_m$. It is important to note that grating contrast does not depend on the value of L_m. It is possible to have the same contrast at many different L_m levels. Also, contrast is unrelated to the spatial frequency. Grating B in Figure 6.7 has a lower contrast than grating A but has the same spatial frequency.

In general, the luminance profile of a sine-wave grating is given by

$$L(x) = L_m[1 + c\sin(2\pi Fx + \phi)] \qquad \text{Eq. 6.3}$$

where *L(x)* is the luminance at position x, L_m is the mean luminance, *c* is the contrast, *F* is the spatial frequency in cycles per unit of x, *x* is the horizontal position in the image, and ϕ is the spatial phase. The *phase* refers to the position of a sine-wave grating with respect to a reference point or another grating. It is sufficient here to mention that the perception of spatial phase information by the visual system is not well understood, although it is important and an active area of research. Spatial phase is not further considered in this chapter.

Spatial contrast sensitivity functions have a band pass shape characterized by a cutoff high frequency at the resolution acuity limit, a peak sensitivity at intermediate frequencies, and a low frequency rolloff

Contrast sensitivity is defined as the inverse of the contrast threshold. Thus, if a subject has a **threshold contrast** of 0.01, this would convert to a contrast sensitivity of 100. Contrast sensitivity, like contrast, is a dimensionless number that varies from 1 to some large value that depends on the stimulus conditions.

When the contrast of a grating is 0, L_{max} equals L_{min}, so no grating can be seen. As the contrast is gradually increased, as it does from the top to the bottom of Figure 6.8, a pattern of light and dark emerges at some threshold contrast. In this figure, the contrast at which the pattern becomes visible varies along its width as the spatial frequency increases from left to right. The highest

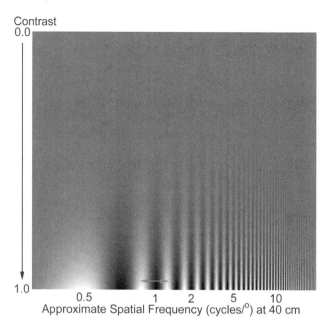

Contrast
0.0

1.0

0.5   1   2   5   10
Approximate Spatial Frequency (cycles/°) at 40 cm

FIGURE 6.8   *Contrast pattern designed to demonstrate the shape of the human spatial contrast sensitivity function. In this illustration, the contrast is 0 at the top of the figure and increases logarithmically to 1 at the bottom of the figure. The spatial frequency increases continuously from left to right. The double arrow at the bottom of the figure subtends 1° at 40 cm, making the horizontal scale approximately correct at that distance.*

points in the figure at which the bars can be detected are the contrast thresholds at each spatial frequency. At a viewing distance of 40 cm (approximately 16 in.), it should be possible to detect the bars nearer to the top of the figure in the region of 3–10 cycles per degree, which indicates that the contrast threshold is lowest in this region. For the lower and higher spatial frequencies, higher contrasts are required to detect the grating, as indicated by the fact that the bars are visible only closer to the bottom of the figure.

In Figure 6.8, one spatial frequency gradually becomes another across the figure and therefore is not a precise measure of contrast sensitivity. It is, nevertheless, possible to see the general inverted U-shape of the **spatial contrast sensitivity function (spatial CSF)**. This can be done by marking the highest points at which the contrast can be detected and connecting the points with straight lines.

To determine the CSF properly, the contrast threshold should be measured using sine-wave gratings at single spatial frequencies and standard psychophysical methods for measuring thresholds. Figure 6.9 shows a typical result from this kind of experiment. The line through the data points represents the boundary between grating contrasts where the bars are visible (below the line) and where they are invisible (above the line).

For humans viewing gratings with a high L_m (approximately 100–1,000 cd/m^2), the spatial CSF shows a characteristic skewed, inverted U shape with the

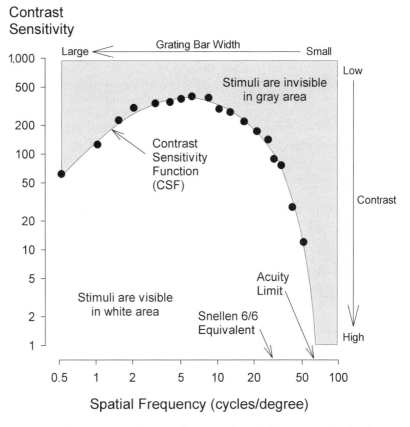

FIGURE 6.9   *Contrast sensitivity as a function of spatial frequency. All the characteristics of a typical spatial contrast sensitivity function are illustrated. See text for details.*

highest contrast sensitivity in the intermediate range from approximately 3 to 10 cycles per degree. The subject whose data are shown in Figure 6.9, had a **peak contrast sensitivity** at approximately six cycles per degree. At this point, the threshold contrast was approximately 0.0025, which corresponds to a sensitivity of 400.

The overall shape of the spatial CSF, with a peak contrast sensitivity in the intermediate spatial frequencies and progressively lower contrast sensitivities at lower and higher spatial frequencies, is characteristic of a **band pass filter**. This means that of all the possible spatial frequencies, only a select range (or band) is detected.

The gradual decrease in sensitivity at low spatial frequencies is called the **low spatial frequency rolloff**. The highest spatial frequency that can be detected at maximum contrast (1) is called the **cutoff high spatial frequency**. The cutoff occurs at approximately 30–60 cycles per degree when, even at the maximum contrast of 1, the bars cannot be detected because the grating widths are too small to be resolved by the visual system. In the example shown in Figure 6.9, the cutoff high spatial frequency was approximately 60 cycles per degree.

The shape of the spatial contrast sensitivity function is the same for many species but the peak contrast sensitivity occurs at different spatial frequencies

The spatial CSF for many species shows band pass filtering similar to that of humans but the peak sensitivity occurs at different spatial frequencies (Figure 6.10). There is a correlation between spatial frequency ranges that can be easily detected by various species and the spatial dimensions of the visual objects that they encounter in their daily life. For instance, falcons detect small animals from high in the sky (high spatial frequencies). It is no surprise that their spatial CSF is shifted toward higher spatial frequencies than the human spatial CSF and that their cutoff high spatial frequency is higher. The spatial CSF for macaque monkeys is nearly identical to that of humans (De Valois et al. 1974).

The cutoff high spatial frequency approximately matches the minimum angle of resolution

As described in Chapter 5, high-contrast square-wave gratings (see Figure 6.6D and Chapter 5, Figure 5.6) can be used to measure the MAR. For a high-contrast square-wave grating in which the black bars and white bars

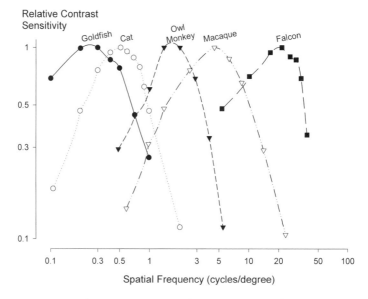

FIGURE 6.10 *Spatial contrast sensitivity functions measured psychophysically of several species of animals. The data for each species have been plotted so that the peak contrast sensitivity is normalized to a value of 1 and other contrast sensitivity values are given the appropriate relative values. (Modified from KK De Valois, RL De Valois. Spatial Vision. New York: Oxford University Press, 1988.)*

each subtend 1', a cycle is one black bar and one white bar, so a cycle would occupy 2'. In a degree (60'), there are 30 cycles of black-white pairs of bars, so a person with 1' resolution acuity should have a cutoff frequency of approximately 30 cycles per degree.

As was shown in Chapter 5, Figure 5.10, people often can resolve smaller strokes than 1'. For a person with a MAR of 0.5' (i.e., a visual acuity of 6/3 or 20/10), the upper limit should be 60 cycles per degree (see the acuity limit in Figure 6.9). For a variety of reasons, there is not an exact correspondence between MAR and the cutoff high spatial frequency. Nonetheless, one should know that the cutoff high spatial frequency for human observers for either square wave or sine-wave gratings is usually between 40 and 60 cycles per degree.

Optical defocus affects mainly the cutoff high frequency of the spatial contrast sensitivity function

As expected from the fact that the cutoff high spatial frequency approximates the MAR, the cutoff high spatial frequency is significantly affected by defocus, although not as severely as is letter acuity (see Chapter 5, Figure 5.7). Defocus produces a redistribution of light in the image on the retina such that it reduces the contrast. For the high spatial frequencies at which the low and high luminance bars are close to each other, this defocus reduces the contrast to below threshold. For low spatial frequencies, however, in which the high and low luminance bars are more widely spaced, defocus does not have a big effect on the contrast (Westheimer 1966). Thus, the contrast sensitivity for low spatial frequencies is relatively unaffected by defocus.

The limit imposed by the optics of the eye on the cutoff high spatial frequency at the fovea approximates the limit imposed by photoreceptor spacing

The ability of an optical system to transmit spatial frequencies is described by its modulation transfer function (MTF). The MTF is simply the ratio of image contrast to object contrast as a function of spatial frequency. If an optical system were to produce a perfect image, the MTF would have a value of 1.0 at all spatial frequencies. A typical optical system generally transmits low spatial frequencies at an MTF of nearly 1.0. At higher spatial frequencies, the MTF decreases gradually up to a cutoff high frequency. The eye's optics follow this pattern and demonstrate two important points. First, the low spatial frequency rolloff in the spatial CSF is not due to the optics of the eye because the MTF of the optics remains high at low spatial frequencies. Second, the MTF of the human eye's optics has a cutoff high spatial frequency of approximately 60 cycles per degree (Woodhouse & Barlow 1982). There is no image information present at spatial frequencies higher than the usual cutoff high spatial frequency seen in the spatial CSF.

Given that there is no image information conveyed to the retina above the optical cutoff high spatial frequency, there is no need to have photoreceptors small enough, or spaced closely enough together, to detect spatial frequencies more than 60 cycles per degree. Two basic concepts predict the photoreceptor spacing needed at the fovea to detect the highest spatial frequencies present in the image. The first concept is that, because photoreceptors have a finite size, they cannot detect the continuous changes in the retinal illuminance in a grating; they can only sample retinal illuminance and average the illuminance changes that occur within the light-capturing area of their outer segments. The second concept is the Whittaker-Shannon sampling theorem. This states that, to reconstruct a continuous function out of uniform samples, the sampling rate must be at least twice the highest frequency present in the original function. In other words, two samples per cycle of the highest spatial frequency present on the retina are necessary to detect that frequency. Thus, to detect a spatial frequency of 60 cycles per degree, there must be 120 photoreceptors per degree of visual angle. Because one degree of visual angle spans approximately 300 µm on the retina, photoreceptors need only to have a center-to-center spacing of 2.5 µm. This agrees quite well with measurements of cone spacing in the human retina as is shown in Chapter 5, Figure 5.5 (Oyster 1999). There is thus a remarkably good match between the upper spatial frequency limit of the eye's optics and the size and spacing of foveal cones.

At low and intermediate spatial frequencies, bypassing the optics of the eye has little effect on the spatial contrast sensitivity function

Using laser interferometry, it is possible to measure the spatial CSF while bypassing the eye's optics (Campbell & Green 1965). Laser interferometry involves imaging two spots of light from a laser on the entrance pupil of the eye. The two spots act as a source of secondary spherical wave fronts that traverse the axial length of the eye and create an interference pattern on the retina. This pattern is a sine-wave grating with a spatial frequency that depends on the separation between the two spots of light. By varying the luminance of the points of light, it is possible to vary the contrast of the interference pattern on the retina. Using this technique, Campbell and Green (1965) confirmed that the optics of the eye do not normally limit the human spatial CSF. However, cataract and other conditions affecting the optics of the eye can seriously reduce the contrast sensitivity for middle and low spatial frequencies under ordinary imaging conditions, as discussed later in this chapter.

Underlying the spatial contrast sensitivity function are individual neurons, each with a spatial contrast sensitivity function

A spatial CSF determined psychophysically measures the contrast sensitivity of the visual system as a whole. The performance of the whole visual system depends on the responses of individual neurons in the retina and the rest of the visual pathway. The spatial CSFs of individual neurons have been measured in the retina, the lateral geniculate nucleus (LGN), and the primary visual cortex (V1) in a variety of species by recording the activity of the neurons through a microelectrode and then measuring the contrast threshold (or the responses) of the neurons for a cat to sine-wave gratings of various spatial frequencies.

As shown for a cat in Figure 6.11, individual retinal and LGN cells have spatial CSFs that superficially resemble the spatial CSF of the whole visual sys-

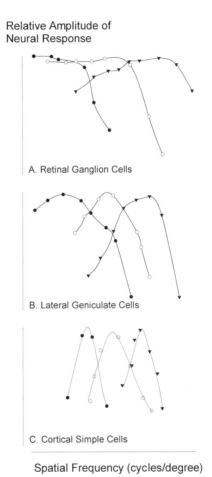

Relative Amplitude of Neural Response

A. Retinal Ganglion Cells

B. Lateral Geniculate Cells

C. Cortical Simple Cells

Spatial Frequency (cycles/degree)

FIGURE 6.11   *Responses of cat* **(A)** *retinal ganglion cells,* **(B)** *lateral geniculate nucleus neurons, and* **(C)** *simple cells in the primary visual cortex to sine-wave gratings of different spatial frequencies and contrast. The relative amplitude of neural response is a neurophysiological analog of sensitivity. Thus, a high amplitude of response (upward on the y-axis) would indicate a high contrast sensitivity for the cell. All nine cells had receptive fields located in the same general part of the retina, close to the center of gaze. Cells with smaller receptive fields have a peak contrast sensitivity and high frequency cutoff at higher spatial frequencies than cells with larger receptive fields. (Modified from L Maffei. Spatial Frequency Channels: Neural Mechanisms. In R Held, H Leibowitz, M Teuber [eds], Handbook of Sensory Physiology: Perception [vol. 8]. Berlin: Springer-Verlag, 1978;39–66.)*

tem measured psychophysically (see Figure 6.10). Each cell's spatial CSF has a peak contrast sensitivity, a cutoff high spatial frequency, and, in most cases, a low spatial frequency rolloff so that each cell operates as a band pass filter. The neurons in V1, through which information on conscious vision must pass, (see Figure 6.11C) are narrowly more band pass than LGN cells. That is, they respond to a much narrower range of spatial frequencies than does the entire visual system (compare Figure 6.11C with the spatial CSFs shown in Figure 6.10). Similar results also have been found for other species.

Thus, it appears that the psychophysically measured spatial CSF is composed of the spatial CSFs of a variety of neurons, each providing contrast sensitivity to a different narrow band of spatial frequencies. This point is considered again after a section that describes how the spatial CSF of individual neurons in the retina can be produced by their center-surround receptive-field organization.

A retinal cell's center-surround receptive-field organization produces a spatial contrast sensitivity function for that cell

To understand how an individual retinal ganglion cell can have a band pass spatial CSF, consider the response of a ganglion cell with an on-center, off-surround receptive field to sine-wave gratings of different spatial frequencies (Figure 6.12A). The left side of Figure 6.12A shows the map of just such a circular on-center receptive field. The right side shows the profile representing the relative number of action potentials that would be produced in response to a small spot of light flashed at a variety of positions across the receptive field. The horizontal line represents its spontaneous firing rate. An on-center receptive field responds most vigorously to a light turned on precisely in the center of the receptive-field center. In the off-surround region, the cell responds most vigorously when a light is turned off (or to the onset of darkness). The left sides of Figures 6.12B–D show sine-wave gratings of three different spatial frequencies superimposed on the receptive field. The right sides show the luminance profiles of the gratings with different spatial frequencies superimposed on the response profile of the receptive field.

As was demonstrated in Figure 6.5, the cell responds maximally when its center is exposed to high luminance and the surround is exposed to low luminance or no light at all. Thus, the receptive field in Figure 6.12A responds maximally to the spatial frequency shown in Figure 6.12C because the spatial frequency of the sine wave matches the receptive-field size exactly. It is positioned such that the highest luminance falls on the center of the receptive field on-center producing an on response, and the lowest luminance falls on the surround producing an off response. These summate to produce a very strong response.

In general, it has been found that the spatial frequency that produces the strongest response from a cell is also the stimulus that has the lowest threshold contrast. Thus, if one reduced the contrast of the gratings in Figures 6.12B–D, the cell would have the lowest contrast threshold (highest sensitivity) to the grating in Figure 6.12C. The fact that the high-luminance bar that activates the center would also extend into the antagonistic surround (i.e., the grating has

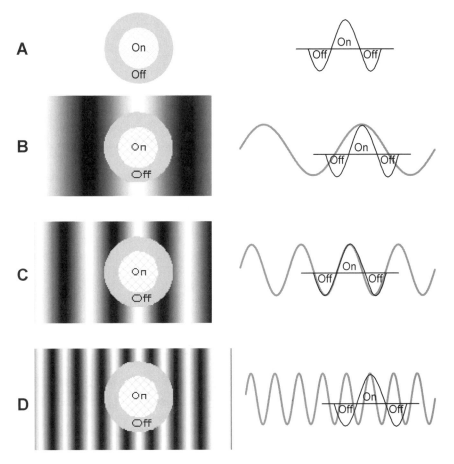

FIGURE 6.12   *Illustration of how sine-wave gratings of different frequencies can produce strong and weak responses in an on-center retinal ganglion cell. See text for details. (Modified from JM Wolfe. An Introduction to Contrast Sensitivity Testing. In MP Nadler, D Miller, DJ Nadler [eds], Glare and Contrast Sensitivity for Clinicians. New York: Springer-Verlag, 1990;5–23.)*

long bars of high and low luminance, and the receptive field is round) would not alter the fact that this spatial frequency would provide a higher contrast sensitivity than any other spatial frequency.

Now consider a grating with a high spatial frequency relative to the receptive field's size (see Figure 6.12D). Here the central high-luminance bar only covers a portion of the receptive-field center, with the low-luminance bars producing an averaging effect within the center. Similarly, high- and low-luminance bars would fall in the surround, also producing averaging effects there. The result would be a weak response to a high contrast grating. If the contrast threshold were measured, it would require a high contrast to reach threshold, which means that the contrast sensitivity would be low. It has been found that the cutoff high spatial frequency for individual retinal neurons is inversely related to the size of the cell's receptive-field center. When the spatial frequency is twice the optimum frequency, the receptive-field center and surround are equally stimulated by high- and low-luminance bars, so that the signals from the receptive-field center and surround are nearly equal and opposite, effectively canceling the receptive field's response and producing the cutoff high spatial frequency.

Finally, when the spatial frequency is low (see Figure 6.12B), the light bar is so wide that it stimulates both the center and the surround. This produces a small response, because the surround response to light subtracts from the center response. The net result is a weak response (because the center is stronger than the surround) even though the contrast of the grating is high. As a result, the contrast sensitivity is low.

From this analysis, which also applies to thresholds for off-center cells when a low-luminance bar is centered on its receptive field (Maffei 1978), it is evident that center-surround cells would be generally band pass. The degree to which a retinal ganglion cell has a low spatial frequency rolloff is related to the strength of the surround relative to the strength of the center. When the surround is weak, in comparison to the center, a cell has little or no low spatial frequency rolloff (see examples in Figure 6.11A). For reasons that are not considered here, cells in the LGN tend to be more strongly band pass (Norton & Godwin 1992) than retinal ganglion cells (compare Figure 6.11A with Figure 6.11B). Cells in the visual cortex are still more narrowly band pass (see Figure 6.11C).

Cells with a variety of receptive-field sizes provide the basis for the behaviorally measured spatial contrast sensitivity function

The preceding section showed that for a particular receptive-field–center size, there is a corresponding peak spatial frequency that requires the least contrast to evoke a threshold response, and the cells have a higher threshold (lower contrast sensitivity) to higher and lower spatial frequencies. What has not been discussed is that, at every retinal location, there are some ganglion cells with smaller, and some with larger, receptive-field centers. This variability in the size of the receptive field results primarily from variations in the amount of convergence from photoreceptors onto bipolar cells and from bipolar cells onto ganglion cells (Rodieck 1998). As shown in Figure 6.11, the peak contrast sensitivity and cutoff high spatial frequency for different cells occur at different spatial frequencies. Cells with smaller centers have a peak contrast sensitivity at a higher spatial frequency. Cells with larger centers have a peak contrast sensitivity at a lower spatial frequency.

In primates, ganglion cells with smaller receptive fields at any given retinal location tend to be a part of a parallel afferent pathway from the retina to the cortex (the **parvocellular [P] pathway**). These cells appear to be responsible for the ability to detect high spatial frequencies and discern color. Cells at the same retinal eccentricity with large receptive fields tend to be part of another parallel pathway (the **magnocellular [M] pathway**) (Casagrande 1994). These cells seem to be responsible for detecting low spatial frequency stimuli, particularly when the stimuli are moving or flickering (Merigan & Maunsell 1993).

In V1, where the cells usually are orientation selective, cells only respond when a grating of the appropriate spatial frequency is also aligned properly

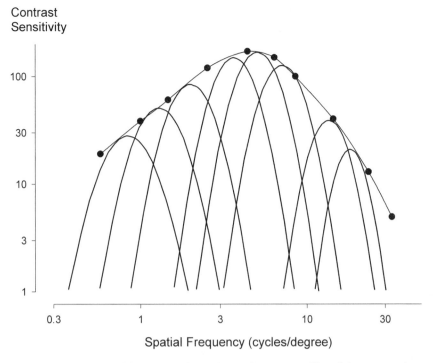

Contrast
Sensitivity

Spatial Frequency (cycles/degree)

FIGURE 6.13   *Spatial frequency channels, as characterized by Blakemore and Campbell. The upper solid line is a human spatial contrast sensitivity function (CSF), as shown in Figure 6.9. The narrow bands under the spatial CSF are idealized spatial frequency channels, each sensitive to a narrow range of spatial frequencies. The spatial CSF connects the most sensitive regions of the channels, forming the envelope (upper limit) of the individual channel sensitivities. (Modified from KK De Valois, RL De Valois. Spatial Vision. New York: Oxford University Press, 1988.)*

with their optimal stimulus orientation. Presented with such an oriented grating, the cells have a peak contrast sensitivity at some spatial frequency and a rather sharp decline in sensitivity at higher and lower spatial frequencies. This makes the cells narrowly band pass, such that each cell resembles one of the **channels** shown in Figure 6.13.

Contrast adaptation demonstrates that there are multiple spatial frequency channels in the visual system

Even before single cell data were available, Campbell and Robson (1968), as well as others, hypothesized that the visual system might contain a number of groups of independent, band-pass filters based on groups of cortical cells (see Figure 6.11C) that are more narrowly band pass than the overall spatial CSF. As suggested in a previous section, the spatial CSF would be the upper envelope of sensitivities of all of these channels, as illustrated in Figure 6.13. The concept of a channel implies a filtering mechanism that selectively responds to (passes) a narrow band of spatial frequencies and does not respond to (filters out) all other spatial frequencies present in a visual stimulus. The width of each channel gives an estimate of the range of spatial frequencies to which the channel responds.

Blakemore and Campbell (1969) provided the first demonstration that spatial frequency channels exist in the human visual system. First, they measured the spatial CSF using standard psychophysical methods. The result is shown as the solid line in Figure 6.14A. Then they took advantage of a phenomenon known as **contrast adaptation**. Exposure to a high-contrast grating of a particular spatial frequency temporarily raises (adapts) the threshold for detecting that grating—that is, contrast sensitivity is depressed. Thus, they exposed the observer to a high-contrast grating with a spatial frequency of 7.1 cycles per degree to produce contrast adaptation. They reasoned that if the human spatial CSF were mediated by neurons that were broadly responsive to the entire range of spatial frequencies seen by the person, then the adaptation to the 7.1 cycles per degree would affect all the neurons and reduce the contrast sensitivity to all spatial frequencies. If, on the other hand, the multiple-channel model were correct, then adaptation to the 7.1–cycle-per-degree grating would reduce the observer's sensitivity to only this spatial

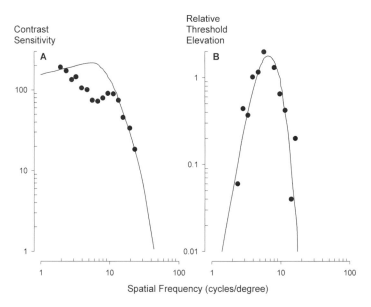

FIGURE 6.14   *Contrast adaptation of the human visual system to a single spatial frequency affects the contrast sensitivity to a narrow range of spatial frequencies.* **A.** *The solid line is the subject's normal contrast sensitivity function. The circles show the contrast sensitivity after adapting with a high-contrast grating with a spatial frequency of 7.1 cycles per degree.* **B.** *The reduction in contrast sensitivity calculated as the difference between the line and the circles in* **A.** *The peak reduction was at 7.1 cycles per degree. As the tested spatial frequency differed increasingly from 7.1 cycles per degree, the amount of reduction in contrast sensitivity decreased. The solid line in* **B** *represents the shape of the channel that was affected by adaptation at 7.1 cycles per degree. When the eye was adapted to other spatial frequencies, other similarly shaped channels were found. (Modified from C Blakemore, FW Campbell. On the existence of neurons in the human visual system selectively sensitive to the orientation and size of retinal images. J Physiol [Lond] 1969;203:237–260.)*

frequency and a small range around this frequency. Neurons that did not respond to the adapting stimulus would show no change in their contrast sensitivity. The result would be a dip in the spatial CSF centered on 7.1 cycles per degree. This is precisely what they found, as shown by the data points in Figure 6.14A.

Figure 6.14B shows the relative threshold elevation derived from the differences between the solid line and the data points in Figure 6.14A. Note that the peak is at the adapting frequency and falls off rapidly. The overall envelope of Figure 6.14B is narrower than the CSF shown in Figure 6.14A. These results are consistent with the characteristics of the animal cortical cells that were shown in Figure 6.11 and support the hypothesis that the overall spatial CSF is the envelope of the contrast sensitivity profiles of relatively independent groups of neurons that form the channels.

The spatial contrast sensitivity function varies with illuminance

Measuring a contrast threshold using a grating is similar to measuring an increment threshold, as described in Chapter 3. Recall that the increment threshold for spots of light on a large background changes with the background luminance such that the threshold $\Delta L/L$ becomes larger as the background luminance decreases (see Chapter 3, Figure 3.2). An increase in the Weber fraction is the same as an increase in the contrast needed to detect the spot. Thus, it should not be surprising that the threshold contrast rises in the human spatial CSF as mean retinal illuminance decreases, though not uniformly at all spatial frequencies, as is explained in the following discussion.

Figure 6.15 shows that, at high photopic retinal illuminance levels, the spatial CSF in a human observer peaks at approximately eight cycles per degree and the cutoff high frequency is approximately 50 cycles per degree. The spatial CSF changes in three ways as the mean retinal illuminance of the grating is reduced. First, the spatial frequency at which the peak contrast sensitivity occurs shifts toward lower spatial frequencies. Second, regardless of illuminance, a sharp high-frequency cutoff is always present, but the cutoff occurs at a lower spatial frequency with lower mean retinal illuminance. A shift in peak spatial frequency from eight to two cycles per degree and a drop in the cutoff can easily be explained by the transition from photopic, cone-driven (small) receptive fields to scotopic, rod-driven (large) receptive fields (De Valois et al. 1974). Third, as the retinal illuminance decreases, the low spatial frequency rolloff becomes less prominent, until it completely disappears. This is related to the inactivation of the receptive-field surround under conditions of very low luminance (Barlow et al. 1957).

The spatial contrast sensitivity function shifts toward lower spatial frequencies with retinal eccentricity

Because receptive fields become larger with distance from the fovea, and because the size of receptive fields dictates the peak spatial frequency and

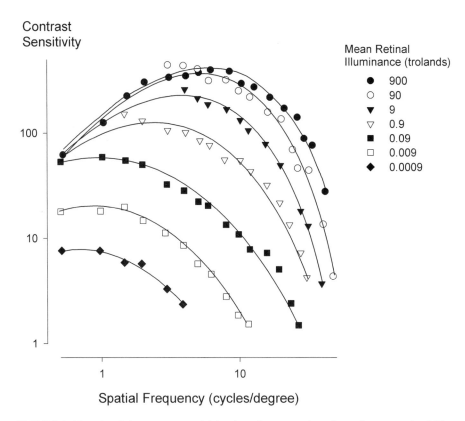

Contrast Sensitivity

Mean Retinal Illuminance (trolands)

● 900
○ 90
▼ 9
▽ 0.9
■ 0.09
□ 0.009
◆ 0.0009

100

10

1

1   10

Spatial Frequency (cycles/degree)

FIGURE 6.15   *Spatial contrast sensitivity functions as a function of mean retinal illuminance. (Modified from RL De Valois, H Morgan, DM Snodderly. Psychophysical studies of monkey vision. 3. Spatial luminance contrast sensitivity tests of macaque and human observers. Vision Res 1974;14:75–81.)*

the cutoff high spatial frequency (see Figure 6.12), it follows that the spatial CSFs generally are shifted toward lower spatial frequencies as a function of increased retinal eccentricity. As described in previous chapters, the size of the receptive field depends on the number of photoreceptors that converge on a bipolar cell and the number of bipolar cells that converge on a ganglion cell. Both types of convergence increase with eccentricity. In addition, the amount of cortical area devoted to representing the periphery (i.e., the cortical magnification factor) decreases with eccentricity. It has been hypothesized that the decrease in spatial CSF with eccentricity can be quantitatively explained by the reduced cortical representation. If one scales the size and spatial frequency of the grating patch used to measure spatial CSF such that it compensates for the reduced representation of the visual field in the cortex, then the spatial CSF functions become fairly similar (Rovamo et al. 1978). Nonetheless, it is evident from Figures 6.15 and 6.16 that the amount of spatial information that can be processed by the visual system decreases with decreasing retinal illuminance and increasing retinal eccentricity. Another way of looking at these stimulus-induced changes in the CSF is in terms of the change in area under the CSF function. Such an index or

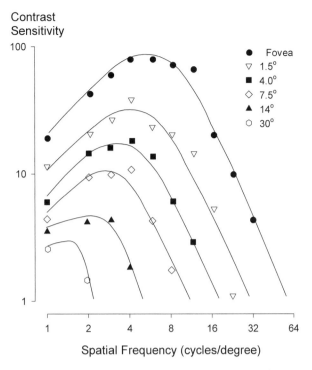

Contrast
Sensitivity

- ● Fovea
- ▽ 1.5°
- ■ 4.0°
- ◇ 7.5°
- ▲ 14°
- ○ 30°

Spatial Frequency (cycles/degree)

FIGURE 6.16   *Spatial contrast sensitivity functions measured at different eccentricities from the fovea. (Modified from J Rovamo, V Virsu, R Nasanen. Cortical magnification factor predicts the photopic contrast sensitivity of peripheral vision. Nature 1978;271:54–56.)*

metric is the subject of current research interest and may prove to be a sensitive measure of change in contrast sensitivity in disorders of vision.

All spatial luminance patterns can be decomposed into the sum of sine-wave gratings of particular spatial frequencies and contrasts

The images produced on the retina by objects in the real world normally contain many spatial frequencies and contrasts. Consider a cityscape such as is shown in Figure 6.17. If a light meter were moved horizontally from left to right across the middle of the scene, its output would vary as it encountered areas of higher and lower luminance, and the resultant luminance distribution would be a complex waveform, as shown at the bottom of the figure.* Approximately two centuries ago, a French mathematician,

*A complex waveform also would occur if the image were scanned in any other direction, but, for simplicity, this chapter considers spatial frequencies in only one dimension.

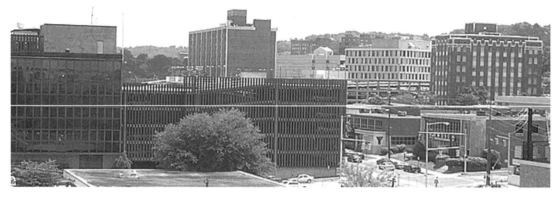

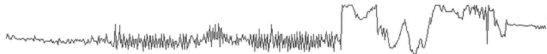

FIGURE 6.17   *Photograph illustrating the presence of a variety of vertically oriented contrast variations in a city scene. The trace at the bottom of the figure represents the relative intensities that were measured at the level of the white line in the scene. The contrast changes at the boundaries of the buildings introduce low spatial frequencies to the scene, whereas the building details, especially the parking deck in the center, introduce much higher spatial frequencies.*

Jean Baptiste Joseph Fourier, discovered that any such complex waveform can be decomposed into the sum of multiple spatial frequencies of different contrasts.*

As an example, Figure 6.18 shows how a square-wave grating (see Figure 6.6D), with its abrupt changes in luminance, can be synthesized by adding up a series of smoothly varying sine waves. A high-contrast sine wave, at what is called the *fundamental frequency* (F), establishes the spatial frequency of the square wave. This sine wave has the same mean luminance (L_m) as the final square wave, and an amplitude that is 1.27 ($4/\pi$) times the amplitude of the square wave. Each subsequent sine wave that is added to the fundamental has a frequency that is an odd-integer multiple of the fundamental frequency, for example, 3F, 5F, 7F, and so on. Their mean luminances are the same as that of the fundamental, but their amplitudes are equal to the amplitude of the fundamental divided by the integer, for example, 1/3, 1/5, 1/7, and so on. Each of these smaller sine waves is called a *harmonic*. As more harmonics are added, the sum more closely approximates a square wave. The synthesis of a square wave with an ampli-

---

*Applied to sound waves (which follow the same rules as sine-wave gratings), **Fourier analysis** has been used to learn the particular sound frequencies (harmonics) present in musical instruments and the amplitudes of these frequencies (the auditory equivalent to contrast). Once the component frequencies and amplitudes are known, **Fourier synthesis** can be used to combine pure sine waves to create the same complex pattern, as in electronic keyboards.

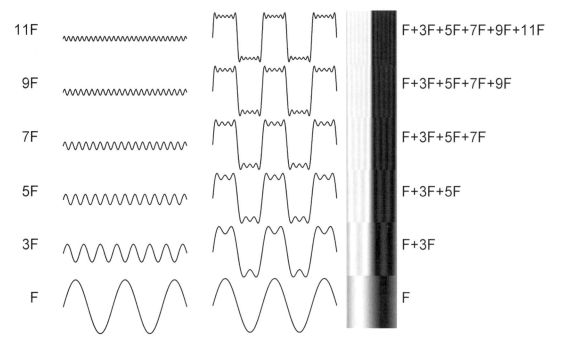

FIGURE 6.18   *An example of Fourier synthesis. Starting at the bottom and moving to the top, the left side of the figure shows a sine wave of a fundamental frequency (F) and harmonic sine waves that are 3, 5, 7, 9, and 11 times F. The contrast of the harmonics is less than the contrast of F, such that the third harmonic has one-third of the contrast, the fifth harmonic has one-fifth of the contrast, and so on. The middle set of waveforms shows that summing the harmonics with the F produces a pattern that increasingly resembles a square-wave luminance profile. The right side of the figure shows the appearance of the grating.*

tude of 1 and a fundamental frequency of F can be expressed mathematically as

$$\frac{4}{\pi}\left[\sin(F) + \frac{1}{3}\sin(3F) + \frac{1}{5}\sin(5F) + \frac{1}{7}\sin(7F) + ... + \frac{1}{n}\sin(nF)\right] \qquad \text{Eq. 6.4}$$

where *n* is a very large odd integer. It is the nature of a square wave that only the odd harmonics and sine components are required for its synthesis; more complex waveforms require the even frequencies and cosine components as well.

Notice in Figure 6.18 that the first trough of the lowest harmonic (3F) coincides with the peak of the fundamental (F). The effect of adding these two waveforms is to reduce the peak luminance of F. Notice also that when the two peaks of the lowest harmonic are added to F, the summed profile begins to look like the profile of the square wave with more rapid transitions from light to dark and the appearance of corners. The addition of sine waves at the higher harmonics gradually produces a summed luminance profile that has a perfectly square corner. The top line in Figure 6.18 approximates the square wave and is the result of adding Fourier components up through the eleventh harmonic. To smooth the waveform to a perfect square wave, an infinite number of sine waves would have to be added together, but the figure shows that a good approximation of a square-wave grating can be synthesized using the

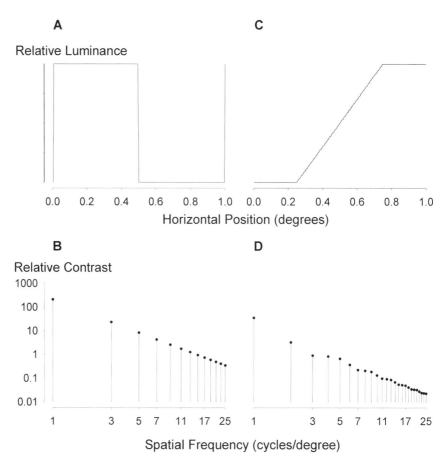

A

Relative Luminance

C

Horizontal Position (degrees)

B

Relative Contrast

D

Spatial Frequency (cycles/degree)

FIGURE 6.19   *Fourier analysis of two simple waveforms.* **A.** *Luminance profile of a square-wave grating.* **B.** *Fourier components of the grating showing the relative amount of contrast at each of the spatial frequencies present in the grating from the fundamental through the twenty-fifth harmonic.* **C.** *A ramp luminance profile with low luminance on the left, rising luminance in the middle, and high luminance on the right.* **D.** *Fourier components of the ramp luminance profile.*

fundamental and only five harmonics. The small, high-frequency contrast changes in the peaks and troughs are barely visible.

The example of constructing a square wave from a series of sines waves with certain frequencies and amplitudes shows that the sharp luminance boundaries produced by objects in the world can be constructed from the addition of a series of spatial frequencies of defined contrasts. Conversely, one may apply Fourier analysis to determine the component spatial frequencies and contrasts of any luminance profile. Figure 6.19B shows the Fourier analysis of the square-wave grating shown in Figure 6.19A. Again, only the odd frequencies are present as harmonics. The Fourier components (see Figure 6.19D) of the ramp function (see Figure 6.19C) are different in that they include the even as well as the odd harmonics. Not shown is that both sine and cosine components are present. It is important to realize here that, even though the perception of a square-wave or ramp change in luminance appears smooth, the perception is actually the result of the combined output of all the tuned spatial frequency channels transmitting a signal that is proportional to the frequency content of the image. The visual system acts, in many ways, like a Fourier analyzer. This is demonstrated in the next section.

The human spatial contrast sensitivity function, with its peak sensitivity in intermediate spatial frequencies, predicts Mach bands

The appearance of Mach bands at contrast boundaries was explained in an earlier section in terms of the relative firing rates of cells that were dependent on where their receptive-field centers and surrounds were located with respect to the boundary. Mach bands can also be explained in terms of the band pass nature of the spatial CSF. Figure 6.20 shows a series of steps leading to the conclusion that Mach Bands should occur if the visual system performs a spatial frequency analysis of the visual scene.

Figure 6.20A shows a step change in luminance that is the same as that in Figure 6.19A. Figure 6.20B shows the Fourier components of this stimulus that are the same as those shown in Figure 6.19B. Note that the spatial frequencies present in the stimulus with the highest contrast are in the range of 1–15 cycles per degree. The spatial CSF (see Figure 6.20) shows that the visual system is most sensitive to spatial frequencies at 6–11 cycles per degree. When the spatial frequency components of the stimulus are filtered by the human spatial CSF, their relative contrasts (amplitudes) are changed, as shown in Figure 6.20D. Because humans do not see low spatial frequencies as well as intermediate spatial frequencies, there would be an attenuation of the contrast of low spatial frequencies relative to the intermediate spatial frequencies. The high spatial frequencies above the spatial CSF cutoff frequency are completely filtered out. These effects can be seen by comparing the relative contrasts in 6.20B and 6.20D. The attenuation of the low spatial frequencies is, in effect, an accentuation of the intermediate spatial frequencies that are present in the stimulus. Finally, panel E shows the result of performing a Fourier synthesis of the spatial frequency components that are passed by the visual system. The resulting brightness profile is a classic Mach band with a bright band on the left and a dark band on the right. Thus, both spatial frequency analysis and receptive-field analysis (see Figure 6.5) can account for the brightness enhancement of Mach bands.

Low and middle spatial frequencies are critically important for detecting and recognizing objects

As described in previous sections, a visual scene contains many spatial frequencies, and the visual system contains neurons (channels) that respond to relatively narrow ranges of spatial frequencies. The natural visual environment is abundantly rich in midrange spatial frequencies that are well matched to the peak contrast sensitivity of the human spatial CSF and cortical neurons (Field

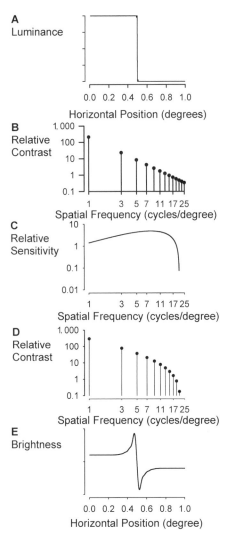

FIGURE 6.20   *Spatial frequency filtering by the visual system can produce Mach bands.* **A.** *Luminance profile of a stimulus that has high luminance on the left and low luminance on the right.* **B.** *Fourier components of the stimulus.* **C.** *The human spatial contrast sensitivity function.* **D.** *Fourier components after filtering by the human spatial contrast sensitivity function.* **E.** *The brightness profile that is produced by adding all the Fourier components in a manner similar to that shown in Figure 6.18. (Modified from TN Cornsweet. Visual Perception. New York: Academic, 1970.)*

1987). One might wonder, then, whether the spatial frequencies to which the visual system is most sensitive are the most important ones for spatial vision.

To answer this question, observers are asked to identify objects in images that have been optically or digitally filtered so that they contain only a selected range of spatial frequencies. It has been found that spatial frequencies in the intermediate range of 1–15 cycles per degree are critically important for much of what is called "seeing objects" in everyday vision. These spatial frequencies are much lower than the cutoff high spatial frequency.

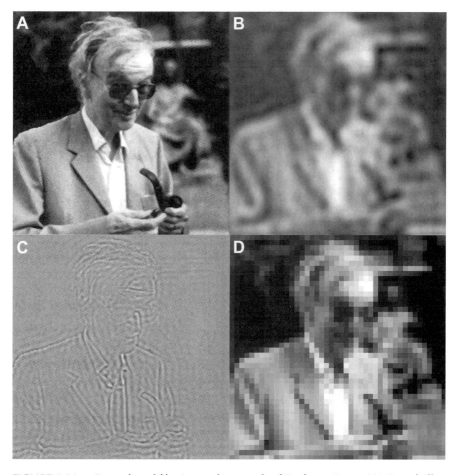

FIGURE 6.21   *Examples of filtering a photograph of Professor Fergus W. Campbell to limit the spatial frequency content of the image. **A.** The original image. **B.** The original image filtered to pass only the medium and low spatial frequencies. **C.** The original image filtered to pass only high spatial frequency information. **D.** The original image that was spatially quantized, so that intermediate and low spatial frequency information is present, but masked by the spurious high spatial frequencies present at the sharp boundaries between the large squares. If the image in **D** is blurred, the sharp boundaries are removed, allowing the face to become more visible because of the predominance of the intermediate and low spatial frequency information. (Modified from A Bradley, L Thibos, Y Wang, et al. Imaging FWC. Ophthalmic Physiol Opt 1992;12:128.)*

Consider, for example, Figure 6.21A, which is a photograph of Professor Fergus W. Campbell, a pioneer in the application of spatial frequency analysis to human vision and whose spatial CSF is shown in Figure 6.14A. Figure 6.21B was produced by filtering out all high spatial frequencies, leaving only the middle and low spatial frequencies that are in the range of the human peak contrast sensitivity. This panel appears as a rather blurry image of a person that might be recognizable as F. W. Campbell by someone who knew him or was familiar with the photograph. The more important point, however, is that the image is clearly recognizable as a human face. On the other hand, if one filters out all low and medium spatial frequencies, leaving only high spatial frequencies, it is difficult to see what the figure contains (Figure 6.21C). If this image were to be optically defocused, thereby removing the high frequencies, all information would vanish.

Figure 6.21D shows an image that has been spatially quantized. This is a form of low pass filtering that replaces all luminances over some spatial distance with the average of all the luminances. This process actually creates spurious high-frequency information at the sharp boundaries between the squares. If this image is defocused to remove the high spatial frequencies, it actually resembles the image in panel B. Also, it is easier to identify the object in an image with this kind of filtering at a distance, rather than close up, because viewing at a distance diminishes the effect of the high spatial frequencies.

From results like these, it is clear that spatial vision is possible with medium and low spatial frequencies. In some instances, high spatial frequencies can even mask low spatial frequency images (see Figure 6.21D). Early studies that asked subjects to identify faces that had been filtered to limit the spatial frequencies present reported that low spatial frequencies are sufficient for face recognition (Harmon 1973). Other studies, however, have found that midrange spatial frequencies also are important for recognition of faces, with neither range being absolutely essential for face recognition (Sergent 1986). As might be expected, high spatial frequencies are necessary for recognizing details.

The ability of subjects to recognize objects with low and intermediate spatial frequencies is useful, because these spatial frequencies are less affected by degradation of image quality due to defocus. However, people who experience a loss of contrast sensitivity at middle and low spatial frequencies can have a great deal of difficulty seeing, especially in low contrast situations, even if their MAR, as measured under high-contrast conditions, is relatively unaffected.

Charts designed to measure spatial contrast sensitivity functions clinically are based on what is important for recognizing objects

As clinicians have become increasingly interested in learning whether patients have a loss of contrast sensitivity at particular spatial frequencies, it has become necessary to devise ways to measure contrast sensitivity quickly in a clinical setting. The first measurements of the human CSF (Bodis-Wollner 1972; Campbell & Green 1965; DeLange 1958) used sine-wave gratings that were produced on an oscilloscope screen. More recently, gratings on computer monitors have been used to examine the spatial CSF of humans and other species in laboratory settings. Neither of these tools is readily adapted to clinical measurements in which speed of measurement is important, and specialized equipment can be intimidating to patients. Arden and Jacobson (1978) published photographic plates that contain specific spatial frequencies on which the contrast decreases across the card (see Figure 6.8). A way was provided for patients to indicate the lowest contrast that they could detect. There are now a wide variety of clinical spatial CSF cards that use sine-wave gratings available (see Patorgis 1991 for a review and description of various charts).

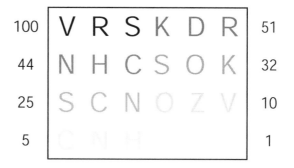

	V	R	S	K	D	R	
100							51
44	N	H	C	S	O	K	32
25	S	C	N	O	Z	V	10
5							1

FIGURE 6.22   *Representation of the contrast-reduction strategy used in the Pelli-Robson chart. The numbers outside the box indicate the contrast of the letters. If viewed at a distance of 57 cm (approximately 22.5 inches), the letters are 0.5° high. (Modified from DG Pelli, JG Robson, AJ Wilkins. The design of a new letter chart for measuring contrast sensitivity. Clin Vision Sci 1988;2:187–199.)*

In addition to charts that use sine-wave gratings, low-contrast letter wall charts have been developed for clinical testing. As described in Chapter 5, Roman letters are a familiar measure of recognition threshold for many patients. The **Pelli-Robson chart** (Figure 6.22) is based on research on reading (Pelli et al. 1988) and assumes that detection of letters at contrast threshold is determined by the contrast sensitivity at two cycles per letter. A second assumption is that the most useful part of the spatial CSF to measure is the spatial frequencies near the normal peak contrast sensitivity (3–10 cycles per degree). The chart consists of three-letter sets, or triplets, drawn from 10 equally visible letters. All of the letters in the chart are the same size, subtending 0.5° in height at 3 m. Each triplet has the same contrast. As one moves to the right and down the chart, the contrast, but not the size of the letters, decreases, such that each set of three letters on the right half of the chart has a slightly lower contrast on a logarithmic scale than the triplet on the left.

Patients read the letters as they do an acuity chart. A scoring system, based on the number of misses, is used. This is similar to the scoring system used with logMAR acuity charts. The Pelli-Robson chart is currently the only wall chart that has individual calibrations of contrast. For low-vision patients, the chart can be used at 1 m, where the spatial frequencies are one-third of that when the chart is used at 3 m, to assess contrast sensitivity at low spatial frequencies.

Clinical measurements of the minimum angle of resolution and the spatial contrast sensitivity function complement each other

From the preceding sections, it should not be surprising that a patient can have a best-corrected MAR of 1' but still complain that he or she does not see well. This is because the MAR measures the cutoff high spatial frequency, which depends only on the neurons with the smallest receptive fields in the fovea; it does not assess the functioning of most of the neurons in the retina or the rest of the visual system. Conversely, a patient may have poor best-corrected acuity but be relatively unimpaired on visual tasks that do not involve reading or detecting other fine details in the visual environment. Such a discrepancy between visual acuity and the ability to function in the visual environment is relatively rare because the most prevalent ocular pathologies affect the spatial CSF in the range from intermediate to high spatial frequencies. When a discrepancy does occur, it is a reminder that the spatial CSF and measures of the MAR assess different aspects of vision. It is conceivable that a patient could read the letters on a Snellen chart but could have difficulty seeing a truck looming out of a fog.

It has been suggested (Patorgis 1991) that visual acuity provides a measure of visual "quantity," whereas the spatial CSF provides a measure of visual "quality." This is not strictly true, because contrast sensitivity is assessed quantitatively, but it does make the point that in patients with visual impairments, such as cataract, age-related macular degeneration (ARMD), and glaucoma, the spatial CSF can be a useful predictor of daily visual functioning over and above measures of resolution acuity.

The spatial contrast sensitivity function is sensitive to many ocular disorders but does not have high specificity for any particular disorder

Although many forms of ocular pathology, including glaucoma, ARMD, diabetic retinopathy, cataract, and keratoconus, affect the spatial CSF of patients, no unique patterns of spatial CSF loss have emerged that are of use in differential diagnosis of a particular condition. In addition, contrast sensitivity has been no more useful than MAR in detecting ocular disease in screenings of clinic-based populations (Ariyasu et al. 1996). Most of these conditions depress the contrast sensitivity at high spatial frequencies, so that these conditions are also detected by simple measures of the MAR.

In conditions that affect the central visual pathway, a dissociation can occur between the MAR and the spatial CSF. Patients with multiple sclerosis, for example, often have a loss of contrast sensitivity at low spatial frequencies but retain contrast sensitivity at high spatial frequencies, so that the MAR is unaffected (Regan 1991). On the other hand, patients with strabismic amblyopia typically have a reduction in the spatial CSF at middle to high spatial frequencies, resulting in a reduction in the cutoff high spatial frequency that is routinely detected with an acuity measure. Because losses in contrast sensitivity have not proven to be generally useful for diagnosing pathology, measures of spatial CSF are generally used to explain vision losses experienced by patients and not as a first-line diagnostic tool. They are more useful in assessing the effects of vision problems on quality of life.

Consider the basic issue of mobility. Elderly patients with visual impairment due to ARMD are more frequently encountered in clinical practice as people live to increasingly older ages. Kuyk and Elliot (1999) found that contrast sensitivity measured with the Pelli-Robson chart was an important predictor of the time ARMD patients took to walk through courses that contained visual obstacles and the number of collisions with the obstacles. Along with a logMAR acuity of worse than 0.18, the presence of a 1 log unit loss in contrast sensitivity at six cycles per degree was significantly associated with patients who had two or more falls over a 12 month period (Ivers et al. 1998). Owsley and Sloane (1987) found that detection of low and intermediate spatial frequencies correlated well with recognition of real world targets, such as faces and road signs.

In cultures in which reading is an important life activity, loss of spatial contrast sensitivity, along with resolution acuity, plays a prominent role in quality of life measures in patients with visual impairment (Hart et al. 1998). Reading speed in normal observers is relatively tolerant of substantial reductions in contrast (as would be suggested by Chapter 5, Figure 5.15). Contrast had to be reduced to a value of 0.06 to decrease reading speed to one-half its maximum value when normal observers read text composed of letters approximately 2.5 times the size of ordinary newsprint.

Contrast effects on reading are closely related to a low-vision patient's contrast sensitivity losses (Legge et al. 1987). An overall reduction in a patient's spatial CSF has a greater effect on reading performance than do small depressions in sensitivity at particular spatial frequencies. Rubin and Legge (1989) have described low-vision observers as having contrast attenuation due either to optical factors, such as intraocular scattering in eyes with cloudy media, or to a reduction in effective contrast in eyes with visual field losses. If contrast is scaled appropriately for low-vision patients' contrast sensitivity losses, it appears as though the effect of contrast on reading is the same as in normal observers. This implies that one can determine which low-vision observers will benefit from contrast-enhancing low-vision aids. Two people with equal visual acuity could have different spatial CSFs, and the person with poorer spatial CSF experiences a greater visual disability. In low-vision patients with unequal impairment in the two eyes, it has been found that spatial CSF, rather than visual acuity, determines which eye is preferred in situations in which only one eye can be used. This information can be helpful in deciding which eye to fit with low-vision aids.

The visual complaints of low-vision patients include difficulty recognizing faces. It has been suggested that face recognition might be improved for patients with a loss of contrast sensitivity at intermediate and low spatial frequencies by enhancing the contrast of facial features using computerized image-processing techniques. The purpose is to raise the contrast of the spatial frequencies that are critical for face recognition to a level such that the low-vision patients can detect the important facial features. As video cameras and computer hardware become smaller, patients might wear a system that displays the enhanced images in front of their eyes, compensating for their spatial contrast sensitivity losses. Several contrast enhancement schemes have been devised and are being evaluated in low-vision patients (Omoruyi & Leat 2000; Peli 1992; Peli et al. 1994), although it has not yet been demonstrated that this strategy can provide significant benefits to visually impaired patients.

Other applications of the spatial CSF include predicting visual performance when changes are made to the dioptric power of the human eye (e.g., intraocular lenses, radial keratotomy, contact lenses). Lakshminarayanan et al. (1995) have described a method to predict relative changes in clinical performance for a given change in the optics of the eye by using a simple model of the patient's spatial CSF and the in vitro MTF of the eye's optics. This method has been applied successfully to predicting visual performance in patients who were implanted with multifocal intraocular lenses.

Study Guide

1. Describe why spatial luminance difference (contrast) is an important cue for seeing objects in the world.
2. Describe the phenomenon of brightness constancy.
3. Describe the phenomenon of simultaneous contrast, and explain how it depends on contrast.
4. Describe assimilation.
5. Describe a stimulus situation that produces Mach bands.
6. Explain how the center-surround organization of the receptive field of retinal ganglion cells can underlie Mach bands.
7. Define spatial frequency.
8. Define Michelson contrast, and explain why the maximum value is 1 and the minimum value is 0.
9. Be able to draw and label a typical human spatial CSF; include the peak contrast sensitivity, cutoff high spatial frequency, low spatial frequency rolloff, and the corresponding spatial frequencies and contrast sensitivities.
10. Show the correspondence between a MAR of 1' and the cutoff high spatial frequency.
11. Explain the effects of defocus, illuminance, and retinal location on the spatial CSF.
12. Describe how the center-surround receptive-field organization explains a cell's spatial CSF (see Figure 6.12).
13. How did Blakemore and Campbell show that different neurons mediate the detection of low and high spatial frequencies?
14. Describe the basic idea behind Fourier analysis and Fourier synthesis.
15. Explain how the human spatial CSF, coupled with the spatial frequency content of a visual stimulus, could produce Mach bands.
16. What is the importance of low and middle spatial frequencies for seeing?
17. Describe a Pelli-Robson chart.
18. Why has the spatial CSF not become a useful diagnostic test for ocular pathology?

Glossary

Assimilation: the brightness of a stimulus co-varies with the brightness of a surrounding stimulus.

Band pass filter: a band pass filter transmits frequencies within its band, and removes ("filters out," does not transmit) frequencies outside of its band.

Brightness constancy: the brightness of objects, which is determined largely by relative local contrast, is relatively invariant, even though the absolute luminance varies widely.

Channels: independent band pass filters narrower than the overall spatial CSF that respond to a limited range of spatial frequencies.

Contrast (between target and background): $(L_T - L_B)/L_B$, where L_B is the luminance of the background and L_T is the luminance of the object.

Contrast (Michelson contrast for gratings): Contrast = $(L_{max} - L_{min})/(L_{max} + L_{min})$ where L_{max} is the maximum luminance of the grating and L_{min} is the minimum luminance of the grating.

Contrast adaptation: an increase in contrast threshold (decrease in contrast sensitivity) produced by exposure to a high-contrast stimulus (usually a grating).

Contrast sensitivity: the inverse (reciprocal) of the threshold contrast.

Cutoff high spatial frequency: the highest spatial frequency that can be detected at maximum contrast.

Fourier analysis: a mathematical tool devised by Jean Baptiste Joseph Fourier that is useful for determining the component spatial frequencies and contrasts of visual stimuli.

Fourier synthesis: a mathematical tool devised by Jean Baptiste Joseph Fourier that is useful for constructing visual stimuli from component spatial frequencies and contrasts.

Lateral inhibition: the effect of the connections from photoreceptors via horizontal cells to bipolar cells that produce the receptive-field surround.

Low spatial frequency rolloff: the gradual decrease in contrast sensitivity at spatial frequencies below the spatial frequency at which the peak contrast sensitivity occurs.

Mach bands: regions of increased or decreased brightness that are caused by the response of the visual system to luminance boundaries.

Magnocellular (M) pathway: a pathway in which the parasol retinal ganglion cells synapse in the magnocellular laminae of the LGN, which, in turn, synapse in layer IVcα in V1. The neurons in this pathway appear anatomically and functionally distinct from neurons in the P pathway.

Mean luminance (L_m): average luminance or $(L_{max} + L_{min})/2$.

Parvocellular (P) pathway: a pathway in which midget retinal ganglion cells synapse in the parvocellular laminae of the LGN, which, in turn, synapse in layer IVcβ in V1. The neurons in this pathway appear anatomically and functionally distinct from neurons in the M pathway.

Peak contrast sensitivity: the frequency at which the highest contrast sensitivity occurs in a CSF.

Pelli-Robson chart: a wall chart with letters of identical size (i.e., spatial frequency content) and decreasing contrast that is used to quickly and easily assess contrast sensitivity at intermediate and low spatial frequencies in patients.

Simultaneous contrast: the brightness of an object is increased when viewed against a background with which the stimulus has positive contrast and is reduced when the stimulus has negative contrast relative to the background.

Spatial contrast sensitivity function (spatial CSF): a graph of the contrast sensitivity (y-axis) measured at various spatial frequencies (x-axis); both axes usually are scaled logarithmically.

Threshold contrast: the minimum contrast required for detection of a grating or target.

7 Temporal Factors in Vision

Nancy J. Coletta

Overview

In nearly all the measurements of visual function described in previous chapters, stimulus duration was either controlled while a measurement was made or varied to test its effect on the dimension that was being measured. Temporal changes on the retina are needed for spatial vision to occur. There are at least five categories of psychophysical measures involving time-dependent effects on visual function that can be studied in their own right: temporal acuity, the temporal contrast sensitivity function, temporal summation, masking, and motion (real and apparent) detection.

Analogous to spatial resolution acuity, temporal resolution acuity is the smallest time interval that can be resolved as flickering light. The minimum interval of temporal resolution is measured psychophysically by determining the critical flicker frequency (the CFF). This is the frequency at which a flickering is detected as flickering 50% of the time and as fused (steady) 50% of the time. The time-averaged luminance of a fused flickering light determines its brightness. The CFF is directly proportional to the log of the stimulus luminance (the Ferry-Porter law). At high luminance levels, the CFF increases with increasing eccentricity from the fovea. The CFF is directly proportional to the log of the area of a flickering stimulus (the Granit-Harper law). Flickering lights with equal luminance at different wavelengths have equal CFFs. The CFF increases with the level of light adaptation.

The temporal contrast sensitivity function (temporal CSF) gives a complete description of temporal vision. Like the spatial CSF, the temporal CSF has a band pass shape with a peak contrast sensitivity, a cutoff high temporal frequency, and a low temporal frequency rolloff. The low temporal frequency rolloff of the temporal CSF may be explained by center-surround interactions in retinal receptive fields.

The visual system does not distinguish the temporal shape of light flashes shorter than a critical duration. For flash durations where Bloch's law holds, the product of the threshold luminance times the stimulus duration is constant, and the threshold number of quanta is constant. The Broca-Sulzer effect describes the fact that suprathreshold flashes of short duration appear brighter than a steady light of the same luminance.

Masking occurs when the detection of a test stimulus is reduced by another visual stimulus, presented before, during, or after the test stimulus. The masking flash may interfere with the detection of a test flash when the stimuli physically overlap, are spatially separated by a small amount, or are presented to similar positions in each eye. Masking may play a role in the decreased sensitivity to visual stimuli that occurs during eye movements.

The ability to detect motion is limited by the temporal resolution of the visual system. Apparent motion can occur when stationary stimuli are presented discontinuously if their duration and spacing is similar to that produced by real motion. Direction-selective neurons may account for direction-specific adaptation and motion aftereffects. Neurons in the middle temporal (MT) region of cortex in macaque monkeys have similar thresholds for detecting motion as the monkey itself.

Five Categories of Time-Dependent Effects on Vision

The visual system, like the nervous system in general, exists in part to inform its owner of changes in the environment. Chapter 6 examined perceptual responses to *spatial* luminance changes and discussed their possible neural basis.

Spatial vision is not possible unless the retinal image changes with time

The visual system also requires at least some change in luminance over time to maintain responsiveness. Eye movements add temporal modulation to the spatial retinal image even when the eye is trying to look at a stationary target. It is normal that when one fixates a stationary target, small involuntary eye movements continue to occur. These include microsaccades, slow drifts, and a high-frequency physiological tremor of the eye. The amplitudes of these movements are measured in minutes of arc and are not noticed consciously; they are difficult to observe even when looking at another person's eye. The effect of these small temporal transients is to improve visibility of spatial patterns.

If a specialized optical system is used to stabilize images on the retina, so that there is no change in the retinal image over time, the images fade in a few seconds, but they return instantly if the images are allowed to change (Riggs et al. 1953; Kelly 1979a). Even without completely stabilizing an image, there can be temporary and irregular fading (i.e., disappearance) of a contour in the visual field during steady fixation. As described in Chapter 4, this is known as the Troxler effect. This phenomenon is easy to produce if an edge with a gradually changing luminance boundary is placed in the peripheral visual field while the fovea is aimed at a fixation point. Steady fixation of a low-frequency spatial sine-wave grating causes it to fade, but its image is refreshed by repetitively flashing the grating or voluntarily moving the eyes back and forth across a few cycles.

Visual resolution acuity is the same for stabilized and unstabilized images, provided, of course, that the stabilization is brief. Because the square-wave gratings that are used as acuity targets contain high spatial frequencies, the slight tremor of the eye ensures that their visibility is maintained during periods of steady fixation.

In the real world, lights appear, disappear, and flicker; objects move, people move, and the eyes move, so that the pattern of images on the retina constantly changes over time. This chapter examines five time-dependent phenomena: temporal acuity, temporal CSF, temporal summation, masking, and real and apparent motion.

Temporal Resolution Acuity

The critical flicker frequency is a measure of the minimum temporal interval that can be resolved by the visual system

In Chapter 5, the minimum angle of resolution for spatial vision was described as the smallest spatial interval that the eye can detect. In the time domain, one can measure the minimum temporal interval between two flashes of light that the eye can detect as two flashes rather than one. This can be measured with pairs of light flashes but is usually measured with rapidly alternating luminances over time, a temporal analog of a spatial square-wave grating. Figure 7.1A shows a temporal square-wave pattern, so called because the transitions from the minimum luminance (L_{min}) (100 units in this example) to the maximum luminance (L_{max}) (300 units) and back to L_{min} are instantaneous. Such patterns of alternating luminance can be produced easily by rotating a windmill-like disk with alternately clear and opaque vanes (an **episcotister**) in front of any light source.

By using rotating polarizing filters, cathode ray tubes, or computer monitors, it is possible to produce sine-wave patterns like those shown in Figure 7.1B. Sine-wave modulation is a way of presenting a pure temporal frequency. Recall from the discussion of Fourier analysis in Chapter 6 that a square-wave stimulus can be constructed by summing a fundamental sine-wave frequency and many additional harmonic frequencies of specific amplitudes. Just as in the spatial domain, a temporal sine-wave stimulus contains only the fundamental frequency, without any harmonics. For a sine-wave and square-wave stimulus, the **period** is the length of time for one complete cycle of light and dark, and the **flicker rate**, or **flicker frequency**, is the number of cycles per second (measured in hertz [Hz]).

When the alternating, repetitive cycle of low and high luminance of a temporal square-wave stimulus is viewed by an observer, the light appears to flicker if the flicker rate is low. If the flicker rate is increased sufficiently, the light appears to be steady rather than flickering. The flicker frequency at which the stimulus is seen as flickering 50% of the time and as steady, or fused, 50% of the time is called the **critical flicker frequency** or the CFF.

The CFF is a measure of the temporal resolving capacity of the visual system. This minimum interval of resolution, the **temporal acuity**, is analogous to the minimum angle of resolution in the spatial domain. Thus, the CFF is a temporal analog to grating acuity in the spatial domain; both measure the upper limit of the visual system for detecting the presence of alterations between light and dark with a high-contrast stimulus.

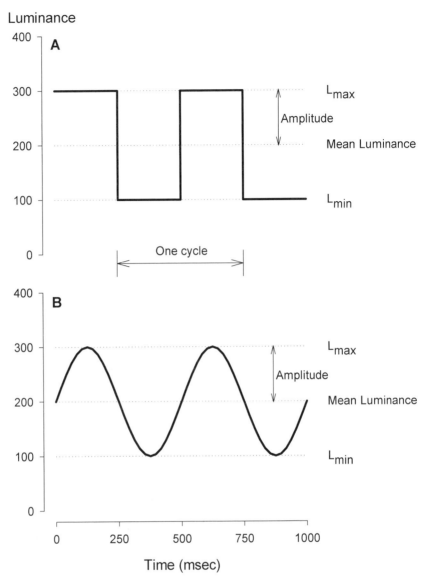

FIGURE 7.1   *Luminance profiles as a function of time for square-wave (**A**) and sine-wave (**B**) lights flickering at 2 Hz. See text for details.*

The time-averaged luminance of a flickering light determines its brightness at flicker rates above the critical flicker frequency (Talbot-Plateau law)

When a fused flickering light (a light flickering faster than the CFF) is compared with a steady light, it matches a steady light whose luminance is the same as the time-averaged luminance of the flickering light. This match between the time-averaged luminance and the luminance of a steady light is referred to as the **Talbot-Plateau law**, and the time-averaged luminance is called the **Talbot brightness**.

Calculating the Talbot brightness is simple when the **duty cycle** is 1 to 1; that is, the time the light is on equals the time it is off. It is the mean of L_{max} and L_{min}. In Figure 7.1, the mean would be 200 units. For any duty cycle, the general formula is

$$\text{Talbot brightness} = L_{min} + ([L_{max} - L_{min}] \times f) \qquad \text{Eq. 7.1}$$

where f is the fraction of time that L_{max} is present during the total period. To convert duty cycle to f, divide the first number of the duty cycle by the sum of the two numbers. For example, for a duty cycle of 1 to 1, $f = 1/(1 + 1) = 0.5$.

Thus, for the square wave shown in the top of Figure 7.1, the Talbot brightness is $100 + ([300 - 100] \times 0.5)$, which equals 200 units. In this case, each luminance level is present half of the time. If the square wave shown in the top of Figure 7.1 were altered so that the L_{max} lasted 125 milliseconds, and the L_{min} lasted 375 milliseconds instead of the 250 milliseconds shown, it would have a duty cycle of 1 to 3, f would equal 0.25, and the Talbot brightness would be $100 + ([300 - 100] \times 0.25)$, or 150 units. Conversely, if the higher luminance were on for 375 milliseconds and the lower for 125 milliseconds, then f equals 0.75, and the Talbot brightness would be 250 units.

Note that in these examples, the duty cycle was changed without changing the period and, hence, without changing the frequency of the flickering light. Changing frequencies with duty cycles other than 1 to 1 becomes a complicated experimental change, because the mean luminance (L_m) changes. It is thus more difficult to interpret the experimental results.

At flicker rates slightly below the critical flicker frequency, brightness is enhanced (the Brücke-Bartley phenomenon)

If one views a flickering light and the flicker rate is varied without changing the time-averaged luminance, the brightness of the flickering light appears to be enhanced at certain frequencies. This is called the **Brücke-Bartley phenomenon**. The flickering light appears brighter than a steady light with equal L_m, and it can even appear brighter than a steady light equal to the L_{max} of the flicker. The maximum brightness enhancement occurs for flicker rates well below the CFF, typically in the 5–20 Hz range (Bartley 1938; Wu et al. 1996).

The neural basis of the critical flicker frequency is the modulation of firing rates of retinal neurons

Some properties of the CFF are probably determined at an early stage of visual processing. Neurophysiological recordings in photoreceptors and outer retinal neurons exhibit the same relationship between the CFF and light intensity as that is obtained from human psychophysics (Tyler & Hamer 1990). Studies of monkey retinal ganglion cells and lateral geniculate neurons indicate that their temporal acuities for luminance flicker are in the same general range as human psychophysical CFFs (Lee et al. 1989; Derrington & Lennie 1984).

Figure 7.2 illustrates the concept of the CFF as it might be measured if a flickering light is presented in the on-center region of a retinal ganglion cell receptive field. When the flicker rate is low, each portion of the light-dark cycle produces distinct responses from neurons in the retina. These, in turn, are conducted through the lateral geniculate nucleus to the primary visual cortex (V1) in the form of bursts of action potentials. The visual system detects that there is an alternation between more (L_{max}) and less (L_{min}) light by detecting the difference in the firing rates of neurons during the two periods.

The responses for a low, a medium, and a high rate of flicker are shown in Figures 7.2A, 7.2B, and 7.2C, respectively. When the stimulus is presented at a low rate of flicker, there is an increase in the firing rate of the cell during L_{max} and a decrease during L_{min}. Note two important things about the response to L_{max}, however: In response to the onset of the L_{max}, the neuron produces a burst of action potentials that has a latency and takes a finite amount of time to cease even after the luminance has dropped to L_{min}. Thus, when the time interval during which L_{min} is presented is very short, as in panel C, the neurons do not have time to stop responding to the cycle's L_{max} before the next L_{max} arrives.

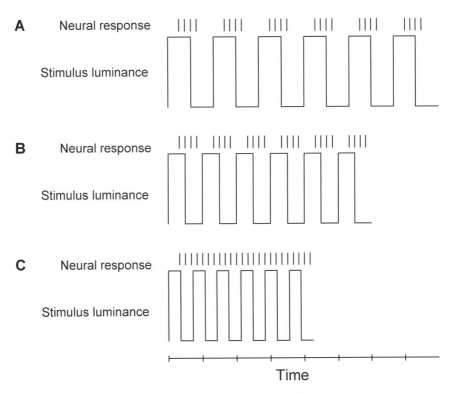

FIGURE 7.2   *Neural explanation for the critical flicker frequency (CFF). When each flash in the flickering light is far apart in time (**A**), each burst of action potentials is distinct. When the flicker rate increases, as in **B** and **C**, a rate is reached at which there is no gap between bursts, and the neural response becomes a continuous series of action potentials.*

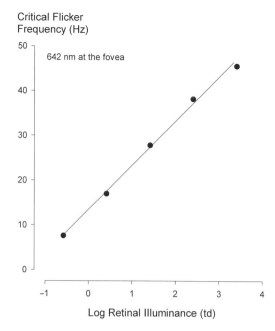

Critical Flicker Frequency (Hz)

642 nm at the fovea

Log Retinal Illuminance (td)

FIGURE 7.3   *Critical flicker frequency as a function of log retinal illuminance of the flickering stimulus. The stimulus was red (642 nm) and 0.5° in diameter and was centered on the fovea. The straight-line relationship is the Ferry-Porter law. (Modified from CW Tyler, RD Hamer. Analysis of visual modulation sensitivity. IV. Validity of the Ferry-Porter law. J Opt Soc Am A 1990;7:743–758.)*

In addition, when the duration of L_{max} is very brief, the stimulus is removed before the neuron reaches a high rate of firing. Thus, at high flicker rates, not only is the signal that L_{min} is present lost, but the average firing rate is less than could be produced by L_{max}. This averaging also helps to explain the Talbot brightness of the fused flickering stimulus.

The critical flicker frequency is directly proportional to the logarithm of stimulus luminance (Ferry-Porter law)

Temporal resolution acuity improves (i.e., smaller time intervals can be detected) as the luminance level of the flickering stimulus increases. As shown in Figure 7.3, the CFF increases linearly with the log of the stimulus luminance. This relationship is known as the **Ferry-Porter law** and can be written as

$$CFF = k\log L + b$$

Eq. 7.2

where k is the slope of the function, b is a constant, and L is the luminance of the flickering stimulus.

In Figure 7.3, the stimulus was a 0.5° diameter round, red spot that was presented on the fovea. The flickering light thus was detected primarily by the cone photoreceptors. In this instance, the slope (k) was approximately 10, meaning that for every 1 log change in luminance, there was a 10 Hz change in the CFF. The foveal results demonstrate that the Ferry-Porter law holds over a

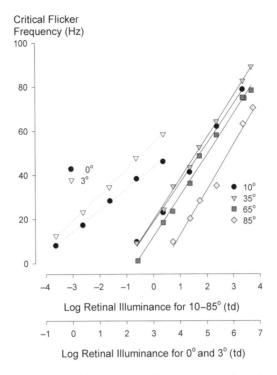

Critical Flicker Frequency (Hz)

FIGURE 7.4 *Effect of retinal location on the Ferry-Porter law. A 642 nm target was presented at the fovea and at eccentricities of 3°, 10°, 35°, 65°, and 85°. The upper x-axis scale shows the retinal illuminance for the stimuli 10°–85° from the fovea. To prevent the foveal data from being covered up by the peripheral data, the retinal illuminance values for the stimuli that were presented at 0° and 3° from the fovea are plotted on a lower scale, which shifts the data 3 log units to the left. (Modified from CW Tyler, RD Hamer. Eccentricity and the Ferry-Porter law. J Opt Soc Am A 1993;10: 2084–2087.)*

range of approximately 4 log units. Its limit is the maximum CFF of approximately 50 Hz, which is reached at high levels of retinal illuminance.

The critical flicker frequency is highest in the midperipheral retina at high luminance and nearly constant across the retina at low luminance

As shown in Figure 7.4, the Ferry-Porter law holds when the stimulus is presented at many retinal locations. The slope of the CFF luminance function is steeper outside the fovea, changing from a k of approximately 10 Hz per log unit at the fovea to almost 20 Hz per log unit by 10° eccentricity. The steeper functions in the periphery may indicate that the peripheral retinal neurons are able to respond with greater **temporal acuity** than those that serve central vision. The ability to follow faster temporal frequencies in the peripheral retina may be due to the larger diameters of the peripheral cone outer segments (Tyler 1985).

Computer screens or fluorescent lights that appear steady in central vision can sometimes appear to flicker if they are viewed with the peripheral retina. For this to occur, the CFF must increase in the periphery. The data in Figure 7.5

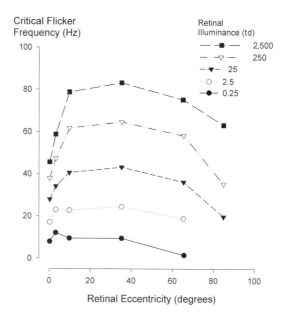

FIGURE 7.5   *Data from Figure 7.4 redrawn to show the critical flicker frequency (CFF) as a function of eccentricity for five luminance levels. The CFF is higher in the periphery at high-luminance levels. At low-luminance levels, there is not much change in the CFF with retinal location. The diameter of the target was 0.5° when presented at the fovea, and was increased in size with eccentricity to stimulate approximately a constant number of cones at each location. (Modified from CW Tyler, RD Hamer. Eccentricity and the Ferry-Porter law. J Opt Soc Am A 1993;10:2084–2087.)*

support this observation. The maximum CFF, measured at 35° from the fovea, is approximately 90 Hz, almost twice as high as the foveal CFF. To control for the decrease in the number of cones as the target is moved into the periphery, the flickering stimulus was enlarged with eccentricity to keep the same number of cones stimulated by flicker at each retinal location. Not shown in the figure is the fact that the CFF is also higher in the lower visual field. The high peripheral CFFs are mainly a feature of vision at high luminance. When luminance is low, the CFF remains fairly constant with retinal location.

The critical flicker frequency is directly proportional to the logarithm of the area of the flickering stimulus (Granit-Harper law)

The CFF increases (temporal resolution acuity improves) as the flickering stimulus is enlarged (Granit & Harper 1938). The CFF has been reported to increase linearly with the log of the area of the flickering stimulus; this relationship is known as the **Granit-Harper law** and can be written as

$$CFF = k \log A + b$$ Eq. 7.3

where k and b are constants, and A is the area of the flickering stimulus. The Granit-Harper law holds for approximately a 3 log unit range of luminance for

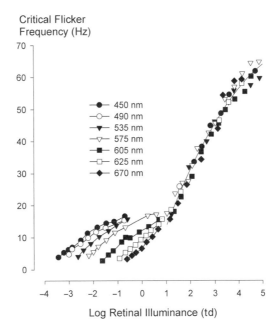

Critical Flicker Frequency (Hz)

FIGURE 7.6   *Critical flicker frequency as a function of retinal illuminance for mono-chromatic lights of different wavelengths. The stimulus was 19° in diameter, centered on the fovea. The coincidence of the curves at high illuminance values indicates that the critical flicker frequency does not depend on wavelength when the different wavelengths stimulate all cones equally; the fanning out of the curves at low illuminance values is attributable to the effect of the different wavelengths on the rods. (Modified from S Hecht, S Shlaer. Intermittent stimulation by light. V. The relation between intensity and critical frequency for different parts of the spectrum. J Gen Physiol 1936;19:965–979.)*

stimuli presented in the fovea and up to approximately 10° from the fovea. At a given retinal location, increasing the stimulus area shifts the overall Ferry-Porter function upwards, but the slope of the Ferry-Porter relationship does not change. Thus, in Figure 7.3, increasing the stimulus area would move the line upward on the graph. Note, in Figure 7.3, that if the flicker rate were fixed and the stimulus area were increased, shifting the Ferry-Porter relationship upwards on the graph, then the CFF would occur at a lower luminance level.

Flickering lights with equal photopic luminance but different wavelengths have equal critical flicker frequencies

Figure 7.6 shows the CFFs for different wavelengths that were presented as 19° diameter targets centered on the fovea. The different wavelength stimuli were matched in photopic luminance; that is, they were equally effective in stimulating cones (see Appendix, Figure A.1). The results show two regions with different spectral sensitivities. As expected, for intensities in the photopic range greater than 1 log troland, the CFFs are independent of wavelength, because the CFFs were mediated by cones. At a given low stimulus intensity where rods are used to detect flicker the CFFs were highest for the shorter wavelengths. Because rods absorb better at those wavelengths, the stimulus was effectively of higher intensity. The maximum CFF of scotopic vision is approximately 20 Hz and has led many to believe that rods are unable to follow flicker at higher frequencies. However, other studies conducted under carefully controlled conditions show that rods can detect flicker up to approximately 30 Hz (Conner & MacLeod 1977).

Rod monochromats, who lack cone photopigments, also exhibit a two-branched CFF-intensity curve in which the low-intensity limb reaches a maximum CFF of 16 Hz, and the high intensity limb reaches a maximum CFF of 27 Hz (Hess & Nordby 1986). The CFF is apparently determined by a slow pathway that operates at low-luminance levels and a fast pathway that operates at higher-luminance levels; the slow pathway receives input from rods, whereas the fast pathway probably has access to rod and cone signals. In a rod monochromat, the sole input to the fast pathway is from the rods, yet the pathway still mediates a higher level of the CFF. Mammalian retinal circuitry indicates that rod signals can travel to retinal ganglion cells via two separate pathways: either via rod bipolar cells to all amacrine cells to cone bipolar cells, or via gap junctions with cones to cone bipolar cells (Sterling et al. 1986; DeVries & Baylor 1995). These two pathways may be the neural substrate for the slow and fast rod pathways evident in studies of **flicker sensitivity** (Stockman et al. 1991).

Flicker sensitivity increases and then decreases during dark adaptation

The previous sections have shown that the CFF at a given luminance level is sensitive to the location of the stimulus on the retina, its area, and its wavelength. Given the relative densities of rods and cones in different retinal areas, their different wavelength sensitivities, and their neural interactions, it is not surprising that the effects of dark and light adaptation can be complex. Generally, the CFF is highest when the eye is light adapted or when a uniform background of light surrounds the flickering stimulus. Consequently, a flickering stimulus at a fixed intensity can appear to be flickering when the eye is light adapted, and fused (i.e., steady) when the eye is dark adapted (Lythgoe & Tansley 1929; Goldberg et al. 1983; Alexander & Fishman 1984; Coletta & Adams 1984). These adaptation effects on flicker are evident at frequencies higher than 15 Hz.

The effects of dark adaptation on flicker visibility can be demonstrated by measuring either the CFF for a fixed-luminance stimulus, or by measuring the luminance threshold for seeing flicker of a fixed-frequency stimulus. In the latter case, the luminance threshold at which flicker is seen at the threshold called the *flicker threshold* and the inverse of flicker threshold is *flicker sensitivity*. Recall that if a small amount of luminance is needed to see a target, then the threshold is low and the sensitivity is high. Likewise, if the flicker threshold occurs at a low luminance level, flicker sensitivity is high.

Figure 7.7 shows the flicker threshold (triangles) for a 3 second stimulus flickering at a constant 25 Hz over 25 minutes of dark adaptation. The figure also shows a typical dark adaptation curve (circles) that is measured as the threshold for detecting a 500 millisecond flash of light for comparison. Both measurements were made at 20° eccentricity, using a white stimulus with a diameter of 1.75°. The thresholds for detecting the 500 millisecond flash follow a standard dark adaptation curve.

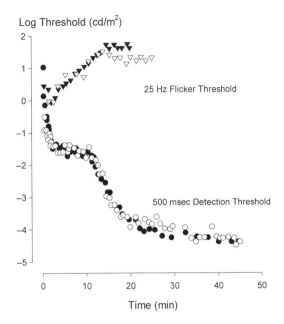

Log Threshold (cd/m^2)

25 Hz Flicker Threshold

500 msec Detection Threshold

Time (min)

FIGURE 7.7   *Thresholds for detecting a 500 msec test flash* (circles) *and for detecting flicker in a 3 second presentation of a 25 Hz flickering stimulus* (triangles) *as a function of time in the dark. Data are for two subjects* (open and filled symbols). *Each stimulus was a 1.75° diameter white light that was located at 20° from the fixation point. (cd = candela.) (Modified from K Alexander, G Fishman. Rod-cone interaction in flicker perimetry. Br J Ophthalmol 1984;68:303–309.)*

The flicker threshold decreased (i.e., flicker sensitivity increased) during the first 2 minutes of dark adaptation in parallel with the decrease in the threshold of the cone branch. As the cone detection threshold plateaus, the threshold luminance to detect flicker begins to rise (i.e., flicker sensitivity decreases). It continues rising, by almost 2 log units, during the cone plateau region and levels off approximately 15 minutes after time zero. Thus, flicker becomes more difficult to detect (higher luminance is needed to see the flicker), even though the observer has increasing sensitivity to detect the presence of a light during dark adaptation. Moreover, change in flicker threshold occurs after the cones have fully dark adapted, suggesting that it is the dark adaptation of the rods that causes the decrease in the cones' ability to detect 25 Hz flicker.

The effects of rod adaptation on cone-mediated flicker sensitivity originate in the outer neural layers of the retina

Adaptation effects of rods on cone-mediated flicker sensitivity can be demonstrated neurophysiologically. Figure 7.8 shows the adaptation effect on the flicker response of a horizontal cell from a cat retina. In the lower trace, the small-amplitude oscillations depict the time that a red (650 nm) stimulus flickering at 16 Hz was presented. In the middle of that trace, the downward deflection indicates the period during which a violet (423 nm) background light was turned on. The upper trace is the membrane potential recorded

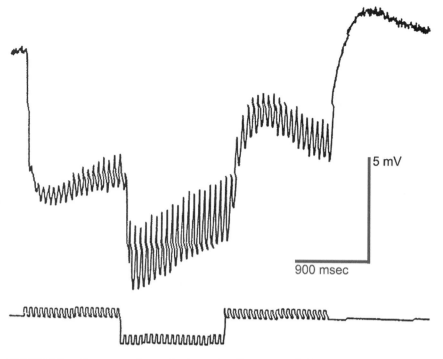

FIGURE 7.8 *Response of a cat horizontal cell to 16 Hz flicker (upper trace), showing the enhancement of the flicker response in the presence of a background light that light adapts rods (middle of trace). The lower trace is a photocell recording of the stimulus; the onset of flicker is marked by oscillation in the lower trace. The result is an overall hyperpolarization of the cell's membrane potential. When rods are dark adapted, the horizontal cell's flicker response is decreased in amplitude relative to when the rods are light adapted. (Reprinted from R Pflug, R Nelson, PK Ahnelt. Background-induced flicker enhancement in cat retinal horizontal cells. I. Temporal and spectral properties. J Neurophysiol 1990;64:313–325.)*

from the horizontal cell with a microelectrode. Recall that horizontal cells hyperpolarize (downward deflection) in response to light. Each oscillation of the horizontal cell membrane potential occurs in response to the flickering light. When the additional (violet) light is turned on, the horizontal cell hyperpolarizes further. Of interest is the amplitude of the rapid oscillations of the horizontal cell membrane potential, which clearly shows an increase when the background is present. Turning off the background results in an almost immediate reduction in flicker response amplitude.

In this particular stimulus configuration, the red 25 Hz flicker favors detection by the cones that connect to this horizontal cell. The violet background light adapts rods more strongly than cones. Thus, before and after the violet light is present, the rods are relatively dark adapted, and the cone-mediated oscillations of the horizontal cell are small. When the rods become more light adapted in the center, the cone-mediated response increases. This experiment is consistent with the psychophysical evidence that dark-adapted rods suppress cone flicker sensitivity. When the rods are light adapted, as in the center of the figure, the horizontal cell responses increase in amplitude. The decreased response amplitude would suggest that the flicker would be harder to detect, so that a more intense light would be needed to detect the flicker when the rods are dark adapted. Under certain conditions, light adaptation of rods has been shown to improve cone flicker sensitivity in psychophysical measurement of human subjects (Coletta & Adams 1984).

The adaptation effect on flicker sensitivity can be used to locate the site of pathology in patients with retinal disorders

As shown in Figure 7.8, the rod-cone interaction on flicker sensitivity appears to be organized in the outer plexiform layer of retina in which the horizontal cells provide feedback onto cones (Frumkes & Eysteinsson 1988; Pflug et al. 1990). If the flicker adaptation effect is absent, it implies that a retinal disorder occurs very early in the pathway from the photoreceptors. Indeed, light adaptation has no effect on flicker sensitivity in patients with photoreceptor disorders such as retinitis pigmentosa. In contrast, in patients with inner retinal disorders, such as dominant optic atrophy and congenital stationary night blindness, flicker sensitivity improves by a normal amount when an adapting background is present (Alexander & Fishman 1984).

Some individuals exhibit an adaptation effect on flicker sensitivity that is greater than normal in magnitude. These patients complain of problems in seeing at night, although they have apparently normal vision on standard diagnostic tests. The problem is believed to be an exaggerated rod suppression of cone flicker sensitivity, although its exact origin is unknown (Arden & Hogg 1985; Lange & Frumkes 1992; Falcao-Reis et al. 1991).

Temporal Contrast Sensitivity

The temporal contrast sensitivity function is a complete description of temporal vision

The temporal acuity limit, as measured by the CFF, described in the previous sections, describes the highest temporal frequency that can be detected at a fixed high contrast; it does not tell how the visual system responds to different combinations of temporal frequencies and contrasts. As was discussed for spatial vision, the spatial CSF gives a complete picture of the visual response over the entire range of visible spatial frequencies. The temporal sine wave shown in Figure 7.1 is analogous in many ways to the spatial sine-wave gratings described in Chapter 6, except that the luminance changes over time rather than over space. Both have a mean luminance (L_m) around which the luminance varies between a maximum (L_{max}) and a minimum (L_{min}). One can thus measure a CSF for temporal vision by finding the threshold contrast at each of a series of sine-wave temporal frequencies, and taking the reciprocal of the threshold contrast.

The **contrast** of a temporal sine wave is defined in the same way as the contrast of a spatial sine-wave grating:

$$\text{Contrast} = \frac{(L_{max} - L_{min})}{(L_{max} + L_{min})} \qquad \text{Eq. 7.4}$$

In Figure 7.1, L_{max} is 300, and L_{min} is 100, so contrast equals $(200)/(400)$, which equals 0.5.

The mean or average luminance is defined as

$$\text{Mean Luminance} = L_m = \frac{(L_{max} + L_{min})}{2} \qquad \text{Eq. 7.5}$$

$L_{max} - L_m$ is the **amplitude**. Another term, the **modulation ratio** (abbreviated as *m*), is sometimes used to describe sine-wave flicker and may be used interchangeably with contrast. It is defined as the ratio of the amplitude to L_m. Hence, contrast and the modulation ratio can also be expressed as

$$\text{Contrast} = m = \frac{(L_{max} - L_m)}{L_m} \qquad \text{Eq. 7.6}$$

Referring again to the sine wave at the bottom of Figure 7.1, the L_m is 200 units, the amplitude is 100, and the contrast therefore is 0.5. Contrast is independent of the luminance level; if the L_m were 2 units and the amplitude were 1 unit, the contrast also would be 0.5. As was the case for spatial sine-wave gratings, *contrast sensitivity* is defined as the inverse of the threshold contrast.

Temporal contrast sensitivity functions have a band pass shape characterized by a cutoff high frequency at the temporal acuity limit, a peak contrast sensitivity at intermediate frequencies, and a low frequency rolloff

Figure 7.9 shows a set of temporal CSFs that were measured at different levels of L_m. These temporal CSFs have several features in common with the spatial CSFs shown in Chapter 6, Figures 6.9 and 6.15. The CSFs have the same general **band pass shape** that includes (1) a **peak contrast sensitivity** that occurs at an intermediate frequency; (2) a **cutoff high temporal frequency** at the limit of temporal acuity, above which flicker cannot be resolved even when the contrast is 1.0; and (3) a reduction in sensitivity at low frequencies (**low frequency rolloff**).

The temporal peak contrast sensitivity shifts from approximately 5 to 20 Hz as the L_m increases. The cutoff high temporal frequency shifts from 15 to 60 Hz as the L_m increases. A plot of these cutoff frequencies against L_m generates a function similar to Figure 7.3, which demonstrates the Ferry-Porter law. Notice that the low frequency rolloff in the temporal CSF is absent at the lowest luminance level.

Because the visual system has a lower contrast sensitivity at low luminance (e.g., 0.06 td), people can only see low temporal frequencies of medium to high contrast. As the luminance level increases, humans can perceive temporally modulated stimuli with lower contrast over a wider band of temporal frequencies.

The visibility of low frequency flicker is enhanced by the presence of spatial edges

The stimulus used to measure the temporal CSFs in Figure 7.9 was a large flickering field with blurred edges (Kelly 1961). If a sharp-edged field is used, temporal contrast sensitivity is higher at low temporal frequencies by as much as 1

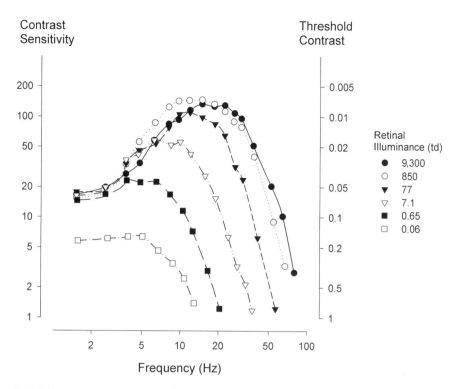

FIGURE 7.9   *Human temporal contrast sensitivity functions for several mean luminance levels. The left ordinate is the contrast sensitivity, and the right ordinate is the
threshold contrast. (Modified from DH Kelly. Visual responses to time-dependent stimuli. I. Amplitude sensitivity measurements. J Opt Soc Am 1961;51: 422–429.)*

log unit. Thus, the presence of spatial edges or spatial detail in the target
improves the visibility of flicker at low temporal frequencies (less than 5 Hz).

If the temporal CSF is measured with a target composed of a flickered sine-
wave grating instead of a field of uniform luminance, the shape of the temporal
CSF changes from its characteristic band pass shape to a low-pass shape in
which the low frequency rolloff is absent (Robson 1966). The use of a flickering grating stimulus does not change the shape of the high temporal frequency
side of the temporal CSF other than to reduce the sensitivity as the grating spatial frequency is increased to near the spatial high-frequency cutoff. A similar
effect is also observed if the spatial CSF is measured using flickering stimuli at
various temporal frequencies: Sensitivity to spatial frequencies less than 3
cycles per degree is improved by flickering the gratings at 6 Hz. This is because
cells in the magnocellular (M) pathway respond well to both low spatial frequencies and to flicker.

Center-surround interactions may account for the low frequency rolloff in the temporal contrast sensitivity function of individual neurons

As explained in Chapter 6, the center-surround receptive-field organization
in retinal ganglion cells accounts for the presence of the low frequency

rolloff in the spatial CSF. The band pass shape of the temporal CSFs of individual neurons may also result from center-surround interactions (Figure 7.10A). For explanatory purposes, it is simpler to think of the temporal low frequency rolloff as an enhancement of the intermediate frequencies, although it amounts to the same thing either way: The contrast sensitivity is lower at low temporal frequencies than it is at the intermediate of temporal frequencies.

The center and the surround of a bipolar cell shift membrane potentials in opposite directions in response to light. Those photoreceptors that connect directly to an on-center bipolar cell (forming the receptive-field center) produce a depolarization of the bipolar cell in response to light (second traces in Figures 7.10B and 7.10C). This response is delayed slightly by the processing time and synaptic delay (Enroth-Cugell & Lennie 1975; Nye & Naka 1971), so the response of the bipolar cell lags slightly behind the change in the luminance incident on the photoreceptors.

The photoreceptors that connect indirectly to an on-center bipolar cell via horizontal cells (i.e., the cells forming the receptive-field surround) move the membrane potential of the bipolar cell in the opposite direction (toward hyperpolarization) in response to an increase in luminance. This surround-mediated input to the bipolar cell lags significantly behind the arrival of the center signal because of the extra synapse and the additional distance traveled. The delay between the arrival of the center signal at the bipolar and the arrival of the surround signal at the bipolar is indicated by *d* in Figure 7.10C.

When the flicker rate is low (approximately 1 Hz), the difference in the arrival time of the center signal and the surround signal is inconsequential. As shown in Figure 7.10B, the two opposite influences are summed by the bipolar cell (the vertical line indicates a pair of points that are summed), which results in a small signal. The bipolar cell membrane has a low-amplitude response that is synchronized with the center input, because, in fact, the center input is usually a bit stronger than the surround input. The cell thus responds weakly to low-frequency flicker. The way to increase the response of the bipolar cell so that it gives a criterion amplitude of response is to raise the contrast of the grating. The neuron can then respond more strongly to this low temporal frequency stimulus, but it would require a high contrast to reach a criterion amplitude and, consequently, would have a low contrast sensitivity.

When the flicker rate is higher (5–30 Hz), the delay, *d*, between the arrival of the center signal and the arrival of the surround signal becomes a significant factor. As shown in Figure 7.10C, if the center-surround delay is equal to half a cycle (e.g., if the delay is 25 milliseconds, and the flicker rate is 20 Hz), the surround signal arrives exactly half a cycle behind the center signal. This would cause the depolarization that is produced by the surround to occur at the same time as the depolarization that is produced by the center. Thus, rather than canceling each other, they would add. When the bipolar cell sums the two inputs (again, the vertical line aligns points that are summed), a large signal is produced by a contrast that was

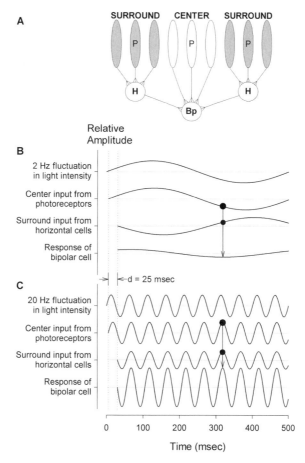

FIGURE 7.10   *Illustration of how the longer latency of the receptive-field surround may account for the low temporal frequency rolloff.* **A.** *Connections of photoreceptors (P) and horizontal cells (H) to bipolar (Bp) cells that comprise center and surround components of a receptive field.* **B.** *Component responses when the flicker rate is slow. It is of no consequence that signals arriving at the bipolar cells via the horizontal cells have a slightly longer latency than the signals arriving via the direct photoreceptor input.* **C.** *The effect on the bipolar cell response when the flicker rate is fast enough that the delay (d) of the surround signal, in comparison to the latency of the center signal, is equal to a half cycle. The combination of center and surround signals now dramatically boosts the response of the bipolar cell.*

relatively ineffective at low temporal frequencies. In this case, the contrast could be reduced to reach a criterion amplitude; contrast sensitivity therefore would be high. Whether the example in Figure 7.10 is viewed as an enhancement at intermediate frequencies or a low temporal frequency rolloff (preferred because it preserves the analogy with the spatial CSF), it is the interaction between the center and the surround of the receptive field that produces this change.

Temporal contrast sensitivity is affected by some retinal disorders

Temporal contrast sensitivity is becoming an important diagnostic test for retinal disorders, such as glaucoma. The rationale for the use of flicker testing in glaucoma is that the retinal neurons that are most sensitive to stimuli of low spatial and high temporal frequencies are believed to be impaired at an early stage in glaucoma (reviewed in Drum 1989). These neurons are most likely neurons in the M pathway, because monkeys with lesions that selectively remove the M pathway have losses in sensitivity for low spatial frequency and high temporal frequency patterns (Merigan et al. 1991). This idea is consistent with the finding that retinal ganglion cells with large diameter axons (a property of M pathway neurons) are impaired at an early stage in glaucoma (Quigley et al. 1987).

Elevated intraocular pressure (IOP) is somehow linked to a reduction in flicker sensitivity, even in normal subjects (Tyler et al. 1984). An artificial increase in IOP causes a temporary loss of flicker contrast sensitivity but no effect on the CFF (Van Toi et al. 1990). Although the mechanism that links IOP and flicker sensitivity may be different in normal and glaucomatous eyes, temporal contrast sensitivity is reduced in patients with glaucoma and in those with ocular hypertension (elevated IOP but no field loss on standard perimetric tests) (Tyler 1981). The loss of flicker sensitivity in patients with ocular hypertension implies that the flicker contrast threshold may be a more sensitive test in the detection of neural damage from elevated IOP than the standard increment threshold measure used in automated perimetry.

The frequency-doubling perimeter has been introduced recently as a rapid screening test for the early diagnosis of glaucoma (Johnson & Samuels 1997). The device measures the patient's contrast threshold for a 0.25 cycle per degree grating that flickers at 25 Hz. It is named for the frequency-doubling illusion, in which a low spatial frequency grating appears to double in spatial frequency when it is counterphase flickered at a rapid rate. A counterphase stimulus is one in which the grating's light bars become dark and vice versa at a certain temporal rate. A particular subset of the M pathway neurons, the MY cells, may be responsible for the frequency-doubling illusion (Maddess et al. 1998). Recall from Chapter 3 that standard visual field testing only reveals deficits when a large fraction of the retinal ganglion cells have already been damaged by glaucoma. Because MY cells are a small subset of retinal ganglion cells, a reduction in their numbers may affect the threshold measured with frequency doubling, making it a more sensitive diagnostic test.

In addition to glaucoma testing, temporal contrast sensitivity is also of diagnostic value in age-related macular degeneration. Eyes at risk for developing exudative age-related macular degeneration show reduced modulation sensitivity to flicker over a frequency range from 5 to 40 Hz (Mayer et al. 1992; Mayer et al. 1994). Flicker sensitivity may be useful as a screening test, because sensitivity at just two frequencies, 5 and 10 Hz, can discriminate pre-exudative eyes from normal older eyes.

Temporal Summation and Bloch's Law

The visual system sums light flashes shorter than a critical duration regardless of the timing with which they strike the retina

The discussion in Chapter 2 of the stimulus values that were selected for measuring the absolute threshold of vision introduced the concept of **temporal summation**. The visual system summates visual inputs over brief time periods in a consistent manner, as described by **Bloch's law**:

$$L \times t = C \qquad \text{Eq. 7.7}$$

where L is the threshold luminance of the flash, t is its duration, and C is a constant (Figure 7.11). It was noted that Bloch's law holds for flashes that are shorter than a **critical duration** (t_c) of approximately 30–100 milliseconds, depending on the conditions that are described in the following discussion. During the presentation of these brief flashes, the visual system adds together the effects of absorbed quanta regardless of the temporal pattern in which they arrive.

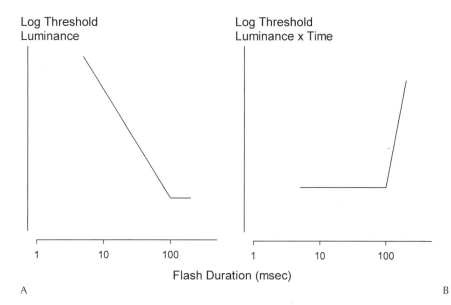

A   B

FIGURE 7.11   *Two different ways of illustrating Bloch's law. Both graphs show Bloch's law holding for flash durations shorter than 100 milliseconds (the critical duration [t_c] in this example).* **A.** *The threshold luminance needed to see the flash as a function of the flash duration.* **B.** *The threshold expressed as luminance times duration, as a function of flash duration. As noted in Equation 7.8, the product of the luminance times the duration yields quanta per area, but the area of the stimulus is held constant. When temporal summation is perfect, that is, when Bloch's law holds, the number of quanta that are needed to see the flash is independent of flash duration (horizontal portion of* **B**).

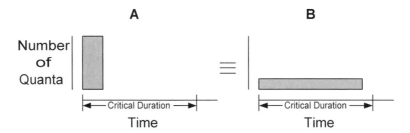

A   B

FIGURE 7.12   *Two stimulus configurations that present the same number of quanta in a period of time, shorter than the critical duration (t_c). The temporal presentation patterns of a brief, more intense flash on the left and a longer, less intense flash on the right are not distinguishable by the visual system. If the flash shown on the left is at threshold, then the one on the right also would be at threshold.*

Equation 2.2 in Chapter 2 states that the luminance (*L*) of a flash is directly proportional to the number of quanta (*Q*) in the flash and inversely proportional to the duration (*t*) and area (*A*) of the flash, or

$$L = \frac{Q}{t \times A}$$
Eq. 7.8

If the number of quanta delivered in a flash and the flash area are kept constant, then *L* must decrease when *t* increases (descending line in Figure 7.11A). For flashes shorter than the t_c, the threshold is reached when a certain number of quanta are delivered in the flash. For flashes longer than the t_c (the horizontal line of Figure 7.11A), the rate at which quanta are delivered (luminance) needs to be constant. This means that the number of quanta at threshold is actually increasing in direct proportion to the flash duration, as indicated by the ascending portion of Figure 7.11B (see also Chapter 2, Figure 2.5).

Figure 7.12 illustrates the fact that when a flash is shorter in duration than the t_c, the visual system does not distinguish the temporal shape of the stimulus. Both of the stimulus patterns yield the same threshold because the total number of quanta that are delivered in the brief period are the same; the shaded areas under the curves are equal.

Bloch's law is a consequence of the temporal filtering properties of vision

A short flash of light is comprised of many temporal frequencies that are added together, just as a square-wave grating or square-wave flicker contains a fundamental frequency with selected harmonics. Chapter 6 described how the spatial CSF can predict Mach bands based on the filtering of the component spatial frequencies present in the stimulus by the human spatial CSF. Similarly, the temporal CSF represents the way in which the visual system filters visual stimuli that flicker at various temporal frequencies: Stimulus frequencies near 8–10 Hz are reduced the least during processing by the visual system, whereas low and high temporal frequencies are relatively more attenuated. Hence, some of the intermediate temporal frequencies in a brief flash of light are more visible to an observer than are other frequencies.

The prediction is that the intermediate temporal frequencies should be the most important frequencies in the detection of the flash at threshold luminance. Cornsweet (1970) showed that when flashes of various durations, all containing an equal number of quanta, are filtered by the temporal CSF, the flashes that are shorter than the t_c all have the same temporal frequency spectrum. In other words, the flashes shorter than the t_c all contain the same information across temporal frequency, and, hence, all should appear equally visible. In comparison to the short flashes, flashes longer than the t_c contain less amplitude at intermediate temporal frequencies after filtering by the temporal CSF and would need more quanta to be visible.

The critical duration decreases as the luminance of a background light or area of the test flash increases

The studies of the temporal summation seen in Bloch's law typically involve measurement of an increment threshold (see Chapter 3): detection of a brief increment flash (a ΔL) presented against a background luminance (L). Bloch's law holds for brief flashes that are detected against a wide range of background luminances. In Figure 7.13, each curve is the threshold flash lumi-

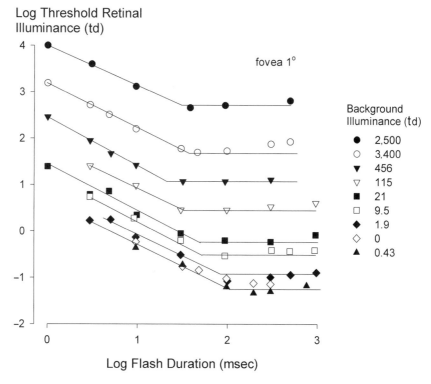

FIGURE 7.13   *Flash threshold illuminance as a function of flash duration for different retinal illuminance values. The stimulus was a 1° diameter circular spot of white light that was imaged at the center of the fovea. In each data set, the critical duration occurs at the point where the downward sloping segment (Bloch's law; slope of –1) intersects the horizontal line segment (no summation). This intersection moves to shorter flash durations as the luminance is increased. (Td = troland.) (Modified from JA Roufs. Dynamic properties of vision. I. Experimental relationships between flicker and flash thresholds. Vision Res 1972;12:261–278.)*

nance plotted against flash duration at a certain level of background luminance. Bloch's law holds over the descending slope of each function; this slope is –1 on the log threshold luminance versus log duration plot, indicating the reciprocity of these variables.

The data in Figure 7.13 tend to follow the model in Figure 7.11 rather well. There is an abrupt transition in the region from where Bloch's law holds to the horizontal region of the curve. Notice, however, that as the background luminance increases, the t_c occurs at progressively shorter durations. When the background luminance is approximately 2 trolands, Bloch's law holds for flashes as long as approximately 100 milliseconds. When the background luminance is approximately 25,000 trolands, Bloch's law only holds for flashes up to approximately 30 milliseconds.

The existence of a shorter t_c at higher background luminance means that the visual system shortens the period over which it sums quantal events in determining the threshold. This is useful because it makes the visual system better able to distinguish when events occur in time. A shorter t_c is indicative of having increased temporal resolution (as was also shown for the CFF). On the other hand, when luminance levels are scotopic, one of the trade-offs that the visual system makes to obtain greater sensitivity is to sacrifice temporal resolution in favor of summing over a longer period.

The t_c also depends on the flash area. As the area of the flash is increased, the t_c decreases. When the stimulus diameter is 1.5–2.0', Bloch's law holds for flash durations up to approximately 100 milliseconds. When the test flash diameter increases to approximately 5°, Bloch's law only holds for flashes up to approximately 30 milliseconds in duration (Roufs & Meulenbrugge 1967).

The brightness of a suprathreshold flash depends on its duration (Broca-Sulzer effect)

Turning from studies that deal with determining the increment threshold (objective measures) to studies that measure the perceived stimulus brightness (subjective measures), one encounters another example of the fact that the brightness of a stimulus is not always predicted by its luminance. The **Broca-Sulzer effect** is just such a phenomenon: The brightness of a suprathreshold flash depends on its duration (Broca & Sulzer 1902). One simple way to demonstrate this effect is to have an observer adjust the luminance of a test flash until its brightness matches that of a continuous light of a fixed luminance. In the range of flash durations of 50–100 milliseconds the adjusted luminance will be at a minimum, meaning that the flash appeared brighter than the continuous light and had to be dimmed to match it. Flash durations shorter and longer than the 50–100 millisecond range produce less brightness enhancement. The effect becomes stronger and the peak brightness occurs at shorter durations with increasing luminance levels (Aiba & Stevens 1964).

A possible neural basis for the Broca-Sulzer effect can be found in the responses of photoreceptors in the monkey and human retina. Individual primate cones elicit a maximum response (largest peak amplitude) when the flash duration is approximately 50 milliseconds (Schnapf et al. 1990), which matches the flash duration that produces the maximal subjective brightness under photopic conditions. As the adaptation state is lowered more toward scotopic levels, maximal brightness occurs for flash durations in the range of 200–400 milliseconds, which also is consistent with the flash duration that elicits a maximal human rod response (300 milliseconds) (Kraft et al. 1993).

Temporal Interactions between Visual Stimuli

The visual thresholds discussed thus far in this chapter have occurred in response to individual stimuli that change in intensity over time. This section deals with the issue of how a stimulus that occurs at one point in time can affect the response to a second stimulus that occurs close to the first in time. Recall that in spatial vision, a perceptual response, such as brightness, is influenced by stimuli that illuminate adjacent areas of the retina. Similarly, the response to a temporally modulated stimulus is not simply dependent on its intensity but also on the effects of preceding and succeeding visual stimuli, as described in the next section.

Masking is any situation in which detection of a test stimulus is reduced by another stimulus presented before, during, or after the test stimulus

The effects of **masking** occur within a time interval measured in milliseconds. Masking effects therefore should be distinguished from adaptation, in which the adapting stimulus exerts an effect on the test threshold over a longer period of time. There are three general stimulus configurations used in masking studies: (1) masking of light by light, (2) masking of a pattern by light, and (3) masking of a pattern by a pattern.

Figure 7.14 illustrates the masking of one light by another light. In this study, the 250 millisecond masking flash was presented once each second, and the brief test flash was presented at a variety of times relative to that onset of the masking light. Over many trials, the luminance needed to see the test flash at threshold was determined. When the test flash was presented approximately 100 milliseconds before the masking flash, the threshold for detecting the test flash was relatively low. When the test flash was presented during the presentation of the masking flash, its detection threshold was elevated by more than 2 log units. This is a basic phenomenon of masking: It is harder to detect the test flash when another stimulus is presented at the same time. Masking that occurs when the test and masking flash are both present is called *simultaneous masking*. Note, however, that the effect of the masking flash is not the same throughout its duration. It produced the most masking during the 100 millisecond period just after it was turned on.

The effects of a masking stimulus may persist after it is turned off and may actually precede its onset

One might expect that the effect of the masking flash on the test flash threshold would end immediately when the masking flash is turned off. This, however, is not the case. As seen in Figure 7.14, the test flash threshold was still elevated after the masking flash had been turned off (from 250 to approximately 500

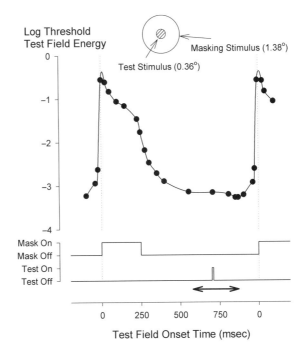

FIGURE 7.14   *Masking of a small (0.36°), 40 millisecond test flash by a larger (1.38°), 250 millisecond high-luminance (50 footlambert) masking flash. The abscissa indicates the onset time of the test flash within the 1 second cycle of masking flashes. The ordinate is the log intensity of the test flash threshold. The last seven data points are the same as the first seven. Backward masking is the rise in threshold just before the masking flash onset, simultaneous masking is the pronounced rise in threshold during the 250 millisecond masking flash presentation, and forward masking is the continued elevation of the test flash threshold for nearly 250 milliseconds after the masking flash is turned off. (Modified from G Sperling. Temporal and spatial visual masking. I. Masking by impulse flashes. J Opt Soc Am 1965;55:541–559.)*

milliseconds on the abscissa). Masking that occurs after the masking flash is turned off is called **forward masking**. Even more interesting is the elevation of the test flash threshold that occurs just before the masking flash is presented (see the data points just to the left of 0 in Figure 7.14); this is called **backward masking**. Backward masking raises the question of how something that occurs later in time can affect something that has already occurred.

Simultaneous and forward masking are signal detection problems

It is not surprising that, when retinal neurons are responding to the high-luminance large masking flash, they have increased difficulty in detecting the small amount of neural activity produced in response to the smaller near-threshold test flash. This is a situation in which a signal must be detected against a background of noise. When there is little noise (no response to the masking flash), the neural signal produced by the test flash is more easily detected. When there are many action potentials occurring in the same retinal neurons, as happens when the test flash and masking flash are superimposed, the few additional potentials produced by the test flash are hard to detect, unless the test flash intensity is raised sufficiently. Indeed, in Figure 7.14, the peak masking effect shortly after the onset of the masking stimulus resembles the overshoot of a photoreceptor response at high flash intensities, which produces a burst of action potentials in ganglion cells.

The explanation for forward masking seems to be the persistence of a neural response to the masking flash after it is turned off. This creates a signal detection situation similar to that which occurs when the test flash is presented while the masking flash is on. The amount of masking is smaller, however, because the neurons are not responding as rapidly to the masking flash, so the "noise" against which the test flash must be detected is less.

Backward masking may be explained by the response latency and duration of the test flash

Backward masking may be accounted for (1) by the duration of the response to a near-threshold test flash, similar to the explanation given for the rise in threshold for detecting a test flash just before the adapting light is turned off (see Chapter 4, Figure 4.10), and (2) by the fact that the response to a near-threshold test flash has a longer latency than the neural response to the intense masking flash. Such latency differences of neural responses are apparent in the early stages of the visual pathway. Thus, by the time the response to the test flash has occurred, the neural response to the higher-intensity masking flash has also occurred and the response to the test flash is again buried in noise.

Masking effects may occur when the test and mask are spatially separated

Metacontrast and **paracontrast** are types of masking in which the test flash and the masking flash do not overlap spatially on the retina. Masking effects—backward in the case of metacontrast and forward with paracontrast—diminish as the spatial separation between the test and mask increases. The distance between the test and masking stimulus cannot be more than 1–3°, or no masking occurs (Alpern 1953). This suggests that the test and masking flash cause masking by activating the same population of retinal or cortical neurons with receptive fields located near each other. With a larger separation between the test and mask, separate populations of neurons are activated, and the test flash signal does not have to compete with the masking flash response to be detected.

A masking stimulus presented to one eye affects detection of a test stimulus at a corresponding retinal location in the other eye

Dichoptic masking occurs when the test flash is presented to one eye and the masking flash is presented to the other eye. For dichoptic masking to occur, the flashes must stimulate *corresponding retinal points* in each eye. These are points on the retinas of the two eyes that are approximately the same distances and directions away from their respective foveas. Consequently, the receptive fields at these points are stimulated by roughly the same image elements. The signals from the cells located at corresponding retinal points converge on binocular cells in the primary visual cortex (V1) that respond to stimulation from both eyes. Because this convergence of signals first occurs in the visual cortex, the masking process must also occur at that level of the visual system.

Masking effects play a role in the decreased sensitivity to visual stimuli that occurs before, during, and after saccadic eye movements (saccadic suppression)

The rapid eye movements that occur when the eyes move voluntarily from one stationary visual target to another, are called *saccadic eye movements*. The eye can move 10–20° in 30–80 milliseconds and can reach peak velocities of 200 degrees per second or more. During such a high-velocity movement, the images of the scene move rapidly across the retina, and, yet, motion is not generally noticed. If one looks in a mirror and tries to observe one's own eye movements, it is not possible to see the eyes move. These phenomena suggest that something interferes with vision during saccades. Indeed, several experiments have confirmed the existence of **saccadic suppression**, defined as a reduction in sensitivity to visual stimuli that occurs before, during and after a saccade.

The retinal image is smeared during a saccade in the same way that a photograph is blurred if the camera is moved during an exposure. Retinal smear due to rapid motion of a scene would be expected to decrease the visibility of high spatial frequencies, but it should enhance the visibility of very low spatial frequencies that are otherwise invisible when stationary (see Chapter 6). However, the main reduction in spatial contrast sensitivity during a saccade is at spatial frequencies less than 1 cycle per degree (Burr et al. 1994). One explanation for this effect is that motion-sensitive mechanisms are selectively suppressed during a saccade, thereby preventing an observer from seeing the world move during the saccade. In other words, the suppression of motion sensitivity serves to stabilize the visual scene during saccadic eye movements. Saccadic suppression may involve extra-retinal signals from the eye-movement control system (corollary discharge or efference copy) that acts selectively on the M visual pathway fairly early in the visual process (Ross et al. 2001).

Visual masking does provide an additional component to saccadic suppression. A stimulus is more difficult to detect when it is superimposed on a rapidly moving background scene, but only if the background is highly patterned (Diamond 2000). The crisp, high-contrast images that are present on the retina just before and after the saccade apparently act to mask detection of the smeared images that occur during the eye movement (Matin et al. 1972; Campbell & Wurtz 1978). Thus, backward and forward masking by a pattern play a role in saccadic suppression.

Motion Detection

Motion is a continuous change in an object's location as a function of time. The ability to sense motion is a fundamental property of all visual systems. Animals can detect moving visual stimuli even if they lack high spatial resolution, color vision, or binocular vision. This ability serves three useful purposes.

First, it enables an animal to detect something moving against a stationary background, for example, a predator or prey. Second, it enables the animal to detect its own motion through the environment. Third, like the ability of the stereoscopic sense of depth perception, the change in object shape with motion allows the visual system to determine the shapes of objects that may otherwise be difficult to detect.

Although motion is a temporal phenomenon and, therefore, appropriate to consider within the context of the temporal characteristics of vision, it really encompasses spatial and temporal interactions. This is because motion, when reduced to its fundamental stimulus elements at any given retinal location, is a change in retinal illuminance that occurs at a rate that is dependent on the speed with which the object moves and its spatial frequency composition. When a stimulus with positive contrast moves past the view of any retinal point, there is a temporary increase in the luminance level at that point. The duration of the increase is related to the size of the object and its velocity. The temporal frequency experienced by a given point on the retina is the product of the velocity of the moving stimulus, in degrees per second, and the spatial frequency, in cycles per degree. For example, a sine-wave grating with a spatial frequency of 30 cycles per degree moving over a retinal point at a constant velocity of 10 degrees per second creates a temporal frequency of 300 cycles per second. A grating with a spatial frequency of 3 cycles per degree moving at the same velocity creates a temporal frequency of 30 cycles per second. A real object that can be decomposed into multiple spatial frequencies (by Fourier analysis; see Chapter 6) creates multiple temporal frequencies when moved at a constant velocity across a retinal point.

The ability to detect motion is limited by the temporal resolution of the visual system

Given a moving stimulus, the psychophysical measurement of interest is the ability to detect that motion is occurring. Figure 7.15A shows the thresholds for stimuli that are moving at different velocities expressed as the contrast sensitivity for detecting the presence of sine-wave gratings of various spatial frequencies that are moving smoothly at the velocities indicated. Stationary gratings give the usual spatial CSF with a cutoff high frequency at approximately 30 cycles per degree, a peak contrast sensitivity at approximately 3 cycles per degree, and a low spatial frequency rolloff. As the grating is moved at increasing velocities, the high spatial frequency cutoff decreases in keeping with the reduced acuity seen with retinal image motion described in Chapter 5. At 800 degrees per second, for instance, the high spatial frequency cutoff is approximately 0.6 cycles per degree. All the CSFs in Figure 7.15A have the familiar shape of the spatial CSF for stationary gratings. All are similar in width (band pass) and have roughly the same peak contrast sensitivity. Increasing the velocity has the effect of moving the CSFs to lower spatial frequencies. In other words, it becomes more difficult to detect higher spatial frequencies as velocity increases.

Figure 7.15B shows the same data transformed by multiplying the spatial frequency by the velocity. For instance, a spatial frequency of 0.06 cycle per degree multiplied by a velocity of 800 degrees per second, yields a temporal frequency of 48 cycles per second. With the exception of the curve for a veloc-

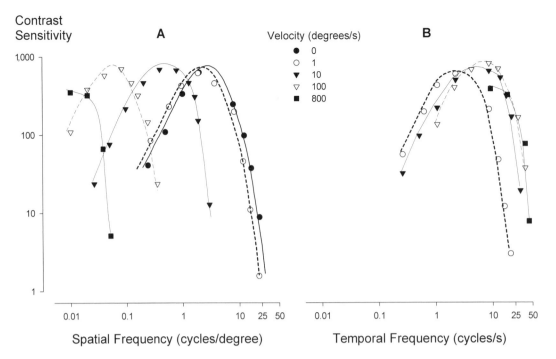

FIGURE 7.15 **A.** *Spatial contrast sensitivity functions for stimuli moving at different velocities.* **B.** *Data from A in which the spatial frequency from A is multiplied by the stimulus velocity to obtain the temporal frequency of the moving stimulus across a single retinal locus. (Modified from D Burr, J Ross. Contrast sensitivity at high velocities. Vision Res 1982;22:479–484.)*

ity of 1.0 degree per second, all of the other temporal CSF curves are nearly coincident when so transformed. The cutoff high temporal frequency is nearly identical for all motion velocities. This means that the temporal CSF (see Figure 7.9) is essentially independent of stimulus velocity. Thus, the limiting factor in motion detection is the temporal resolution of the visual system, not velocity itself. When the stimulus has a low spatial frequency and a high contrast, it is possible to detect motion at several thousand degrees per second.

Direction-selective neurons are responsible for direction-specific adaptation and motion aftereffects

To determine an object's speed and direction of motion, the visual system requires more information than just the temporal luminance modulation at a single retinal point. A mechanism is needed that compares the changing luminance patterns across at least two retinal points. The visual system has solved this problem at the level of the retina and again at higher cortical levels by developing direction-selective cells that respond maximally to stimuli moving in one direction, but weakly or not at all to stimuli moving in the opposite direction (Nakayama 1985).

One consequence of having direction-selective neurons is that the visual system can adapt to constant motion in a particular direction. A moving stimulus can appear to slow down during prolonged viewing, and for a period of time after the adaptation, sensitivity to a low contrast stimulus moving in the adapted direction is impaired. This direction-specific adaptation presumably occurs because the motion-sensitive neurons become fatigued by prolonged stimulation in their preferred direction (Sekuler & Pantle 1967). Another consequence of this adaptation is the **motion aftereffect**: After prolonged viewing of a moving stimulus, a stationary stimulus appears to drift in the opposite direction (Sekuler & Ganz 1963; Pantle 1974). A common example of a motion aftereffect is the **waterfall illusion**: After watching a waterfall for several minutes and then looking away from it, the world seems to drift upward.

Apparent motion is the perception of real motion that can be produced when a stimulus is presented discontinuously

The movement of objects seen on video displays and in motion pictures is **apparent motion**, also called *stroboscopic* or *sampled motion*. In apparent motion, the visual stimulus that creates the perception of smooth motion is produced by sequential presentation of static images that have captured (sampled) real motion at regular intervals.

In its simplest form, apparent motion can be generated with two lights that are slightly displaced from each other and turned on and off alternately. When separated optimally and flashed at an optimal rate, there appears to be one light that moves smoothly across the space between the two positions; this is called the **phi phenomenon**. When strings of lights are flashed in a sequence, as on a movie marquee, the lights appear to move fairly smoothly. Flashing two (or more) lights at any arbitrary combination of time interval and physical separation may or may not produce the phi phenomenon. There are optimal temporal and spatial interval combinations that produce the best appearance of apparent motion of different velocities, as shown in Figure 7.16. For example, to achieve an apparent velocity of 10 degrees per second, the best timing delay between successive flashes is approximately 35 milliseconds, and the optimal distance between the lights is approximately 25'. This is close to the distance (21') in which a real stimulus moving at 10 degrees per second would move during that time. The optimal distances and times for sampled motion tend to lie along curves determined from the peak spatial and temporal frequencies for detecting drifting gratings (Kelly 1979b).

When motion is displayed in a stroboscopic manner, the act of breaking the motion up into snapshots (sampling the motion) introduces more spatial and temporal frequencies to the moving object's frequency spectrum. The additional frequencies would make the apparent motion appear jerky instead of smooth. However, if these additional frequencies are so high that they lie beyond the observer's spatial and temporal frequency cutoffs, the observer will not be able to tell that the motion was sampled—the apparent motion will appear smooth and identical to real motion (Burr et al. 1986; Watson & Ahumada 1985; Watson et al. 1986). Apparent motion will best simulate real motion when, after filtering by the visual system's spatial and temporal CSFs, the information presented by the real and apparent motion is the same.

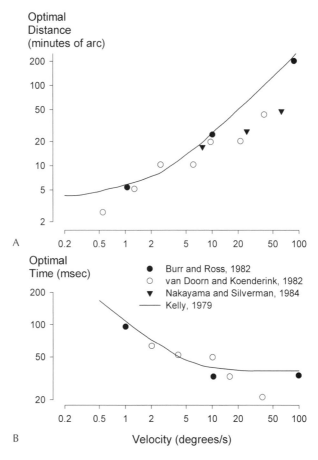

FIGURE 7.16 *Optimal distance (**A**) and optimal time interval (**B**) to achieve a variety of apparent motion velocities. The symbols are from studies of direction discrimination, detection of coherent motion of a random dot display, and maximal distance between dots. The solid lines in each figure are determined from the peak spatial and temporal contrast sensitivity for detection of drifting grating stimuli. (Modified from K Nakayama. Biological image motion processing: a review. Vision Res 1985;25: 625– 660.)*

Detection of motion and sensitivity to direction of motion is achieved in hierarchic fashion in the middle temporal region of the cortex

As mentioned above, there are direction-selective neurons in the retinas of many species. These direction-selective cells respond to a spot that moves in one direction, but not to the same spot when it moves in the other direction. Indeed, they also respond to apparent motion generated by flashed spots, so the phi phenomenon works even at the level of some retinal cells.

In primates, motion detection and the perception of the direction of motion appear to be achieved in the cortex from interactions among neurons in the M and interactions among pathways that are not themselves direction selective as they leave the retina. The processing of motion is hierarchical: Many neurons in the V1 are sensitive to direction, but only to the motion of elongated stimuli that are oriented near the orientation to which the cell is optimally sensitive. If presented with two drifting gratings, each with a slightly different orientation, the perceptual result is that of a plaid stimulus that is drifting in one direction (Marshon et al. 1985). The V1 neurons, however, respond independently to the motion of one of the two gratings.

Some cells in V1 then project to the MT region of the cortex. Neurons in the MT region are specialized to respond to the rate and direction of motion, rather than just the spatial frequency components. MT cells may determine the behavioral threshold for discriminating direction of motion.

A series of studies by Newsome and colleagues (Newsome et al. 1989; Salzman et al. 1992) has found that when an awake monkey performs a motion direction discrimination task, the activity of individual MT neurons correlates well with the monkey's perception of the motion. These investigators first trained a monkey to work for a reward that was presented when the monkey correctly signaled the direction of motion that was presented for a few seconds on a computer monitor display. However, they wanted to do a threshold test of motion detection, so they devised a stimulus consisting of luminous dots that would appear briefly on the monitor panel. During the time that the dots were present on the screen, each dot would move and then disappear to be replaced with another dot somewhere on the panel. As shown on the left side of Figure 7.17, the dots could be programmed to move completely randomly, in which case there is no correlation between the direction of the movement of one dot with the direction of another dot's movement. Alternatively, the dots could be programmed so that they all moved in the same direction. That is, the motion of one dot was 100% correlated with the direction of every other dot's motion (see Figure 7.17, right). The investigators could vary the correlation in the stimulus motion between 0% and 100%. The center panel in Figure 7.17 illustrates 50% correlation.

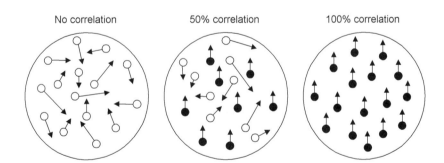

FIGURE 7.17   *Examples of stimuli used by Newsome et al. (1989). Each dot appeared briefly on the monitor, moved in a particular direction, and disappeared. Each dot was then replaced by another dot. If all of the dots always moved in the same direction (**right panel**), the correlation between their motion was considered to be 100%. If the direction of motion of each dot was random in relation to the other dots (**left panel**), correlation was 0%. The center panel shows 50% correlation, where half of the dots are always moving in the same direction at any time. (Modified from CD Salzman, CM Murasugi et al. Microstimulation in visual area MT: effects on direction discrimination performance. J Neurosci 1992;12:2331–2355.)*

The monkeys were trained to signal the direction of motion for high correlation levels at which the direction of motion was clearly visible. Then the correlation was reduced to determine the amount of correlated motion needed at threshold. Many trials were presented using the Method of Constant Stimuli. The resulting psychometric function was obtained, as shown by the filled circles in Figure 7.18B.

The second part of their study was designed to examine the threshold of neurons in the MT region for detecting motion with the same stimulus. While a monkey was working at this task, a single MT neuron's activity was sampled by a microelectrode placed in the cortex next to the cell. The investigators found the neuron's preferred direction and velocity using stimuli with high levels of motion correlation. They then presented trials in which the stimulus contained several levels of correlated motion and recorded how many action potentials the neuron produced when the stimulus was presented (1) in the preferred direction of motion and (2) in the opposite direction.

As shown in the top panel of Figure 7.18A, with 12.8% correlation and movement in the preferred direction, the neuron would sometimes produce more than 100 action potentials (spikes per trial) in response to the stimulus. On other trials it could produce as few as 44 action potentials per stimulus trial. Recall from Chapter 1 (see Chapter 1, Figure 1.3) that there usually is variability in the neuronal responses, even when the same stimulus is presented repeatedly. However, it is clear from the figure that the neuron generally produced more spikes per trial when the motion was primarily in the cell's preferred direction than when the motion was primarily in the opposite direction.

As the amount of correlation in the dots' motion decreased (see the center and bottom panels of Figure 7.18A), the responses of the neuron to motion in the preferred direction and the opposite direction became more similar. Using signal detection theory (see Chapter 1), the investigators constructed a receiver operating characteristic curve (see Chapter 1) and determined the optimal criterion that could be used to maximize the number of correct responses and minimize the number of false alarms. From this, they calculated the number of trials on which the neuron would correctly detect the direction of motion. When this was repeated for a variety of levels of motion correlation, a **neurometric function** could be plotted (see the open circles in Figure 7.18B).

The neurometric function for the neuron shown in Figure 7.18B corresponded closely to the psychometric function that was produced by the monkey at the same time that the neuron's responses were being sampled. In this case, the threshold amount of motion correlation (they set 82% correct as threshold) needed by the neuron was 4.4% for the neuron and 6.1% for the monkey.

The investigators compared the motion detection thresholds of 60 MT neurons with the behavioral thresholds in two monkeys by taking the ratios of the neurometric and psychometric functions shown in Figure 7.18B at threshold. Figure 7.19 shows the numbers of neurons at each ratio. The mode of the distribution is at 1.0, indicating that the neurometric and psychometric thresholds were equal. Some neurons had lower thresholds than the monkey in which they resided, and a few had higher thresholds.

It is not known whether these neurons are actually the ones that cause the monkey to detect the direction of motion because there could be neurons in

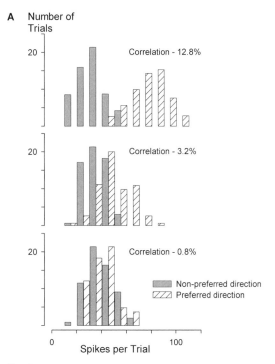

A Number of Trials

Correlation - 12.8%

20

Correlation - 3.2%

20

Correlation - 0.8%

20

■ Non-preferred direction
▨ Preferred direction

0   100

Spikes per Trial

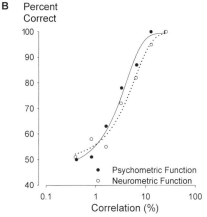

B Percent Correct

100

90

80

70

60

50

40

0.1   1   10   100

Correlation (%)

● Psychometric Function
○ Neurometric Function

FIGURE 7.18   *Psychophysical and neurophysiological data obtained simultaneously from a rhesus monkey. **A.** The responses of a neuron in the middle temporal (MT) area to three different amounts of motion correlation. The hatched bars represent the number of action potentials produced by the neuron on 60 trials with motion in the neuron's preferred direction. Solid bars are the responses on 60 trials with motion opposite to the preferred direction. **B.** Comparison of the monkey's psychometric function for detecting the direction of motion, as a function of the amount of motion correlation (filled circles) with the neurometric function (open circles) derived from the neurons' responses. (Modified from WT Newsome, KH Britten, JA Movshon. Neuronal correlates of a perceptual decision. Nature 1989;341:52–54.)*

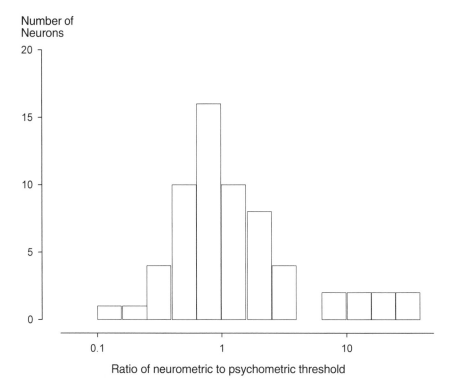

Number of
Neurons

Ratio of neurometric to psychometric threshold

FIGURE 7.19 *Comparison of the psychophysical and neurophysiological thresholds for 60 middle temporal neurons recorded in two monkeys. The histogram shows the ratio of the threshold of the neurons to the monkeys' thresholds. A value of 1 indicates that a neuron and the monkey had the same threshold. Values greater than 1 indicate that the neuron had a higher threshold than the monkey. Values less than 1 indicate that the monkey had a lower threshold than the neuron. (Modified from WT Newsome, KH Britten, JA Movshon. Neuronal correlates of a perceptual decision. Nature 1989;341:52–54.)*

other brain areas with similar thresholds. It is clear, however, that they could provide the information that the monkey needs to detect the motion. These results not only further an understanding of motion processing but also provide a better understanding of the link between neuronal activity and visual perception.

Study Guide

1. What happens when visual stimuli are held stationary on the retina?
2. What is the CFF and how is it determined?
3. Define duty cycle.
4. If the duty cycle is 1:5, what is the value of *f*?
5. Know the Talbot-Plateau law and how to compute the Talbot brightness.
6. Write the Ferry-Porter law.
7. Write the Granit-Harper law.

8. What is the Brücke-Bartley phenomenon, and how is it similar to the Broca-Sulzer effect?
9. What is the definition of contrast for the temporal CSF?
10. Be able to draw and label a "typical" human temporal CSF with approximate values for cutoff high frequency and peak sensitivity.
11. Explain how the difference in latency of the receptive-field center and surround can explain the low temporal frequency rolloff in a cell's temporal CSF.
12. Describe how the human temporal CSF changes as a function of the mean stimulus luminance.
13. Explain the way in which the cutoff high temporal frequency is like the CFF. Compare this to the relationship between spatial resolution acuity and the spatial CSF.
14. What is the Troxler effect, and how is it related to stationary images on the retina?
15. Write Bloch's law.
16. What is meant by the term critical duration (t_c)?
17. What is the retina "counting" during a flash that is shorter than the t_c?
18. Give the approximate range of values of the t_c.
19. How is the t_c affected by background luminance?
20. How is the t_c affected by stimulus diameter?
21. Define and explain the Broca-Sulzer effect.
22. What is the probable neural basis for the Broca-Sulzer effect?
23. Define masking.
24. What is forward masking, and what is a plausible neural explanation?
25. What is backward masking, and what is a plausible neural explanation for how the masking flash "catches up" with the test flash?
26. What is metacontrast, and what is a plausible neural explanation for this phenomenon?
27. What is dichoptic masking, and what is a plausible neural explanation for its existence?
28. Explain why the ability to detect motion is limited by the temporal resolution of the visual system.
29. What is the phi phenomenon?
30. How does one construct a neurometric function?
31. Is it reasonable that some neurons have a lower threshold than the monkey in which they reside? Why or why not?

Glossary

Amplitude (of square-wave or sine-wave flicker): $L_{max} - L_m$

Apparent motion (also called *stroboscopic motion* or *sampled motion*): the perception of a moving visual stimulus that is produced by sequential presentation of stationary visual stimuli.

Backward masking: masking that occurs when the test flash is presented before the masking flash is turned on.

Band pass shape: having higher contrast sensitivity in an intermediate frequency range with lower sensitivity at higher and lower frequencies.

Bloch's law: $L \times t = C$, where L is the threshold luminance of the flash, t is its duration, and C is a constant.

Broca-Sulzer effect: a short-duration (approximately 50 milliseconds) supra-threshold flash can appear brighter than a longer or shorter flash of the same physical intensity.

Brücke-Bartley phenomenon: brightness enhancement in which a flickering stimulus appears brighter than the Talbot brightness at flicker frequencies below the CFF.

Contrast (for square-wave or sine-wave flicker): $(L_{max} - L_{min})/(L_{max} + L_{min})$

Critical duration (t_c): the longest flash duration for which Bloch's law holds.

Critical flicker frequency (CFF): the flicker frequency at which the stimulus is detected as flickering 50% of the time and as fused (steady) 50% of the time.

Cutoff high temporal frequency: the temporal frequency at which flicker cannot be resolved when the contrast is 1; the limit of temporal acuity.

Dichoptic masking: masking that occurs when the test flash and the masking flash are presented to separate eyes.

Duty cycle: the ratio of the time that a temporal square-wave pattern is at L_{max} to the time that it is at L_{min}.

Episcotister: a rotating sectored disk used to produce square-wave flickering stimuli.

Ferry-Porter law: $CFF = k\log L + b$, where k is the slope of the function, b is a constant, and L is the luminance of the flickering stimulus.

Flicker rate (or **flicker frequency**): the number of light-dark cycles per second of a flickering stimulus.

Flicker sensitivity: the reciprocal of the threshold luminance necessary to detect that a flickering stimulus is flickering rather than steady.

Forward masking: masking that occurs when the test flash is presented after the masking flash is turned off.

Granit-Harper law: $CFF = k\log A + b$, where k and b are constants, and A is the area of the flickering stimulus.

Low frequency rolloff: the reduction in contrast sensitivity at low frequencies.

Masking: any situation in which the detection of a visual test stimulus is reduced by another visual stimulus presented before, during, or after the test stimulus.

Metacontrast and **paracontrast:** masking in which the test flash and the masking flash do not overlap spatially on the retina. Metacontrast involves backward masking, whereas paracontrast involves forward masking.

Modulation ratio (m): $(L_{max} - L_m)/L_m$ (numerically equal to Michelson contrast).

Motion: a change in an object's location as a function of time.

Motion aftereffect: after prolonged viewing of a stimulus moving in one direction, a stationary stimulus appears to drift in the opposite direction.

Neurometric function: a function plotting the probability that a neuron can correctly detect a stimulus as a function of some stimulus parameter.

Peak contrast sensitivity: the frequency at which the highest contrast sensitivity occurs in a CSF.

Period: the length of time for one complete cycle of light and dark of a flickering stimulus.

Phi phenomenon: apparent motion that occurs when two dots that are slightly displaced from each other are turned on and off alternately.

Saccadic suppression: a reduction in sensitivity to visual stimuli that occurs before, during, and after a saccade.

Talbot brightness: $L_{min} + ([L_{max} - L_{min}] \times f)$, where f is the fraction of time that L_{max} is present during the total period.

Talbot-Plateau law: the brightness of a fused flickering stimulus is equal to the brightness of a steady stimulus with the same time-averaged luminance.

Temporal acuity: the minimum temporal interval that can be resolved by the visual system.

Temporal summation: the adding together of events that occur at different times.

Waterfall illusion: an example of a motion aftereffect: after watching a waterfall for several minutes and then looking away from it, the world seems to drift upwards.

8   Color Vision

Wayne A. Verdon and Anthony J. Adams

For the Rays to speak properly are not coloured. In them is nothing else than a certain Power and Disposition to stir up a Sensation of this or that Colour.

Sir Isaac Newton, 1730

Overview

In previous chapters, the wavelength of light was either set at a particular value during the measurement of a visual function or varied to test for its effects on a visual function. In these cases either a single wavelength or a mixture of wavelengths was used. The wavelength composition of light produces the perception of color, which is very useful for detecting or distinguishing objects. Hundreds of thousands of different color sensations are possible due to the presence of just three types of cones in the human retina and the color opponent neural pathways to the visual cortex. The cone types differ in the light absorbing photopigment they contain, thus creating short-wavelength sensitive (SWS), middle-wavelength sensitive (MWS), and long-wavelength sensitive (LWS) receptors. At least two photopigment types are required to distinguish at least some colors instead of seeing only in shades of gray. At least three photopigments are required to distinguish the full spectrum of colors. People with an inherited color defect have either an alteration of one pigment (anomalous trichromats) or the absence of one or two pigments (dichromats and monochromats).

Color matching is a fundamental psychophysical measurement of visual function. Any monochromatic, spectral color can be matched by a mixture of three primary colors in color-normal individuals. These primaries do not need to match the peak sensitivities of the three cone types. These matches remain stable over a variety of conditions. The use of a standard set of primaries, along with a standard psychophysical method, provides the basis for specifying any color, including mixtures of wavelengths, using only two coordinates of an internationally recognized chromaticity diagram. The color-matching performance of individuals with color defects can also be mapped on the chromaticity diagram and used to design color vision tests that are specific to the various color defects.

Color matching can be done without consideration of the subjective appearance of a color. The perceptual visual functions of color naming and color ordering can also be measured and specified psychophysically. The subjective appearance of a color can be specified in terms of its hue, brightness, and saturation or in terms of its hue, value (analogous to brightness), and chroma (analogous to saturation) as are used in the Munsell color naming system. When measured psychophysically, the appearance of the hue and saturation of a color depend to a small extent on stimulus luminance (the Bezold-Brücke effect), hue varies somewhat with saturation, hue varies with the color composition of the background against which it is viewed (simultaneous contrast), and hue shifts occur in time when different colors are presented sequentially (successive contrast). Nevertheless, colors seem to be reasonably constant under a variety of lighting conditions in normal viewing.

Threshold measurements indicate that humans can distinguish monochromatic colors of equal luminance with wavelength differences of as little as 1 nm in the middle of the visible spectrum, and as little as 6–7 nm at its limits. The amount of a monochromatic light that has to be added to white before color can be detected is the smallest at about 570 nm and increases with longer and shorter wavelengths.

The existence of opponent color mechanisms was proposed on the basis of the observation that reddish-green or bluish-yellow hues are never observed. Quantitative measurements of hue cancellation at wavelengths across the visible spectrum confirm that there are red-green and blue-yellow opponent mechanisms. Color naming using the technique of magnitude estimation confirms the existence of these mechanisms.

Zone models of color vision based on the existence of trichromatic mechanisms at the photoreceptor level and opponent color processing at various levels in the visual pathway after the photoreceptors have been very successful in accounting for much color vision data. Parallel pathways that begin in the retina carry luminance information (the magnocellular pathway) and color opponent information (the parvocellular pathway). The processing characteristics of these pathways can be distinctly identified in the lateral geniculate nucleus and the primary visual cortex, though some convergence of function can be seen in the cortex.

Although color deficiencies can occur as a result of disease processes, they are most often inherited as an X-linked recessive trait affecting cone photopigments. The absorption spectrum of one of the three photopigments may be altered, or one or two pigments may be entirely absent. Each of these variations, when viewed in the context of the trichromatic and opponent mechanisms, produces predictable results on psychophysical tests of color matching, color confusions, color naming, and color ordering. These are the foundation of diagnostic tests for inherited and acquired color deficiencies.

Humans have the ability to distinguish hundreds of thousands of colors

Previous chapters have dealt with measures of photopic and scotopic vision, some of which included light of differing wavelengths, but have not dealt specifically with **color vision**. Wavelength information provides important cues for detecting objects that may be important for survival or competitive advantage. Examples include distinguishing between ripe and unripe food, identifying one's mate or offspring, and detecting predators. In addition to its utility, color vision enriches life and adds immeasurable beauty, such as the experience of a vivid sunset or the fantastic use of color in impressionist paintings.

Human color vision, like vision in general, is effortless and because of the private nature of individual perceptions, it is perhaps not intuitively obvious how one can even study the phenomenon of color vision. How does one quantitatively compare his or her own color vision with that of a colleague? The goals of this chapter are to show that there are indeed meaningful ways to measure color vision and to provide a framework to understand normal and defective color vision. Along the way, the neural machinery involved in color vision is described, and it is shown how psychophysical measures are used to determine the ability of people to identify or discriminate between different colors. The essence of what makes a surface appear as one color and not another is explained, along with how colors may be specified such that an individual may create a match to any color by a mixture of other colors. The nature of color vision deficiencies (color defective or colorblind) and the psychophysical basis of the clinical tests used to identify them are discussed.

From Photopigments to Trichromatic Vision

The visible spectrum is the small segment of the entire spectrum of electromagnetic radiation to which the eye is sensitive

As described in the Appendix, electromagnetic radiation may be specified by its wavelength. Quanta with wavelengths in the range of approximately 400–700 nanometers (nm) are absorbed by photopigments and can be seen. Color Plate 8.1 represents the wavelengths that can be detected by the normal human visual system: the visible electromagnetic spectrum. **Monochromatic** light* in the visible spectrum produces colors called **spectral colors** or **spectral lights**.

Color processing begins with light absorption by a cone photopigment

The cone photoreceptors of the human retina are the initial neural elements in color processing. Each cone contains millions of molecules of light-absorbing photopigment, but within a single cone, all of the photopigment molecules are the same. There are, in general, three classes of cone photopigments and, therefore, three classes of cones. Each cone class has a characteristic **spectral sensitivity**, which means that each of the three classes of photopigments absorbs light with a different range of wavelengths and with maximum efficiency at a particular wavelength.

One photopigment absorbs maximally at short wavelengths (peak absorption at approximately 425 nm), and the cones containing it are called *SWS cones*. SWS is shorthand for short-wavelength sensitive. Another photopigment absorbs maximally in the middle wavelengths (approximately 530 nm), and the cones are called *MWS cones*. The third photopigment absorbs maximally at somewhat longer wavelengths (approximately 560 nm) and is found in the LWS cones. Historically, these cone classes also have been called *blue* (SWS), *green* (MWS), and *red* (LWS).[†] However, as may be seen by comparing Figures 8.1 and 8.2 with Color Plate 8.1, LWS cones absorb maximally at a wavelength that would be called *yellow-green* by people with normal color vision; wavelengths in this region of the spectrum certainly do not appear as red to people with normal color vision. Therefore, calling photopigments by color names—red, green, or blue—is an unfortunate practice. Furthermore, assigning a color name to a cone type leads to much confusion by surreptitiously leading one to the incorrect but intuitively appealing notion that green cones signal green light, red cones signal red light, and so on. This is a trap. Avoid it!

---

*Technically, monochromatic light is specified as a single wavelength, but in practice, it consists of a narrow band of wavelengths usually less than 5 nm wide.
[†]These are sometimes abbreviated as S, M, and L.

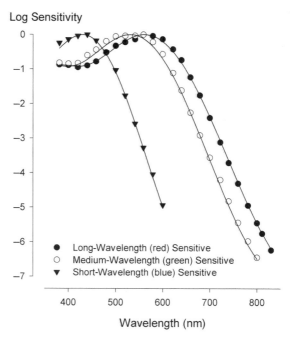

FIGURE 8.1 *Macaque monkey long-wavelength sensitive, medium-wavelength sensitive, and short-wavelength sensitive cone spectral sensitivities (action spectra) measured by the suction electrode technique. (Modified from DA Baylor, BJ Nunn, JL Schnapf. Spectral sensitivity of cones of the monkey Macaca fascicularis. J Physiol [Lond] 1987; 390:145–160.)*

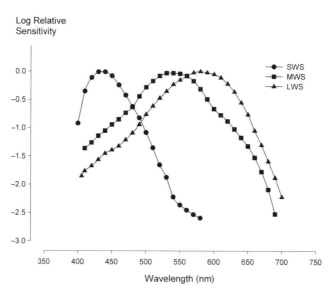

FIGURE 8.2 *Spectral sensitivities of the three cone types measured in two subjects by using a psychophysical technique that uses selective chromatic adaptation. See text for details. (LWS = long-wavelength sensitive; MWS = middle-wavelength sensitive; SWS = short-wavelength sensitive.) (Modified from G Wald. The receptors of human color vision. Science 1964;145:1007–1016.)*

Individual cone spectral sensitivity can be measured using a suction electrode technique

The spectral sensitivity of MWS, LWS, and SWS cones from macaque monkey are shown in Figure 8.1. The data were recorded from isolated cones, using a suction electrode technique. The retina of a freshly excised eye was dissected and an individual cone outer segment was gently sucked into a micropipette that served as an electrode. The electrode recorded membrane currents that were amplified electronically and measured. The outer segment was illuminated with monochromatic light at various wavelengths across the visible spectrum. At each wavelength, the intensity of radiation was altered until a criterion current was recorded. This form of threshold measurement produced a curve known as an **action spectrum**. In Figure 8.1, the action spectrum is shown as a measure of sensitivity (inverse of the intensity needed to produce a criterion change in membrane potential by the photoreceptor). It is clear that MWS and LWS cones respond to light over almost the entire visible spectrum. In addition, at very short wavelengths, both cone types have approximately equal sensitivity and have the same sensitivity in the ultraviolet range (wavelengths shorter than 400 nm). The peak sensitivity of these cones lies close to 530 nm (MWS) and 560 nm (LWS). This is because the **cone opsins** of the photopigments determine which wavelengths are absorbed most efficiently. The absorption spectrum for the SWS cones is shifted toward shorter wavelengths. Although macaque monkey data are shown, the curves for human cones are almost identical (Schnapf et al. 1987).

There are fewer short-wavelength sensitive cones than long-wavelength sensitive and middle-wavelength sensitive cones

The distribution and population of SWS cones are significantly different from those of the LWS and MWS cones. SWS cones comprise only approximately 6–7% of the total cone population. There are twice as many LWS cones as MWS cones in a normal trichromatic retina, giving cone ratios of approximately 10 LWS to 5 MWS to 1 SWS. There may be considerable individual variations in the LWS-to-MWS ratio. Furthermore, although the highest density of LWS and MWS cones is at the center of the foveola, SWS cones are absent from the central 20' (roughly 100 μm). This area is approximately the size of a 20/80 letter on the retina. The highest density of SWS cones is at 1° eccentricity, and beyond 5°, the SWS cone density remains constant at a little less than 1,000 per mm^2.

A possible reason for the absence of SWS cones at the central foveola is to allow optimal packing of LWS and MWS cone types, which might enhance visual acuity or other visual functions. Normal color vision with very small, centrally fixated stimuli is **tritanopic**, because SWS cones are locally absent, and the paucity of SWS cones helps explain the lower absolute sensitivity of the SWS-cone pathway compared to the LWS and MWS pathways.

The optical density of a cone's photopigment can affect its spectral sensitivity function

The spectral sensitivity of a cone type depends not only on the absorption curve of its photopigment (determined by the precise amino acid sequence of each cone opsin), but also on the optical density* of the photopigment in the light path. This, in turn, is dependent on both the concentration of unbleached photopigment and the length of the light path through it. Imagine an extreme example in which a cone outer segment is many centimeters long instead of tens of micrometers. A quantum traveling down such an outer segment would encounter a huge number of pigment molecules, thereby increasing its absorption probability, even if the wavelength of the quantum placed it on the portion of the absorption spectrum where the absorption probability ordinarily would be low. Thus, as a photopigment's optical density increases, the spectral sensitivity function for the cone that contains the photopigment becomes flatter. Normally, the optical density of a cone at the wavelength of peak sensitivity is only approximately 0.3. That means that only one out of every two quanta is absorbed by photopigment at the peak wavelength. At all other wavelengths, the absorption of quanta is less. To the extent that there are hereditary variations, or variations from other causes in the optical density of cone pigments across people, there may be subtle differences in normal color vision.

Chromatic adaptation techniques yield psychophysical measures of the three cone spectral sensitivity functions

Figure 8.2 shows the spectral sensitivity of the three cone types measured in a human subject using the psychophysical technique of selective **chromatic adaptation** (Wald 1964). Nobel laureate George Wald was one of the first scientists to employ this technique to study cone spectral sensitivity. The principle behind chromatic adaptation was described in Chapter 4: It is possible to use long wavelength (red) light to light adapt cones while having little effect on rods. Similarly, by carefully choosing the wavelengths of an adapting stimulus, it also is possible to selectively light-adapt two cone types, thereby decreasing their sensitivity, while leaving the remaining cone type relatively more sensitive.

The ordinate in Figure 8.2 plots the normalized sensitivity of the subject (the inverse of the intensity of radiation incident on the cornea required for a threshold response) as a function of wavelength. Though it involves a lot more neural processing, the threshold determined psychophysically can be considered to be analogous to the criterion photocurrent response in the suction electrode technique described above.

---

*Optical density is log (1/**Transmittance**).

As was shown in Figure 8.1, the cone spectral sensitivity curves overlap across much of the visible spectrum. This means that light at any single wavelength will stimulate more than one cone simultaneously, but one cone class will be more strongly stimulated than the others. For example, to measure the spectral sensitivity of the SWS cones, a subject was chromatically adapted with an intense adapting background field containing all wavelengths longer than 550 nm. The LWS and MWS cones absorb more of the incident quanta in this spectral region than the SWS cones, so they became light adapted and their sensitivity was reduced. Because the SWS cones absorb fewer quanta at these wavelengths, they retain high sensitivity to test flashes with short wavelengths. Thus, when the psychophysical threshold for detecting the presence of a test flash was measured using wavelengths in the range of 400–580 nm (as in Figure 8.2), the SWS cones had the lowest threshold. The resulting curve is thus a plot of their sensitivity.

To measure the spectral sensitivity of LWS cones, a blue-green (or cyan) adapting light containing wavelengths in the range of approximately 430–530 nm was used. This differentially reduced the sensitivity of the SWS and MWS cones relative to the LWS cones. To measure the spectral sensitivity of MWS cones, the adapting light was composed of both wavelengths longer than 645 nm that adapt the LWS cones and of wavelengths shorter than 462 nm to adapt the SWS cones.

Additional estimates of the spectral sensitivities of the three cone classes have been obtained from people who are missing one of the cone classes. In such people, the task of using chromatic adaptation to reduce the sensitivity of one of the other cone classes is made easier because there is less overlap.

The psychophysical spectral sensitivity curves of MWS and LWS cones in Figure 8.2 are a reasonable approximation to the cone spectral sensitivities seen in Figure 8.1. The differences in the exact shape of the curves between the two figures reflect the difficulty, in the intact human subjects, of producing threshold responses that are exclusively determined by a single cone type over a wide range of wavelengths. The spectral transmittance of the preretinal ocular media and nonphotosensitive pigments in the retina also plays a role when psychophysical measures are made in human subjects. Nonetheless, use of this procedure has clearly established the presence of three classes of cones in humans.

Events following light absorption in a photoreceptor are independent of the wavelength of the quantum absorbed (the principle of univariance)

Once the **chromophore** of a photopigment molecule is isomerized by absorption, all subsequent events proceed in an identical manner regardless of the wavelength of the quantum that was absorbed. In other words, all single photopigments and, therefore, the cones in which they reside, are wavelength blind in the sense that they cannot distinguish between quanta of different wavelengths. It is the probability that a quantum may isomerize the chromophore of a photopigment molecule that changes with the wavelength of the quantum. Thus, a photopigment absorption curve, or spectral sensitivity function of a cone, is best thought of as a probability curve because it measures the probability that a quantum may be absorbed as a function of its wavelength. If individual cones cannot code for wavelength, other processes beyond the photoreceptors must be responsible for the varied sensations of human color vision as described later in this chapter. Nonetheless, the nature of cone photopigments influence many functions of color vision, including how colors are specified and the perceptual appearance of mixtures of wavelengths.

A person with only one photopigment cannot discriminate between lights on the basis of wavelength

In a trichromat, each wavelength in the visible spectrum produces a unique level of activation of each of the three cone classes. Through the neural connections of the retina and central structures, this produces a unique sensation of color that appears different from the sensation produced by any other single wavelength (except that wavelengths very close to each other may be difficult to distinguish). This section and the following sections show why three cone types are needed for this to occur.*

Consider the situation that would occur if a person had only one type of photopigment (pigment A) in all the retinal photoreceptors, and such a person was presented with a bipartite field such as is shown in the top of Figure 8.3. This stimulus traditionally is used to test **color matching** (or **color discrimination**) and consists of a foveally viewed 2° diameter field. On the left half of the field is a monochromatic reference light of a fixed wavelength and intensity. On the right half of the field is a test stimulus of monochromatic light whose wavelength and intensity can be changed. When any particular test wavelength is presented, the subject adjusts the intensity of the test stimulus in an attempt to match it to the reference. In the top of Figure 8.3, the reference is a 500 nm light. The subject's task is to adjust the intensity of a 520 nm light on the right to make it match the reference stimulus.

The key to understanding whether the subject achieves a match is to apply the univariance principle: Quanta of all wavelengths, once absorbed, have identical effects on a cone. In the case of a person with only one cone type, this means that if two lights produce the same number of photopigment isomerizations in the cone type, regardless of whether the lights contain many wavelengths or only one, the lights are indistinguishable. To demonstrate how this principle works, the bottom part of Figure 8.3 shows two identical photopigment absorption spectra for photopigment A. These are hypothetical action spectra designed for ease of calculation, with the y-axis expressed in terms of the fraction (f) of incident quanta absorbed. There are two copies of the spec-

---

*The description here follows the logic in Cornsweet 1970.

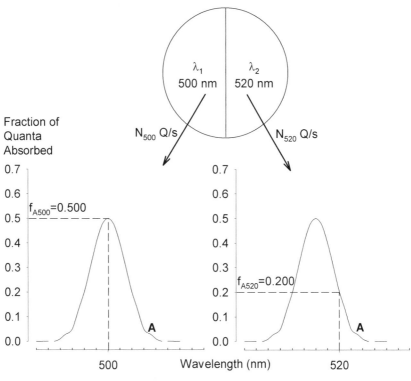

FIGURE 8.3 **Top.** *Representation of a typical bipartite field that can be used for psy-chophysical studies of color matching or color discrimination. The left (reference) hemi-field displays light of fixed wavelength (λ_1 = 500 nm) and intensity (N = 1,000 quanta [Q], per second). The right (test) hemifield displays light of a different, fixed wavelength (λ_2 = 520 nm) and variable intensity. The subject's task is to adjust the intensity of the test stimulus until it matches the reference hemifield.* **Bottom.** *Two representations of an absorption spectrum of a hypothetical photopigment A, expressed as the fraction of quanta absorbed (f) at different wavelengths. The dashed lines show the fractions of quanta absorbed by the photopigment at the reference wavelength (**left**) and the test wavelength (**right**).*

trum to make the point that the two halves of the bipartite field are stimulating two different parts of the retina, each containing cones with the same photo-pigment.

Suppose that the lights from the two hemifields have identical outputs of 1,000 quanta per second, that is, $N_1 = N_2 = 1,000$ (where N is the number of incident quanta per second). The number of quanta per second absorbed for the reference wavelength (where f is 0.5) would be $1,000 \times 0.5 = 500$. For the test wavelength, (where f is 0.2) $1,000 \times 0.2 = 200$ quanta per second would be absorbed, as shown in Table 8.1.

It is easy to see that, to achieve a match to the reference, it is necessary for the subject to increase the number of quanta per second produced by the test (520 nm) hemifield by a factor of 2.5, so that 500 quanta per second are absorbed. Therefore, 2,500 quanta per second at a wavelength of 520 nm match 1,000 quanta per second at a wavelength of 500 nm in this example.

Table 8.1 Quantal absorptions by a single photopigment at different wavelengths

Hemifield	Reference	Test
Wavelength	500 nm	520 nm
Incident quanta/sec (N)	1,000	1,000
Fraction (f) absorbed by pigment A	0.5	0.2
Total quanta/sec absorbed by pigment A	**500**	**200**

Suppose that a second wavelength, say 485 nm, was then added to the right hemifield. According to the absorption spectrum, the photopigment absorbs 30% of the incident quanta at that wavelength. The combination of the two wavelengths (485 nm and 520 nm) could be adjusted to match the left hemifield by setting the 520 nm light to 1,000 quanta per second and the 485 nm light to 1,000 quanta per second, because the sum of the quanta per second absorbed by these two wavelengths would be 500.

To summarize, the two hemifields appear perceptually indistinguishable when they produce identical effects on the visual system at the photoreceptor level. If the two fields are perceptually identical, but they have different **spectral compositions**, as in the previous two examples, the fields are known as **metamers**, and the match therefore is called a *metameric match*. If the hemifields are physically identical (contain the identical wavelengths), they are called **isomers**. In the previous hypothetical example, all single wavelengths and all combinations of wavelengths would be metameric matches to the 500 nm reference if their intensity were adjusted appropriately. Similarly, if any other wavelength were chosen as a reference, the intensity of all other wavelengths could be adjusted to produce a match. For instance, if 520 nm with an N of 1,000 quanta per second were chosen as the reference stimulus, a metameric match at 500 nm would be achieved with an N of 400 quanta per second.

Although the example used here has been hypothetical, it does have a basis in reality. As described in Chapter 3, there are individuals, called *rod monochromats*, who have normally functioning rod receptors but completely lack functional cone vision. Because they possess only one functional photopigment, rhodopsin, they are totally color blind. Objects in the world appear to be varying intensities of gray, similar to the view on a black and white television. In principle, true **color blindness** results whenever there is a single photopigment operating regardless of its spectral sensitivity, even a single cone photopigment. For instance, a SWS-cone monochromat who is light adapted, so that the rods are saturated, views the world with one cone photopigment. All wavelengths appear the same color, differing only in brightness.

Color matching with a bipartite field is a good way of determining whether an individual is able to discriminate lights based on their wavelength composition alone, because the subject is never asked which colors are seen. The sub-

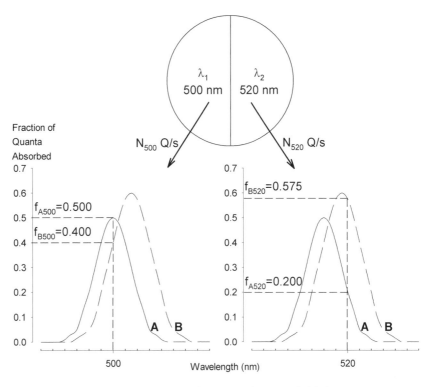

FIGURE 8.4   **Top.** *Representation of the same bipartite field shown in Figure 3.3.* **Bottom.** *Two representations of the absorption spectra of two hypothetical photopigments (A and B), expressed as the fraction (f) of quanta absorbed versus wavelength. The dashed lines show the fractions of quanta absorbed by the photopigments at the wavelengths presented in the two hemifields. (λ = wavelength; N = number of incident quanta per second; Q = quanta.)*

ject's response is limited to either "the hemifields match" or "the hemifields do not match." However, this technique provides little information about how colors appear to the subject.

A person with two photopigments with overlapping absorption spectra is capable of wavelength discrimination

The bipartite stimulus and the photopigment absorption functions for another hypothetical subject, this one with two photopigments (A and B), is shown in Figure 8.4. The stimulus arrangement is the same as that in Figure 8.3. The bottom of the figure now shows two overlapping absorption spectra. These have their absorption peaks at different wavelengths and also absorb different fractions of incident quanta at their peaks. Notice that on the fixed reference side the vertical line at 500 nm now intersects each spectrum at different fractions (A, $f = 0.5$; B, $f = 0.4$). The vertical line at 520 nm also intersects the two spectra at different values (A, $f = 0.2$; B, $f = 0.575$).

Table 8.2   Quantal absorptions by two photopigments at different wavelengths

Hemifield	Reference	Test
Wavelength	500 nm	520 nm
Incident quanta/sec (N)	1,000	1,000
Fraction (f) absorbed by pigment A	0.5	0.2
Total quanta/sec absorbed by pigment A	**500**	**200**
Fraction (f) absorbed by pigment B	0.4	0.575
Total quanta/sec absorbed by pigment B	**400**	**575**

Suppose that, initially, both sides of the bipartite field are set to intensities of 1,000 quanta per second. Table 8.2 shows the results of the simple calculations. For the two hemifields to match, it is necessary to have equal numbers of quanta per second absorbed by both pigments at the test wavelength and the reference wavelength. It is clear from the table that for pigment A, 500 is greater than 200, and for pigment B, 400 is less than 575. At this test wavelength and at this intensity, there is not a match to the reference wavelength. Can they be made to match? Recall that in the example with one photopigment, the sides matched when the intensity of the 520 nm light was increased to 2,500 quanta per second. Table 8.3 shows what happens if that adjustment is made in this case. The total quanta per second absorbed by pigment A is equal on both sides, as expected, but the difference in the total quanta per second absorbed by pigment B is even larger. It should be easy to see that there is no one intensity of the 520 nm light that simultaneously produces absorptions of 500 and 400 quanta per second. If, for example, the intensity of the 520 nm light was adjusted to 695 quanta per second to produce an absorption of 400 quanta per second in pigment B, pigment A would only absorb 139 quanta per second. Thus, in this situation with two overlapping absorption spectra, the subject cannot produce a match of the 520 nm test stimulus to the reference stimulus. It always appears different in some regard. If asked, the subject most likely says that the two hemifields differ in their color. Thus, subjects are capable of distinguishing the test stimulus from the reference stimulus based on the wavelength. In other words, **wavelength discrimination** is possible with two photopigments for at least some wavelengths.

Table 8.3   Another attempt to match the test stimulus to the reference

Hemifield	Reference	Test
Wavelength	500 nm	520 nm
Incident quanta/sec (N)	1,000	2,500
Fraction (f) absorbed by pigment A	0.5	0.2
Total quanta/sec absorbed by pigment A	**500**	**500**
Fraction (f) absorbed by pigment B	0.4	0.575
Total quanta/sec absorbed by pigment B	**400**	**1,438**

However, even with two photopigments, certain pairs of wavelengths may not be discriminable. That is, an intensity for the test wavelength can be found that produces the same number of quantal absorptions as the reference wavelength, and, therefore, the test and reference match. For these wavelengths, the ratios of absorptions of the photopigments are the same at each wavelength, and an intensity can be found that matches the reference stimulus. For a person to achieve wavelength discrimination, the outputs of the two classes of cones must be compared by other classes of neurons at postreceptor levels. Much of this comparison is carried out in the retina itself. Thus, two photopigments with overlapping absorption spectra—dichromatic color vision—provide limited color vision.

Just as in the case of the monochromat, the examples given here have a basis in reality. Although the spectra used in these examples are hypothetical, certain individuals have only two pigments; they are called **dichromats**. The characteristics of these individuals are discussed later in this chapter.

A person with three photopigments with overlapping absorption spectra is capable of wavelength discrimination for nearly all wavelengths

When three spectrally overlapping photopigments are present, each in its own cone type, and a subject is presented with any monochromatic reference stimulus and any monochromatic test stimulus, no test wavelength at any intensity matches the reference outside of a small range (less than 7 nm) close to the reference stimulus wavelength. These test wavelengths always differ from the reference, because each produces a unique pattern of absorption in the three photopigments and, hence, in the three cone types. This difference is detected by other neurons in the retina and in central structures, so that the person can distinguish the different wavelengths as different colors.

Color Matching and Color Specification

For dichromats, two appropriately chosen wavelengths can match any reference wavelength

Although an individual with two overlapping photopigments cannot adjust a single test wavelength to match a reference, a match can be found if he or she is allowed to adjust the intensity of two wavelengths. Figure 8.5 has absorption spectra identical to those in Figure 8.4. The reference stimulus is still 500 nm, and one wavelength on the adjustable hemifield is still 520 nm. The only thing that has changed is the addition to the test stimulus of a second wavelength of 485 nm. The subject's task in this case is to independently adjust the 485 nm and 520 nm lights, until a combination is found that matches the 500 nm light.

Table 8.4 shows how the intensities must be set, in this example, to achieve a match. Note that, on the test hemifield, it is the sums of the quanta per second absorbed for each pigment at the two different wavelengths that

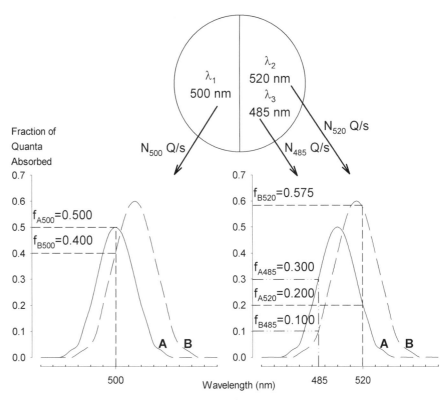

FIGURE 8.5 **Top.** *Representation of the same bipartite field as in previous figures, except that the test stimulus contains two wavelengths (520 nm and 485 nm), each with variable intensity.* **Bottom.** *Two representations of absorption spectra of two hypothetical photopigments (A and B), expressed as the fraction (f) of quanta absorbed versus wavelength. The dashed lines show the fractions of quanta absorbed by the photopigments at the wavelengths presented in the two hemifields. (λ = wavelength; N = number of incident quanta per second; Q = quanta.)*

match the absorptions on the reference hemifield. There is only one combination of intensities in the test hemifield that matches a given intensity of the reference stimulus. The intensities of the wavelengths in the test stimulus that must be used to produce a match can be calculated using the following equations:

$$N_{485} = \frac{N_{500}(f_{B_{520}}f_{A_{500}} - f_{B_{500}}f_{A_{520}})}{f_{B_{520}}f_{A_{485}} - f_{B_{485}}f_{A_{520}}} \quad \text{and} \quad N_{520} = \frac{N_{500}(f_{B_{500}}f_{A_{485}} - f_{B_{485}}f_{A_{500}})}{f_{B_{520}}f_{A_{485}} - f_{B_{485}}f_{A_{520}}}$$

Eq. 8.1

where N_{500} is the number of incident quanta per second in the reference stimulus, N_{485} and N_{520} are the number of incident quanta per second for the two wavelengths in the test stimulus that are required to match the reference stimulus, and f_{Bx} and f_{Ax} are the fractions of quanta of each wavelength absorbed by photopigment A or B.

Table 8.4 Intensities needed to match the test stimulus to the reference

Hemifield	Reference	Test		Total Test
Wavelength	500 nm	520 nm	485 nm	
Incident quanta/sec (N)	1,000	459	1,361	
Fraction (f) absorbed by pigment A	0.5	0.2	0.3	
Total quanta/sec absorbed by pigment A	**500**	92	408	**500**
Fraction (f) absorbed by pigment B	0.4	0.575	0.1	
Total quanta/sec absorbed by pigment B	**400**	264	136	**400**

There is a special case that needs to be considered in this kind of matching study. Notice that in the example in Figure 8.5 and Table 8.4, the two wavelengths in the test stimulus were located on either side of the reference wavelength. Suppose now that the reference wavelength was set at 485 nm (N = 1,000 quanta per second), and the two wavelengths in the test stimulus were set at 520 nm and 500 nm.

Equation 8.1 then yields the result shown in Table 8.5. Note that N, for the 520 nm wavelength, is a negative number, suggesting that some 520 nm light has to be subtracted from the right hemifield for a match to occur. This is clearly impossible, because there cannot be a negative number of quanta per second. In practice, to make the match, it is necessary to add the 520 nm light to the reference 485 nm light. Thus, in matching situations when negative values are found in a table, the implication is that that wavelength and amount are added to the reference stimulus to achieve a match. This procedure appears again in the section on color-matching functions.

For trichromats, any reference color can be matched by a mixture of three primary colors

A logical extension of what was presented in the previous sections is that, in trichromatic vision, any wavelength of light can be precisely matched or spec-

Table 8.5 Matching when both test lights are in the same spectral direction from the reference wavelength

Hemifield	Reference	Test		Total Test
Wavelength	485 nm	520 nm	500 nm	
Incident quanta/sec (N)	1,000	−105	803	
Fraction (f) absorbed by pigment A	0.3	0.2	0.4	
Total quanta/sec absorbed by pigment A	**300**	−21	321	**300**
Fraction (f) absorbed by pigment B	0.1	0.575	0.2	
Total quanta/sec absorbed by pigment B	**100**	−61	161	**100**

ified by mixtures of three suitably chosen colors. Such colors are known as **primary colors**. Red, green, and blue lights are convenient primaries, but any three colored lights can be used as primaries, provided that a mixture of two primaries does not match the third. Note that, although all of the previous examples have used monochromatic lights in the test stimulus, primaries do not have to be monochromatic lights.

Trichromatic color mixing is not necessarily imposed by the number of photopigments

Before cones and cone pigments were studied directly, there was a great deal of psychophysical evidence, primarily from color-matching studies that showed that normal human color vision is trichromatic. It should be noted that trichromatic color mixing is an empirical finding. It implies that there are three fundamental variables or channels that determine color-matching behavior, but it does not require that there be three cone photopigments. There is, in fact, evidence for more than three cone photopigments in some color normal individuals, even though these individuals are trichromatic. What **trichromacy** suggests is that the outputs from the multiple cone types are pooled into three channels.

Three eighteenth and nineteenth century figures were important in developing the trichromatic theory of human color vision. George Palmer (1777) wrote: "The surface of the retina is compounded of particles of three different kinds, analogous to the three rays of light; and each of these particles is moved by its own ray."

He therefore proposed a physiologically based trichromacy in which the three particles were equivalent to the three cone types, but he incorrectly thought that the physical variable of wavelength, or frequency, of light was discrete rather than continuous.

Thomas Young (1802) wrote what is probably the first physiologically and physically accurate account of trichromacy. He argued that there cannot be an infinite number of particles (cones) but that the number is limited to three that are influenced to a greater or lesser extent by light. In a famous quote, he considered and rejected the idea that there are a large number of different cone types:

> As it is almost impossible to conceive each sensitive point of the retina to contain an infinite number of particles, each capable of vibrating in perfect unison with every possible undulation,* it becomes necessary to suppose the number limited; for instance to the three principal colours, red, yellow and blue, and that each of the particles is capable of being put in motion more or less forcibly by undulations differing less or more from perfect unison. Each sensitive filament of the nerve may consist of three portions, one for each principal colour.

*"Undulations" refers to the wavelength (or frequency) of light.

The writings of Thomas Young lay dormant until the German psychologist Hermann von Helmholtz recognized them in 1856–1866 and became a staunch supporter. Helmholtz (1862) promoted Young's ideas, proposed overlapping spectral sensitivity functions, and elaborated on the theory that has since become known as the *Young-Helmholtz trichromatic theory*. The idea is that three different and independent receptors act individually and in concert to mediate color.

Color-Matching Functions

The amounts of primary lights needed to match spectral lights are represented by color-matching functions

James Clerk Maxwell (1855) provided the first quantitative data on human trichromatic color matching. He used a spinning top to additively mix colors and determined the relative amounts of various primaries needed to match a white reference. A more recent approach is to use a fixed set of primaries and to determine the amounts of each needed to perfectly match each visible wavelength. This is simply an expansion of the technique shown in Figure 8.5 to include three colors in the test hemifield.

By using three standard colors, or primaries, it is possible to develop a standard way of specifying any color. In the real world, **color specification** is extremely important because it provides a way for industrial processes around the world to exactly match the color of, for example, a traffic light, wallpaper, ink, and so on.

British physicist W. D. Wright laid the foundation of much of color matching in 1928 by generating color-matching functions (Wright 1946). He chose 650 nm (red), 530 nm (green), and 460 nm (blue) as the primaries. He used a bipartite matching field that was 2° in diameter. The task of the observer was to adjust the intensities of each of the three primaries, until the combination appeared to match precisely the reference wavelength, thus producing a metameric match.

Figure 8.6 shows Wright's color-matching functions. The abscissa shows the wavelength of the reference stimulus. The ordinate shows the **tristimulus values**—the relative amounts of each primary required to match each reference wavelength.*

Across most of the spectrum, the relative intensity of all three primaries can be adjusted in the test stimulus, but sometimes a negative amount of a primary is needed, just as in the hypothetical dichromatic matching that was described previously. A negative value simply means that, to make a match, the observer added that amount of one of the primaries to the reference side to achieve the match. Color matching is like solving simultaneous equations. In this case,

---

*To get the tristimulus values, Wright first found the unique intensities of the three primaries that together match a specific white light stimulus, with a color temperature of approximately 4,800 K (see Figure 8.11). He then defined these intensities as unit amounts. Therefore, white equals 1 R + 1 G + 1 B. The tristimulus values thus reflect the normalized, or relative, coloring power of the primaries.

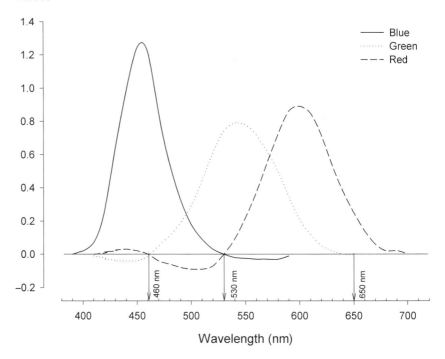

Tristimulus
Values

— Blue
······ Green
--- Red

460 nm
530 nm
650 nm

Wavelength (nm)

FIGURE 8.6   *Wright's color-matching functions. The tristimulus values on the y-axis are the relative amounts of the three primaries required to match the monochromatic wavelength indicated on the x-axis. The arrows indicate the positions of the three primaries used: 460, 530, and 650 nm. Note that the tristimulus values are 0 for two of the three primaries at these positions. Negative tristimulus values indicate that the primary had to be added to the reference side to achieve a color match. (Modified from WD Wright. Researches on Normal and Defective Colour Vision. St. Louis: Mosby, 1946.)*

there are three equations with three unknowns: the intensities of the three primaries. If a solution to an equation turns out negative, that primary is added to the reference wavelength on the other side of the equation.

Note that, at some reference wavelengths, only two primaries are needed to make a match, and the intensity of the third primary is 0. This occurs at the longer wavelengths where the SWS cones are stimulated very little by the reference wavelength (see Figure 8.1). At some wavelengths, a match requires only a single primary. This occurs three times, at wavelengths where the fixed reference light is the same wavelength as one of the primary wavelengths. In addition, for very long reference wavelengths (longer than 680 nm) where the color appears constant for a variety of wavelengths (see Color Plate 8.1), only a small amount of the long-wavelength red primary is needed to achieve a match.

Color matches, once made, remain stable over a range of conditions

Grassman's laws state formally that color mixtures obey some simple rules of algebra. The laws deal with the properties of metameric matches.

1. **Additive law**: When equal radiation is added to both sides of a metameric color match, the match still holds.
2. **Scalar law**: When both sides of a metameric match are changed by the same proportional amount (multiply or divide the reference and mixture by the same number), the match still holds. This can be observed by viewing metameric matches through neutral density filters. The scalar law holds over a wide range of filter densities.
3. **Associative law**: If color A is metameric to color B, then A and B can be used interchangeably in any color match involving the other. For example, if A matches B, and C matches B + D, the associative law says that C matches A + D.

Also, if a metameric match is made and the observer then stares, for example, at a red adapting field for a few minutes and then views the original metameric match, the two hemifields remain matched. Both hemifields, however, now appear a different color than before the adaptation to the red color, a condition known as **chromatic adaptation**. The change in color appearance usually is brief but may persist depending on the intensity and duration of the adapting stimulus. This example illustrates that color matching indicates little about color appearance.

Only one set of color-matching functions corresponds to the spectral sensitivities of the three cone types

Of all the possible equivalent sets of color-matching functions, there is one particular set that corresponds precisely to the action spectra of the three cone pigments in the eye that are responsible for trichromatic behavior—these are called the **fundamental response functions**. Any proposed set of fundamental response curves should be a linear transformation of the small field color-matching data. Therefore, it might be convenient to think of color-matching functions as being functionally equivalent to the spectral sensitivities of the cones. Remember, however, that trichromacy is not imposed solely by three cone photopigments, but that other neural connections in the retina and central visual pathways are involved.

Changing the primaries changes the tristimulus values of the color-matching functions

Compare the color-matching functions shown in the top of Figure 8.7 to those in Figure 8.6. In Figure 8.7, the primaries are 700 nm (red), 546.1 nm (green), and 435.8 nm (blue), whereas in Figure 8.6, they were 650 nm, 530 nm, and 460 nm. One obvious difference is the change in the location of

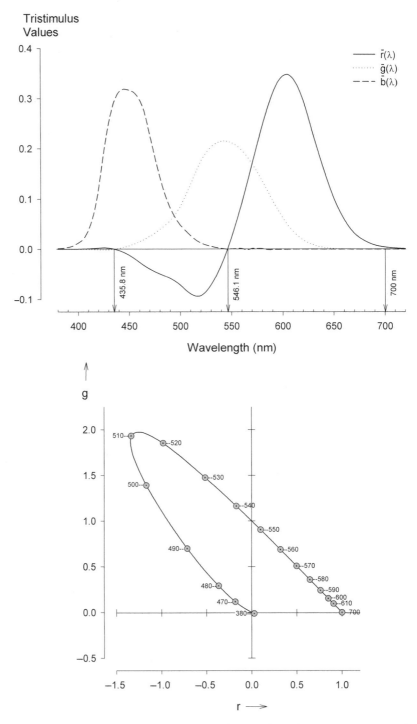

FIGURE 8.7 *Top. The CIE 1931 RGB color-matching functions.* **Bottom**. *The CIE 1931 RGB chromaticity diagram. The RGB system is based on primaries of 435.8, 546.1, and 700 nm. By definition, an equal energy white light plots at (r = 0.33, g = 0.33) on the chromaticity diagram. (λ = wavelength.) (Modified from G Wyszecki, WS Stiles. Color Science: Concepts and Methods, Quantitative Data and Formulae [2nd ed]. New York: Wiley, 1982.)*

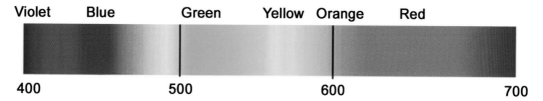

COLOR PLATE 8.1   *A representation of the visible electromagnetic spectrum, the spectral colors, with color names and selected respective wavelengths in nanometers.*

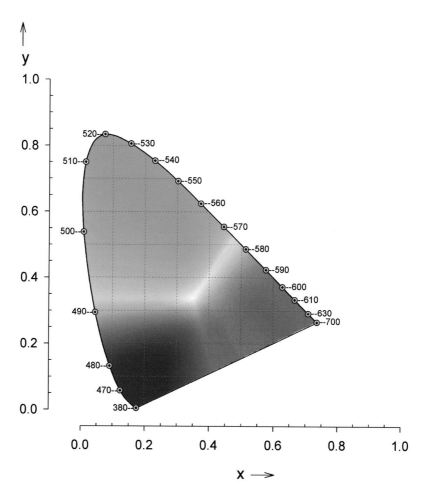

COLOR PLATE 8.2   *Color representation of the CIE 1931 (x, y) chromaticity diagram, similar to the black-and-white representation in Figure 8.8 bottom.*

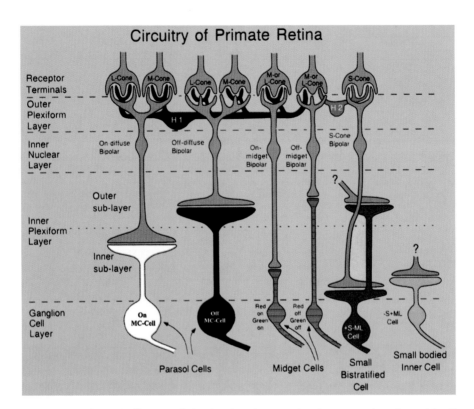

COLOR PLATE 8.3   *Schematic diagram of circuitry in primate retina. Long-wavelength sensitive (L-cone) and middle-wavelength sensitive (M-cone) cones connect to on-center and off-center diffuse bipolar cells on the left of the figure, forming an achromatic receptive-field center. L-cones and M-cones also connect to H1-type horizontal cells, which provide an achromatic receptive-field surround to the bipolar cells. The diffuse bipolar cells connect to center-surround–organized magnocellular cells (on MC-cell and off MC-Cell). At the right center in the figure, on-center and off-center midget bipolar cells receive their receptive-field center input from a single M-cone or L-cone. H1 horizontal cells provide a surround from M-cones and L-cones. The midget bipolar cells connect to the midget ganglion cells. At the right of the figure, short-wavelength sensitive (S-cone) cones provide a receptive-field center to the S-cone bipolar cell, which, in turn connects to the small bistratified ganglion cell. All three cone classes connect to H2 horizontal cells that provide a surround to the bistratified ganglion cell through an off-bipolar cell (shown as a "?"). (Reprinted with permission from BB Lee, DM Dacey. Structure and Function in Primate Retina. In C Cavonius, AJ Adams [eds], Colour Vision Deficiencies XIII: Proceedings of the Thirteenth Symposium of the International Research Group on Colour Vision Deficiencies held in Pau, France, July 27–30, 1995. Boston: Kluwer Academic Publishers, 1997;107–117.)*

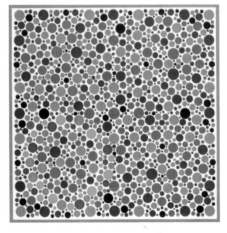

COLOR PLATE 8.4   *Hardy-Rand-Rittler (HRR) plate number 13. (Reprinted with permission from Richmond Products, Boca Raton, FL.)*

the points at which only one wavelength is needed to match the reference wavelength. Again, these occur at the wavelength of each primary. The shapes of the functions are also slightly different, as are the relative heights. The color-matching functions in Figures 8.6 and 8.7 are equally valid in that they specify the intensities of the selected primaries to match any spectral light. However, if every paint factory or television manufacturer, for example, used its own different set of primaries, the tristimulus values for any one color would differ. This means that anyone who tried to produce a particular color would need to know the primaries used by the person with whom they were dealing.

To solve this problem, an international system was adopted in 1931 by the CIE based on the primaries 700 nm (red), 546.1 nm (green), and 435.8 nm (blue). To develop the **CIE 1931 RGB color-matching functions**, shown at the top of Figure 8.7, the CIE combined the color-matching data from 10 subjects tested by Wright with the data from seven additional subjects tested by Guild (1931) as the *Standard Colorimetric Observer*. This was the first step in the derivation of an internationally recognized color system based on human visual performance. The three color-matching functions are designated $\bar{r}(\lambda)$, $\bar{g}(\lambda)$, and $\bar{b}(\lambda)$, each with a bar above the letter to indicate that these are the radiometric amounts (see Appendix) of the primaries needed to match a unit radiometric amount of the reference wavelength.

Any color with a known spectral energy distribution can be characterized by the tristimulus values

Although the CIE color-matching functions were derived by the intensities of the primaries needed to match spectral colors, its greatest utility is that it can be used to provide tristimulus values to match nonspectral colors, that is, colors that are a mixture of wavelengths and contain some amount of white light in addition to spectral colors. To use the color-matching functions to specify any color, first multiply the energy (P_λ) at each wavelength in the reference color sample by each of the tristimulus values at those same wavelengths. At 500 nm, for example, the multipliers would be $\bar{r}_{500} = -0.072$, $\bar{g}_{500} = 0.085$, and $\bar{b}_{500} = 0.048$. Second, separately sum the $P_\lambda\bar{r}(\lambda)$, $P_\lambda\bar{g}(\lambda)$, and $P_\lambda\bar{b}(\lambda)$ products across all the wavelengths present in the reference color. The resulting three sums are a new set of tristimulus values that match the colored sample and are represented as upper case letters R, G, and B. These symbols are without bars. They provide a three-number specification—the tristimulus values—for any colored sample. If the sample were, for example, the entire visible spectrum with equal energy at each wavelength, then R = G = B.

In keeping with Grassman's Associative law, any two colors that have the same tristimulus values appear identical to the Standard Colorimetric Observer, regardless of the spectral content of the colors. In other words, metamers have identical tristimulus values. As a result, if one wishes to do so, other sets of three primaries may be specified in terms of the original RGB system, as was done in the CIE 1931 XYZ system (described later).

Relative tristimulus values represent colors as chromaticity coordinates in a two-dimensional chromaticity diagram

A **chromaticity diagram** is a convenient chart on which to plot colors. The transformation from the tristimulus values of the CIE 1931 RGB color-matching functions, which is shown at the top of Figure 8.7, to the chromaticity diagram, which is shown at the bottom of Figure 8.7, is straightforward, as shown in the following equations, written in terms of the more general tristimulus values (R, G, B):

$$r = \frac{R}{(R + G + B)}$$ Eq. 8.2

$$g = \frac{G}{(R + G + B)}$$ Eq. 8.3

$$b = \frac{B}{(R + G + B)}$$ Eq. 8.4

Here r, g, and b are without bars; they represent the relative *proportions* of the red (R), green (G), and blue (B) tristimulus values. Therefore, it follows that r + g + b = 1. By knowing just two of these three variables, known as *chromaticity coordinates*, the other can be derived. For this reason, only two of the variables, r and g, are typically plotted on a chromaticity diagram, as shown at the bottom of Figure 8.7; the b term is equal to 1 − (r + g). The 700 nm (red) primary is plotted at r = 1, g = 0, the 546.1 nm (green) primary at r = 0, g = 1, and the 435.8 nm (blue) primary at r = 0, g = 0. The b-axis is perpendicular to the page at r = 0, g = 0, and the b primary would plot at a value of 1 on that axis. Calculating chromaticity coordinates throws away information about the total amounts of energy in the color sample, which is related to the sample's luminance. This is justified by the fact that color matches hold over a rather wide range of stimulus intensities.

Spectral lights (single wavelengths) plot around a horseshoe-shaped curve, known as the **spectral locus** (see Figure 8.7). An "equal energy white" light plots at r = 0.333, g = 0.333. It is important to keep in mind that there are three dimensions to this specification and that the plot of only the r and g values represents a projection of that three-dimensional space on a flat plane. All real colors lie on or within that part of the chromaticity diagram that is bounded by the spectral locus and a straight line that connects the chromaticity coordinates of the limits of the visible spectrum (approximately 400 nm and 700 nm). Colors outside the boundary, for example at r = 0.5 and g = 1.0, do not exist for humans.

Note, in both the color-matching functions and chromaticity diagram, that wavelengths longer than 435.8 nm and shorter than 546.1 nm require negative amounts of the 700 nm red primary, and wavelengths shorter than 435.8 nm require negative amounts of the 546.1 nm green primary. As discussed previously, this simply indicates that, for those wavelengths, some of the negative primary had to be added to the reference wavelength to match a mixture of the remaining two primaries. The blue-green color of a wavelength of 490 nm, for example, appears more vivid (more saturated) than a mixture of the blue and green primaries that match the hue of 490 nm and appears a different color. Adding the red primary to 490 nm allows a complete match of both the hue and saturation of the two mixtures (red primary + 490 nm and green primary + blue primary). Which wavelengths require negative primaries depend on the set of three primaries that were chosen, as is seen in the next section.

The CIE 1931 XYZ system of tristimulus values is a mathematic transformation of the CIE 1931 RGB system

Regardless of which real primaries are chosen for a color-matching study, some parts of the spectrum always require a negative amount of one primary to make a trichromatic match. For the purposes of color specification, it would be more convenient to transform the data to a new set of primaries that has only positive chromaticity coordinates. The advantage of a positive system is that computations are simpler, and a direct-read photoelectric **colorimeter** can be used to compute chromaticity coordinates. The downside is that the new primaries must lie outside the spectral locus of real colors. This means that they are unrealizable or **imaginary primaries**. Despite the real possibility of creating confusion with the notion of imaginary primaries, the CIE transformed the RGB system to the **CIE 1931 XYZ system**. As is seen in the following discussion, the chosen transformation offered real advantages.

The transformation of either the color-matching functions or the chromaticity coordinates from one set of primaries to another is a straightforward, matrix algebra problem. The solutions were subject to three constraints. First, the new tristimulus values, X, Y, and Z and the chromaticity coordinates, x, y, and z had to be completely positive. Second, an equal energy white light would plot at x = y = z = 0.33 in the x, y chromaticity diagram. Third, the $\bar{y}$ color-matching function was chosen to match the CIE 1924 V_λ curve, the photopic luminous efficiency function (see Appendix, Figure A.1). This means that the photometric luminance of a color stimulus can be derived by calculating its Y tristimulus value. Thus, two samples with the same Y tristimulus values are defined as having equal luminance, regardless of their Z and X values. The resulting 1931 XYZ color-matching functions and the **CIE 1931 (x, y) chromaticity diagram** are shown in Figure 8.8. Color Plate 8.2 shows the CIE 1931 (x, y) chromaticity diagram in color.

The chromaticity diagram in Figure 8.8 shows the locations of the named wavelengths of the spectral colors along the spectral locus. A straight line that

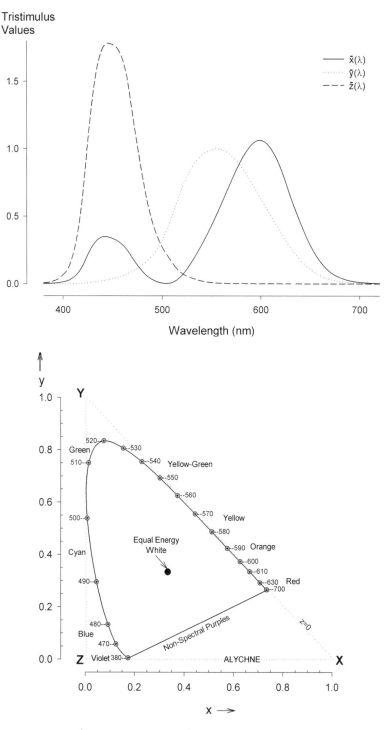

FIGURE 8.8 **Top.** The CIE 1931 (XYZ) color matching functions. **Bottom.** The CIE 1931 (x, y) chromaticity diagram (see Color Plate 8.2 for a color representation of this figure). The XYZ system is based on imaginary primaries located at the apices of the triangle and outside the spectral locus. These primaries are derived from an algebraic transformation of the RGB system shown in Figure 8.7. Equal energy white light plots at (0.33, 0.33) on the chromaticity diagram. (Modified from G Wyszecki, WS Stiles. Color Science: Concepts and Methods, Quantitative Data and Formulae [2nd ed]. New York: Wiley, 1982.)

connects the limits of the spectral locus, together with the spectral locus itself, enclose a subspace of the chromaticity diagram in which all real colors are represented. The colors along the straight line that connects the spectral limits are mostly purples—mixtures of red and violet light. Colors on this purple line and colors everywhere inside the real color space, are therefore **nonspectral colors**.

Notice that the original, real primaries are no longer located at values of 1.0 on this diagram. The 700 nm red primary is located at x = 0.735, y = 0.265, and z = 0, for example. The new primaries, X, Y, and Z, at their respective values of 1.0, thus lie outside the locus of real colors and are therefore physically unrealizable—they can be thought of as imaginary or virtual. Conversely, all real colors must lie on or within the spectral locus and the straight line that connects its limits. Because all real colors lie completely within the triangle of XYZ, all computations are positive, and any real color can be specified in terms of the x, y, and z values, just as it could with the r, g, and b values in the RGB system.

It is important to remember that the point at which z = 1 lies at x = y = 0. z is computed as 1 – (x + y). Therefore, z equals 0 along the line where x + y = 1. That line is tangent to the spectral locus over the range of wavelengths from approximately 545 to 700 nm. Over this spectral region, normal trichromats require only two primaries to make a match. This example illustrates one of the many practical uses of the CIE 1931 XYZ system. An instrument known as an *anomaloscope*, to be described later in this chapter, identifies persons with common, hereditary, color vision deficiencies by asking them to set a mixture of 546 nm and 670 nm lights until the mixture matches a 589 nm light. The mixture matches that are produced by people with color deficiencies differ significantly from those with normal color vision.

As shown in Figure 8.8, in the CIE (x, y) chromaticity diagram there is a line of zero luminance known as the *alychne*. It is the line at which y = 0. Recall that the CIE 1931 XYZ system chose the ȳ color-matching function to be identical to the V_λ curve. If ȳ = 0, then Y = 0 and the luminance is 0. A number of other properties of the CIE 1931 (x, y) chromaticity diagram are discussed with reference to Figure 8.9 in the following section.

Color mixtures, complementary colors, and dominant wavelength can be determined graphically using the CIE (x, y) chromaticity diagram

As noted often before in this chapter, two or more colors can be mixed to produce a new color. If two spectral colors are mixed, the new color lies on a straight line that connects the chromaticity coordinates of the two colors in the CIE 1931 (x, y) chromaticity diagram. Suppose, for example, that the wavelengths λ_1 = 580 nm and λ_2 = 500 nm are mixed in the appropriate amounts to produce the mixture, M, shown in Figure 8.9. The point M could be moved back and forth along the line by increasing and decreasing the relative amounts of the two wavelengths—if more of the 580 nm wavelength were added, M would move toward the yellow-orange color of 580 nm, whereas

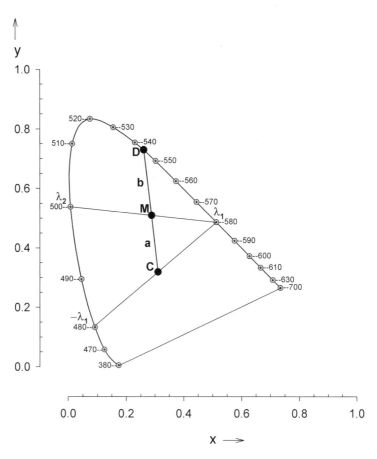

FIGURE 8.9   *The CIE 1931 (x, y) chromaticity diagram on which are shown the locations of points, distances, and directions that can be used to determine the dominant wavelength (D) and the excitation purity (a/[a+b]) for a color mixture (M) created by mixing the appropriate amounts of two wavelengths (λ_1 and λ_2). It also shows two complementary colors (λ_1 and $-\lambda_1$). See text for details. C is the location of the reference white. (Modified from G Wyszecki, WS Stiles. Color Science: Concepts and Methods, Quantitative Data and Formulae [2nd ed]. New York: Wiley, 1982.)*

more of the 500 nm wavelength would move M toward the green-cyan color of 500 nm. It is easy to see that there is essentially an infinite number of lines joining two other points on or within the chromaticity diagram that can be drawn through point M to create that color.

Regardless of what colors are mixed to create M, it has a **dominant wavelength**. The dominant wavelength of a color is defined as the wavelength that can be mixed with a reference white (illuminant C [Figure 8.10], labeled "C" in this example) to give a match to that color. Because of the linearity of the color space, this can be determined graphically by drawing a straight line from the chosen reference white, *C*, through the color, *M*, to a point on the spectral locus, *D*. The wavelength at which the line intersects the spectral locus is the dominant wavelength. It is approximately 545 nm in this example.

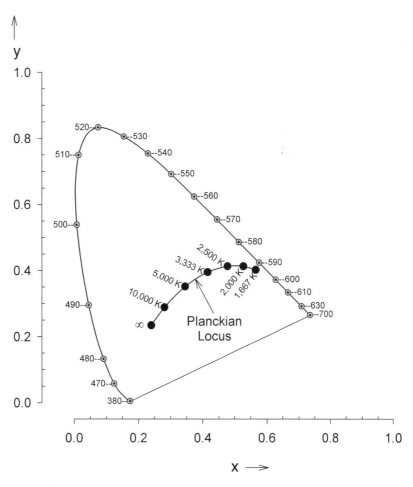

FIGURE 8.10   *The CIE 1931 (x, y) chromaticity diagram on which is shown the black-body radiator locus (Planckian locus) along which standard white illuminants of varying color temperature are represented. (Modified from G Wyszecki, WS Stiles. Color Science: Concepts and Methods, Quantitative Data and Formulae [2nd ed]. New York: Wiley, 1982.)*

Once the dominant wavelength is determined, the **excitation purity** can be calculated. Excitation purity is a measure of the distance of a color from a reference white light. Spectral lights (monochromatic lights) have excitation purities of 1.0 (the maximum possible), whereas pastel colors have low excitation purities and the reference white has a value of zero. Excitation purity is the ratio of the distance from the reference white to the colored sample (*a* in Figure 8.9) divided by the distance from white to the dominant wavelength (a + b).

There is a special case of color mixture in which white is produced. Spectral and nonspectral colors that produce white when mixed in the proper proportions are called **complementary colors**. Figure 8.9 shows that 580 nm mixed with 480 nm can produce white. Note that there is a range of wavelengths from 380 nm to slightly longer than 490 nm over which the complement is a spectral wavelength. There is another range from approximately 570 to 700 nm over which the complement is a spectral wavelength. However, wavelengths from approximately 490 to 570 nm do not have spectral complements.

The locus of blackbody radiators is represented as a curved line near the center of the CIE (x, y) chromaticity diagram

Determining a dominant wavelength and a complementary wavelength requires the specification of a reference white light. The reason for this is that there are many possible white lights. For convenience, a reference often used is an equal energy white, one for which the energy of all wavelengths is equal. It has CIE (x, y) coordinates of (0.33, 0.33). Many other whites can also be specified in terms of the **color temperature** of a **blackbody radiator**. As a blackbody radiator is heated up, it emits electromagnetic radiation. If its temperature is sufficiently high, it emits visible radiation. The locus of points that describes the visible appearance of a blackbody or Planckian body as it heats up is known as the **Planckian locus** and is located as shown in Figure 8.10. At low temperatures, it glows red hot and is plotted near the red corner of the diagram. As is gets hotter, it eventually becomes white hot. As temperature rises further, the color becomes blue hot and is plotted more toward the blue corner of the diagram. Because color is correlated with temperature, points along the Planckian locus represent the **correlated color temperature** of white light. The Planckian locus does not pass through the equal energy point, but it is very close to it when the color temperature is approximately 5,600 K.

A number of standard illuminants can be located along this locus. For example, Standard Illuminant A represents a 100 W incandescent (tungsten filament) lamp and has a correlated color temperature of 2,855.6 K; it is actually fairly red, as anyone who has taken pictures with daylight film in a room lit only with a tungsten bulb can attest. Standard Illuminant B represents direct sunlight and has a correlated color temperature of 4,874 K. **Standard Illuminant C**, which is the standard under which most color vision tests must be performed, approximates light from a overcast north sky and has a correlated color temperature of 6,774 K. Another reference illuminant, Standard Illuminant D65, represents daylight with a correlated color temperature of 6,504 K.

The CIE 1931 Standard Colorimetric Observer is based on data from subjects viewing a 2° field and is recommended for specifying stimuli from 1° to 4°. In 1964, the CIE defined a Standard Colorimetric Observer for 10° diameter (large) fields, and the CIE 1964 (x_{10}, y_{10}) chromaticity diagram was generated. It is recommended that this large field diagram be used for stimuli larger than 4°. A large part of the difference between the 2° and 10° color-matching functions can be accounted for by differences in the effects of the extracellular macular pigment that preferentially absorbs short wavelengths and has a greater influence on the small-field standard observer function.

Color Naming and Ordering

Colors are named consistently across cultures using 11 basic color terms

People assign names to many of the colors that can be distinguished, and, most of the time, people from varied cultures agree with one another on the way colors are assigned into categories (Berlin & Kay 1969). The agreement in the color nomenclature provides support for the belief that the perception of color is similar across people. There are 11 basic color terms, each related to a unique sensation. Three terms describe the achromatic colors: *black*, *white*, and *gray*. Four terms describe primary, "landmark," or unique colors, that is, those chromatic colors that contain no trace of any other color: *red*, *green*, *blue*, and *yellow*. There are four secondary basic terms: *brown*, *orange*, *purple*, and *pink*. These 11 terms are considered basic, because, within and across populations, they are used more consistently than nonbasic terms, there is much higher agreement in their use than in the use of nonbasic terms (e.g., peach or tan), and the response time for naming them is shorter than for nonbasic terms (Boynton & Olson 1990). Anthropologists have shown that these terms, expressed in the appropriate language, are consistently used across diverse populations, even though not all languages use all 11 basic color terms. It is not known what neural activity, if any, is correlated with the use of these terms, but it is possible that there are 11 distinct types of neurochemical activity in the brain that provide this categorical color vision (Yoshioka et al. 1996).

Colors can be logically ordered on the basis of hue, saturation, and brightness

Human color vision is trivariant; colors have three perceptual (subjective) attributes: **hue**, **saturation**, and **brightness**. In addition, if a color belongs to the surface of an object (as do most, but not all, naturally occurring colors) a color may have texture. Colors perceived by reflection from an object are known as *surface* or *object colors*. Colors, such as the blue sky and many colors presented in research optical systems, are known as *aperture colors* or *film colors*. They do not belong to a surface.

Hue is the property of a color most closely associated with the dominant wavelength. The hue of a color is designated by a name, such as blue or red. In casual communication, the terms *hue* and *color* are frequently interchanged. In a strict sense, two colors may differ, for example, in brightness, but they may be of the same hue, for example, green.

Saturation refers to how pastel or vivid a color appears. It is related to the actual and perceived white content of the color. For example, pink is less saturated than red. The monochromatic (spectral) colors are saturated colors, whereas white is a desaturated color. However, not all spectral colors are equally saturated. For example, monochromatic yellow appears less saturated than monochromatic blue or red. The physical variable to which saturation is most closely related is **colorimetric purity**. Note, however, that all spectral colors have equal colorimetric purity.

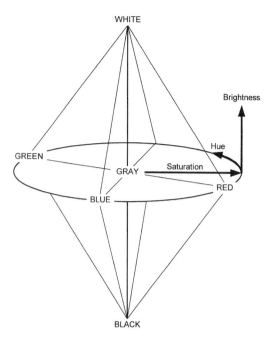

FIGURE 8.11   *Three-dimensional space representation of color perception in which brightness is represented along the vertical axis, hue around the circumference, and saturation along the radius.*

Brightness is the perceptual response that is related to the amount of radiant energy that comes from a color. One can imagine a blue coffee cup that gets brighter when the illumination in a room is increased. The saturation does not change, that is, the blue does not appear more pastel as the lights are turned up, but the brightness has increased.

A logical arrangement of the three perceptual attributes, shown in Figure 8.11, places hue around the circumference of a circle, following the spectral order of red, orange, yellow, green, blue, and violet (ROYGBV) from Color Plate 8.1, with the nonspectral purples linking the two ends of the circle. The center of the circle is gray (an **achromatic color**). As one moves along the radii of the circle from the center to the rim, saturation increases but brightness and hue are constant. Perpendicular to the circle is the brightness axis, with brightness increasing upwards toward white and decreasing downward to black. The arrangement is shown as two cones placed base to base, as in Figure 8.11. At very high brightness, all colors desaturate to white. At very low brightness, colors darken to black. Hence, conical shapes are used to display this concept rather than cylinders.

As Figure 8.11 shows, it is possible to arrange colors in an orderly fashion based on perceptual judgments without knowledge of cone photoreceptor spectral sensitivities and without resorting to actual data, as was used in the CIE color specification system. Several other color-ordering systems are in use, including the Munsell Color System.

The Munsell Color System is a practical application of trivariant color perception useful for making clinical tests of color vision

The Munsell Company produces colored papers that are used widely in clinical tests of color vision. Color samples are labeled using hue (H), **value** (V), and **chroma** (C). There are five major hues, designated by letter codes P (purple), B (blue), G (green), Y (yellow), R (red), and five intermediate hues assigned the symbols RP, PB, BG, GY and YR. Each major and intermediate hue category is further subdivided into 10 steps, designated by numbers from 1 to 10. The maximum number of possible hues therefore is 100. To illustrate specification of hue, suppose that a Munsell color has a hue designated as 5BG. This is a blue-green midway between the major hues of blue (5B) and green (5G).

Value is related to brightness. Samples with a high value are bright, and samples with a low value are dark. Value varies in 11 steps, from 0 to 10 (dark to bright).

Chroma is analogous to saturation. The Munsell Color System uses reflective colored paper samples, and chroma is related to the amounts of colorless pigments (white, gray, or black) that are mixed in with colored pigments to make the color. Chroma is designated by a number scale from 0 to 14, where 0 is achromatic and 14 is maximum color saturation. Maximum chroma can only be achieved for a limited set of hues and values. Samples are designated fully by (H V/C), for example (6Y 9/6). A sample of the same hue and value but one step lower in saturation would be designated by (6Y 9/5).

The Munsell colors are ordered in a manner similar to the perceptual color space in Figure 8.11. Hue is arranged around the circumference of a circle, value (brightness) is on the vertical axis, and chroma (saturation) is represented by the distance from the center of the circle. Munsell colors are designed to be viewed under Standard Illuminant C. Persons with limited color vision cannot distinguish all of the divisions of (H V/C) samples. They therefore make errors when asked to place the hues in correct order. Errors of ordering hue at constant V/C is diagnostic of deficient color vision. The details of how clinical tests of color ordering are designed and constructed are explained more fully in the Testing for Color Vision Defects section of this chapter.

Color Discriminations

Humans can discriminate a change of one nanometer in wavelength in some regions of the spectrum

Early in this chapter, it was stated that, in trichromatic vision, each wavelength produces a unique pattern of excitation of the three cone types, which results in the perceptual experience of a unique color. However, when presented with a bipartite field, as in Figure 8.3, if the test wavelength is very similar to the reference wavelength, a subject with normal trichromatic color vision may not be able to determine that the test wavelength differs from the reference and may judge that it matches the reference wavelength. If the wavelength of the test stimulus is changed, so that it differs from the reference by a greater and greater amount, the subject eventually is able to determine that it does not match the reference. The threshold for determining that the test wavelength differs from the reference wavelength is the **wavelength discrimination threshold**. The wavelength discrimination threshold is not uniform across the spectrum.

The average wavelength discrimination functions of two observers with normal trichromatic vision and other observers with dichromatic color vision are plotted in Figure 8.12. To generate these data, subjects foveally viewed a 2° diameter bipartite field. One hemifield was set at the reference wavelength, for example, 500 nm. The test hemifield was initially set to the same wavelength as the reference hemifield. The subject then adjusted its wavelength until its color became just perceptibly different from the reference hemifield. In this figure, the threshold change in wavelength, Δλ, was averaged for the longer (+Δλ) and shorter (−Δλ) wavelength directions. The threshold Δλ could also be thought of as a just noticeable difference (jnd), the point at which subjects could just detect that the test wavelength was different from the reference wavelength. As the test wavelength was altered, its brightness was automatically adjusted so that it remained as bright as the reference light. In fact, for all but the extreme ends of

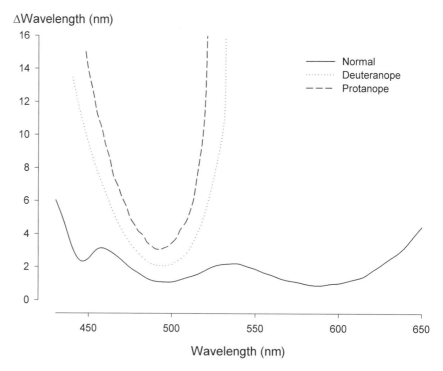

FIGURE 8.12   *The wavelength discrimination function for people with normal color vision (average of two individuals) and for individuals with protanopia (MWS cone function absent) and deuteranopia (LWS cone function absent). (Redrawn from JB Gregg, GG Heath. The Eye and Sight. Boston: Heath, 1964.)*

the spectrum, the color change that is due to a $\Delta\lambda$ is much more salient than the brightness change that is associated with a small shift in wavelength.

The wavelength discrimination function of normal trichromats in Figure 8.12 shows a **W**-shaped function with minima at approximately 490 and 590 nm. At these two spectral locations, the threshold $\Delta\lambda$ is approximately 1 nm. Notice that only at the spectral extremes does the threshold wavelength difference exceed 7 nm. If one starts at the short wavelength end of the spectrum and counts each threshold change in color as a jnd, then by the time one reaches the long-wavelength end of the spectrum, a normal observer has distinguished approximately 150–200 variations in color. For the protanopic and deuteranopic subjects, the wavelength discrimination function is only slightly elevated in the vicinity of 490 nm. The wavelength discrimination threshold rises rapidly for shorter and longer wavelengths, and above 520 nm, discrimination based on wavelength is not possible, making it understandable that people with these forms of color deficiency have problems telling the difference between (have *color confusion* for) colors such as yellow and red. Based on jnds across the spectrum, the dichromatic observers are able to distinguish perhaps 20–30 colors.

Explanations of the shape of the wavelength discrimination function are based on the hypothesis that two putative chromatic channels compare the outputs of the SWS, MWS, and LWS cones and convey these signals from the retina through the lateral geniculate nucleus (LGN) to the cortex. As is discussed in more detail in later sections, one channel, the red-green, compares MWS and LWS cone outputs. The other, blue-yellow, channel compares SWS cone output with the sum of the MWS and LWS cone outputs. Wavelength discrimination thresholds are based on the comparison of the neural output that occurs in response to any wavelength, λ, with the neural output that occurs in response to $\lambda + \Delta\lambda$, with brightness held constant (Kaiser & Boynton 1996). The red-green opponent channel responds in an excitatory manner in the long-wavelength part of the spectrum, and in an inhibitory manner in the middle- and short-wavelength part of the spectrum.* Similarly, the blue-yellow channel operates in an opponent fashion: excited (or inhibited) by short wavelengths and inhibited (or excited) by middle and long wavelengths. The region of the spectrum in which the color opponent channels' responses change most rapidly is the part of the spectrum in which wavelength discrimination is best. The minimum, at approximately 490 nm in the normal and color deficient curves, is due to the rapidly changing response of the blue-yellow opponent channel around this wavelength, and the second minimum, at approximately 590 nm in the normal curve, is due to the rapidly changing responses of the red-green opponent channel. It also must be the case that the ratio of quantal absorptions in the cones that mediate these responses is rapidly changing about these min-

---

*It also is possible that this channel acts in the opposite manner—inhibitory at long wavelengths and excitatory at middle and short wavelengths. In either case, the opponent nature of the channel would be the same.

imum points as well. The dichromat's curves indicate an impaired or absent red-green channel and, therefore, MWS- or LWS-cone function. Impairment in either of these cone types produces a similar wavelength discrimination function because the absorption spectra of the MWS and LWS cones are rather similar (see Figure 8.2). Color opponent channels are more fully explained in the section on Color Appearance and Color Opponency later in this chapter.

The ability to detect that a white light is tinged with color is described by the saturation (colorimetric purity) discrimination threshold

Saturation discrimination is measured by adding spectral light to a reference white light, while luminance is held constant. If very little of a spectral light must be added before the white is visibly tinged with color, the spectral light is considered very saturated. One can think of the spectral light as having a lot of *coloring power*. If a lot of spectral light must be added before the white appears colored, the spectral light is less saturated, and it has little coloring power.

Recall that saturation is a perceptual variable. In the discussion of the CIE 1931 (x, y) chromaticity diagram, the term *excitation purity* was introduced as a measure of the degree to which a color differs from white. The physical variable in the measurement of saturation discrimination is colorimetric purity, and therefore, such studies are best termed *colorimetric purity discrimination studies*. Colorimetric purity (p_c) is defined as

$$p_c = \frac{L_\lambda}{(L_w + L_\lambda)}$$

Eq. 8.5

where L_λ is the luminance of the monochromatic light that is added to the white, and L_w is the luminance of the white. Colorimetric purity is 1.0 when there is no white light added to the spectral color, and it is 0 for a reference white light. The terms *saturation discrimination* and *colorimetric purity discrimination* are often used interchangeably. Figure 8.13 shows a typical colorimetric purity discrimination function. The function is roughly V shaped with a minimum at approximately 570 nm. This means that yellow appears less saturated than blue or red when the lights have equal physical colorimetric purity.

Chromaticity discrimination is described by nonuniform distances in the CIE (x, y) chromaticity diagram

Chromaticity discrimination was briefly mentioned when discussing the CIE 1931 (x, y) chromaticity diagram, and it refers to discrimination of color changes due to changes in dominant wavelength or colorimetric purity, or both. In such measures, brightness is held constant. Whereas wavelength discrimination studies deal with measurements along the spectral locus of the CIE diagram, chromaticity discrimination deals with thresholds to detect differ-

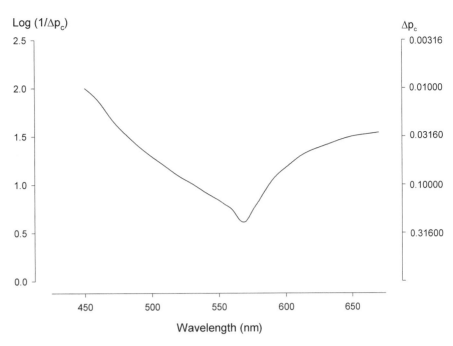

FIGURE 8.13   *Colorimetric purity discrimination relative to a 4,800 K reference white light. Δp_c (right ordinate) represents the change in colorimetric purity (p_c) required to reach the threshold for the detection of color as each wavelength is added to white. Log($1/\Delta p_c$) (left ordinate) creates a scale that is positively correlated with colorimetric purity. Thus, the short wavelengths at the blue end of the spectrum have the highest purity, or saturation, whereas 570 nm has the least. (Modified from G Wyszecki, WS Stiles. Color Science: Concepts and Methods, Quantitative Data and Formulae [2nd ed]. New York: Wiley, 1982.)*

ences in color within the area of the CIE diagram. However, **chromaticity** is continuously variable and it is not practical to measure discrimination at all possible chromaticities or beyond a limited number of directions of change about a reference color. Furthermore, the chosen light level for the studies affects the outcome. Therefore, it has been difficult to globally characterize chromaticity discrimination thresholds.

The name most associated with determining the chromaticity discrimination thresholds is David L. MacAdam, of the Eastman Kodak Company (MacAdam 1942). One reason for his interest in color discrimination was to protect the trademark "Kodak yellow" by obtaining a patent. The problem was to decide when two yellows were visibly equivalent and to establish a reasonable tolerance about this value using CIE tristimulus values. In other words, the task was to determine how much the CIE tristimulus values of a test color could vary in any direction before they would be detectably different from the yellow trademark color. As discussed earlier, it is completely inadequate to specify whether two surfaces appear the same color by using only their physical characteristics—they may have different spectral reflectances but appear identical (i.e., they may be metamers).

Data from one of MacAdam's studies (MacAdam 1942) are shown in Figure 8.14. The x-and y-axes in the top graph are CIE 1931 (x, y) chromaticity coordinates, and the reference color plots at (0.212, 0.550) in the center of the ellipse. The other data points are the standard deviations of repeated attempts by subjects to match the reference sample with mixtures of colors using the Method of Adjustment. The lines connecting the data points indicate the different directions in color space. The ellipse is drawn to fit the standard deviations. The larger the ellipse, the higher the chromatic discrimination threshold. The MacAdam unit of discrimination, designated as M, is one standard deviation of the match distribution. A jnd, the point at which subjects could detect at threshold that the test color was different from the reference, is approximately 3 M units; 5 M units may be an acceptable standard for industrial applications, allowing Kodak and other companies to specify their trademark colors. As shown in the bottom graph of Figure 8.14, MacAdam measured ellipses for 25 regions of color space. The size and the orientation of the major and minor axes of the ellipses varied, depending on the choice of reference color. These results have implications for using the CIE 1931 (x, y) chromaticity diagram to specify perceptual differences between colors, as is discussed in the next section.

The CIE (u', v') chromaticity diagram was created so that equal distances represent equal differences in color

Although the CIE 1931 (x, y) chromaticity diagram faithfully represents color-matching behavior, distances on the diagram are unrelated to chromaticity discrimination thresholds. In other words, two colors that are separated by a fixed distance on the CIE 1931 (x, y) chromaticity diagram might appear similar to each other in one part of the diagram, whereas two other colors separated by the same distance in another part of the diagram may appear dissimilar. In particular, the chromaticity discrimination thresholds (MacAdam ellipse dimensions) are the largest in the greenish region of the diagram, as shown in the bottom of Figure 8.14.

In the **CIE 1976 (u', v') uniform color space diagram** (Figure 8.15), equal distances represent equal perceptual steps along the dimension of chromaticity discrimination. The MacAdam ellipses become circles of approximately equal diameter, as one might expect if equal perceptual differences are represented by equal distances. This was accomplished by a mathematic transformation of the (x, y) color space that is, in turn, a transformation of real color mixture data, the (r, g) space. However, the transformation is nonlinear, which means that mixtures of two colors do not necessarily lie along the straight line that joins them, as was the case with the CIE 1931 (x, y) chromaticity diagram.

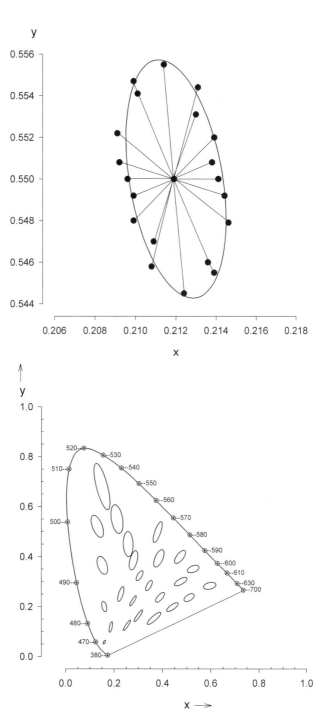

FIGURE 8.14 **Top.** *A chromaticity discrimination ellipse as measured by MacAdam. The precision with which a colored sample could be matched was taken as a measure of chromatic discrimination. The points represent one standard deviation from the mean match setting. The just noticeable difference is approximately three standard deviations.* **Bottom.** *CIE 1931 (x, y) chromaticity diagram that shows MacAdam ellipses at various locations on the diagram. The ellipses are drawn 10 times larger than their actual size. (Modified from DL MacAdam. Visual sensitivities to color differences in daylight. J Opt Soc Am 1942;32:247.)*

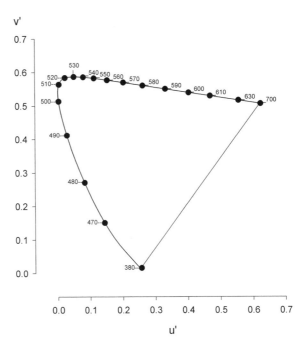

FIGURE 8.15   *The CIE 1976 (u', v') uniform color space diagram. The diagram attempts to represent equal perceptual steps as equal distances along the dimension of chromaticity discrimination. (Modified from G Wyszecki, WS Stiles. Color Science: Concepts and Methods, Quantitative Data and Formulae [2nd ed]. New York: Wiley, 1982.)*

Color Appearance and Color Opponency

Trichromacy at the photoreceptor level and color opponency at postreceptor levels account for color mixture and color appearance data

In the latter part of the nineteenth century, Ewald Hering proposed an opponent color theory to account for the appearance of colors. Hering observed that red and green were never seen simultaneously, as in greenish-red, nor were blue and yellow, as in bluish-yellow. Therefore, he proposed that these color pairs, plus black and white, were processed in an opponent or antagonistic fashion to code for color. This idea eventually led to models of color vision in which the three cone types constituted a first trichromatic stage, as postulated by Young and Helmholtz, and a second opponent-processing stage, postulated by Hering. The first stage accounts for color mixture data and the second stage accounts for the opponent-appearance of colors. It was hoped that such a two-stage model (a *zone model*) would account for more color vision data than either one alone.

A simplified version of a zone model is shown in Figure 8.16. For clarity, the model shows three of each cone type, but it is not meant to represent realistically the anatomical proportion of these cone types in the wiring diagram of the retina. The main features are the opposition of SWS cone signals with a

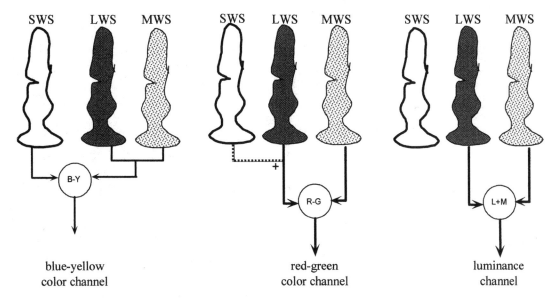

SWS LWS MWS   SWS LWS MWS   SWS LWS MWS

B-Y   R-G   L+M

blue-yellow   red-green   luminance
color channel   color channel   channel

FIGURE 8.16 *A simplified zone model for color vision showing how cone outputs (photoreceptor zone) are combined in a second zone (opponent and nonopponent color) to produce color and luminance signals. Short-wavelength sensitive (SWS) cone signals oppose long-wavelength sensitive (LWS) and middle-wavelength sensitive (MWS) signals (LWS + MWS = Y) to generate a blue-yellow (B-Y) opponent signal. LWS signals (with a SWS input) oppose MWS signals to generate a red-green (R-G) opponent signal. LWS and MWS signals combine additively (LWS + MWS) to generate a luminance signal. The diagram is not anatomically correct, and it simplifies numerous details.*

combination of LWS and MWS cone signals to generate a blue-yellow (B-Y) opponent channel, the opposition of LWS with MWS cone signals (with an input from SWS cones in the same direction as LWS signals) to generate the red-green (R-G) opponent channel, and a luminance channel that sums the outputs of LWS and MWS cones (L + M).

It is important to understand that the model is based on psychophysical evidence and the three identified channels are not necessarily identical to specific neural substrates. For example, luminance signals could be carried by different neural "streams" to the cortex, and the stream responsible for color perception might change, depending on the spatial or temporal frequency of the visual stimuli or other stimulus factors. Similarly, the two color opponent channels of the model may share features with the responses of certain retinal ganglion cell types, but (as is described in the Physiology of Color Vision section) there are some important differences between color opponency in ganglion cells and perceptual opponency.

Psychophysical studies of hue cancellation quantify color opponency

It was more than 50 years from the time that Hering put forward his ideas on opponent colors before Hurvich and Jameson (1955) measured the coloring power of spectral lights. Hurvich and Jameson reasoned that if a light appeared red, and there is a red-green color opponent channel, the redness could be canceled out by adding green to it. The amount of green required to neutralize the red would reflect the strength of the redness. Similarly, if there is a blue-yellow opponent channel, blue light could be used to cancel yellow, and so on.

Hurvich and Jameson tested their hypothesis by determining hue cancellation functions for spectral lights of various wavelengths. The observer was provided with a 1° target that was exposed repeatedly for several seconds. Mixed with the test wavelength was a cancellation wavelength that was a unique blue, unique yellow, unique green, or a long-wavelength red (not unique red, which is nonspectral). First, the radiance of one cancellation wavelength was adjusted until its mixture with the test wavelength produced a light that was neutral in color. *Neutral* was defined as neither blue nor yellow or neither red nor green. For instance, if the cancellation wavelength was green, then neutral would be reached when the test stimulus appeared neither red nor green. The procedure was repeated for each of the remaining cancellation wavelengths until the test stimulus appeared neutral in each case (neither blue or yellow and neither red or green). They called the resulting curves **chromatic valence functions** (Figure 8.17). For the purpose of

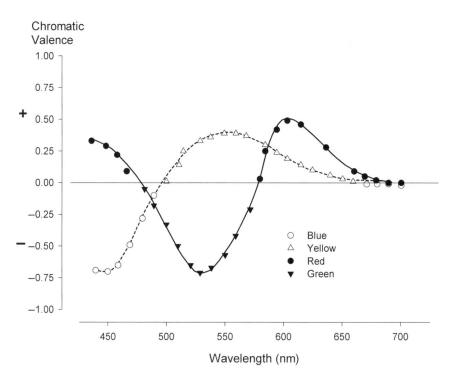

FIGURE 8.17 *Chromatic valence functions that are postulated for the CIE standard observer. The task is to adjust the intensity of three unique hues (blue, green, and yellow) plus long wavelength red to neutralize the color of the test wavelength. At each test wavelength, a positive red value means that the observer added green to neutralize the color. A negative green value means that red was added. Similarly, a positive yellow means that blue was added, and a negative blue value means that yellow was added. (Modified from G Wyszecki, WS Stiles. Color Science: Concepts and Methods, Quantitative Data and Formulae [2nd ed]. New York: Wiley, 1982.)*

more easily visualizing the data in the figure, blue was assigned a negative value and its opponent, yellow, was assigned a positive value. Likewise, red was assigned a positive value and green a negative value. The signs are arbitrary but make the point that subjects never used the two colors in an opponent pair simultaneously to neutralize the test wavelength.

Two examples should help to understand the figure. When the observer was presented with a 600 nm light, which appears orange (see Color Plate 8.1), the observer had to add green light to cancel the red component of the stimulus and blue light to cancel its yellow component. The figure actually plots the opponent colors, that is, the amount of red and yellow that were perceived to be in the test wavelength and had to be canceled to create the neutral appearance. At a short wavelength, such as 440 nm, the observer had to add yellow to cancel the blue component, so the figure shows the amount of blue (plotted as a negative value) present in the stimulus. This short wavelength also appears to have a significant amount of red (plotted as a positive value) because some of the green cancellation stimulus was needed to produce a neutral appearance in the test patch.

The unique hues are those hues that contain no trace of any other hue. They can be found by locating the crossing points for each opponent mechanism. This is the point at which the observer switched from adding green to adding red or from adding yellow to adding blue to neutralize. The red-green mechanism has a zero value at approximately 475 nm (unique blue) and again at approximately 580 nm (unique yellow). The blue-yellow mechanism has a zero crossing at approximately 500 nm (unique green), and it approaches a second zero crossing at very long wavelengths. However, most observers agree that even long-wavelength lights appear to contain a little yellow, and unique red is therefore nonspectral, which is realized by adding blue to a long-wavelength light.

Color naming further supports the opponent nature of color perception

The original observation that colors appear in opposed pairs can be quantified using color naming studies. Using Magnitude Estimation (see Chapter 1), observers were presented with a spectral color and asked to name it using any combination of the terms *red, green, yellow,* and *blue* (Boynton & Gordon 1965; Gordon & Abramov 1977). Sometimes a value for the achromatic content also was required. Despite the fact that no restrictions were placed on which color names could be used together, observers rarely or never used red and green simultaneously or blue and yellow simultaneously. Thus, color-naming functions support the data from the chromatic valence functions.

Stimulus size and retinal location also play a role. When the color of a small target that was presented in the visual periphery was assessed in this manner, it appeared desaturated and of uncertain color. If the target size was increased, a full range of peripheral hues was found, comparable to the range at the fovea. This suggests that peripheral color vision for large stimuli is similar to foveal color vision.

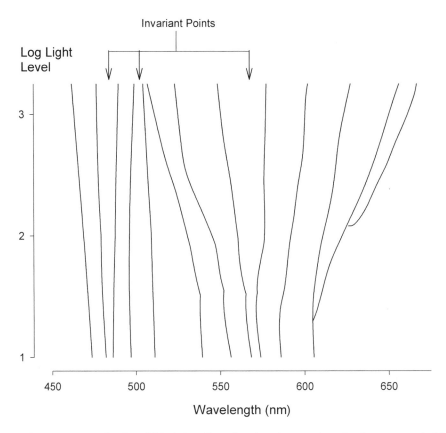

FIGURE 8.18 *The Bezold-Brücke effect showing the wavelengths that are needed for constant hue over a more than 2 log unit change in luminance. For example, starting at a low luminance (log 1), a 605 nm light must be shifted by approximately 15 nm toward longer wavelengths to maintain its hue as the luminance increases. The wavelengths that remain invariant as light level increases (approximately 475, 510, and 570 nm) are indicated by the arrows. (Modified from LM Hurvich. Color Science. Sunderland, MA: Sinauer, 1981.)*

Color Appearance Phenomena

The hue and saturation of a color may depend on its luminance (the Bezold-Brücke effect)

Earlier in this chapter it was stated that hue is the property of a color most closely associated with the dominant wavelength. Despite this close association, as the luminance of a spectral color is changed, its hue can shift somewhat. This is known as the **Bezold-Brücke effect**. It is measured by asking subjects to adjust the wavelength of a test light to match the hue of a reference spot as the intensity of the monochromatic test spot is increased. As shown in Figure 8.18, there is little or no shift for three wavelengths: 475 nm, 510 nm, and 570 nm. These unique spectral hues are similar in wavelength to the unique hues of Hurvich and Jameson (see Figure 8.17). At other wavelengths, the perceived hue changes in a predictable manner. For wavelengths shorter than 500 nm, lights become bluer as luminance increases, and for wavelengths longer than 500 nm, lights become more yellow as luminance increases. In other words, the blueness and yellowness responses increase with luminance faster than the redness and greenness responses, as if the blue-yellow and the red-green opponent systems had different luminance-response functions.

The hue of a color may depend on its colorimetric purity (the Abney effect)

The **Abney effect** refers to the hue shift that is induced by a colorimetric purity change. Recall that colorimetric purity is 1 when there is no white light added to a spectral color, and 0 for pure white light. There is an Abney effect for most color stimuli as the colorimetric purity is changed from 1 to 0. This means that in the CIE 1931 (x, y) diagram, a constant hue would plot along a curved line as one moves from the spectral locus to a reference white light, not a straight line as suggested in Figure 8.9. The exceptions are yellow, which has a dominant wavelength of 570 nm, and nonspectral bluish-purple hues, which follow a straight line. This is another example of a limitation of the CIE 1931 (x, y) color diagram to convey information about color appearance.

Color appearance is affected by surrounding colors or recent exposure to colors (simultaneous and successive color contrast)

The phenomenon of simultaneous contrast was discussed in Chapter 6. For achromatic spatial stimuli, if a central patch is surrounded by a region of lower luminance, the central patch appears brighter than it does if the surrounding region has higher luminance than the central patch (see Chapter 6, Figure 6.1). **Simultaneous color contrast** can be demonstrated by viewing a gray (achromatic) circle surrounded by a colored field. The central gray patch takes on a tinge of color that is the complementary color of the surrounding region. For example, if the surrounding region is red, the circle appears greenish. **Successive color contrast** (or complementary afterimages) can be demonstrated by adapting to a red light for a few minutes, removing the light, and then viewing an achromatic surface. The formerly colorless surface temporarily takes on the complementary color to the adapting light. The spatial and the successive color contrast phenomena reflect the opponent nature of color coding that is mediated by neural connections after the photoreceptors (see Figure 8.16).

Object color is relatively stable under different colored illuminations (color constancy)

The previous examples have shown that color appearance is not solely determined by the photoreceptor quantal catches, particularly under conditions involving rich or complex visual scenes. The Bezold-Brücke effect, the Abney effect, and color contrast effects are examples that color is not rigidly tied to receptor quantal absorptions. Despite these illustrations, as a practical matter, the perceived colors of objects vary little under different illumination conditions. This is called **color constancy**. For instance, as the spectral distribution of light from the sun and sky varies over the course of the day or as one moves an object from a room that is illuminated with tungsten light to one with fluorescent light and then to outside illumination, the spectral distribution that reaches the eye from the object can vary considerably. Colors, however, remain fairly invariant but not perfectly so. For example, people can appear ill because their complexion appears greenish under some fluorescent lights, and rare meat appears more appetizing under tungsten than fluorescent lights. In general, however, color appearance is better predicted from constancy than from the reflected light.

Physiology of Color Vision

The initial processing of color information occurs in the retina

As was illustrated in Figure 8.16, human color vision begins with multiple cone types that signal in a trivariant manner, as was proposed by the Young-Helmholtz trichromatic theory. The outputs from the three classes of cones are processed by subsequent cells in the retina and visual pathways in a way that compares the output of the cone types to create color opponent signals, which is in keeping with the suggestion of Hering. The conceptual model that was shown in Figure 8.16 is gradually becoming understood in terms of the actual synaptic connections that establish the color opponent channels in the retina (Dacey 1996). For color vision to occur and be measured psychophysically in human subjects, the information that is separated into color opponent channels in the retina must be preserved as it travels through the LGN in parallel afferent streams to the visual cortex. Color Plate 8.3 gives an overview of the circuitry in primate retina that converts the trichromacy of the cones into color opponent channels. Note that this is an active area of research, so any summary diagram is soon out of date.

In the retina, cones connect to bipolar cells, which, in turn, connect to ganglion cells, forming a direct or straight-through pathway to the ganglion cells whose axons leave the eye in the optic nerve. In the outer retina (the outer plexiform layer) near the base, or terminals, of the cones, horizontal cells make lateral connections between cones and bipolar cells. In the inner retina (the inner plexiform layer), amacrine cells (not shown in Color Plate 8.3) provide lateral connections between bipolar cells and ganglion cells.

Before discussing the specific connections that transform the color information received from the three cone types, it is important to note that there are several levels of complexity that are superimposed on the retinal circuitry. First, there appear to be distinct cell types that are involved in processing luminance signals and opponent color signals. The luminance and chromatic pathways (groups of cells involved in each type of processing) are carefully segregated and, indeed, remain largely separate up to and within the primary visual cortex (V1). Second, within the color pathway, there are receptor specific connections (although LWS and MWS connections might be wired interchangeably). Third, a center-surround, circular, receptive-field structure appears to be present within each pathway at the level of retinal ganglion cells and possibly earlier. Fourth, each ganglion cell's receptive-field type (whether within the luminance or chromatic pathways) comes in on-center and off-center varieties.

The magnocellular visual pathway can provide luminance information but not color-opponent information

There is anatomical, physiological, and psychophysical evidence for the existence of parallel information streams, or pathways, through the visual system. A single photoreceptor may provide input to more than one of these streams, so that each stream has a view of the same visual world but extracts different information about the visual scene. As shown on the left in Color Plate 8.3, in the **magnocellular (M) pathway**, diffuse bipolar cells receive input from LWS and MWS cones. Both on-center and off-center diffuse bipolar cells exist. Because the receptive-field centers receive input from LWS and MWS cones, they respond to a broad range of wavelengths. The H1 horizontal cells, which form the antagonistic receptive-field surround to the bipolar cells, also receive input from LWS and MWS cones, so the center and the surround respond equally to light of all wavelengths. (Ahnelt & Kolb 1994; Dacey et al. 1996). Because the surround signal through the H1 bipolar cell is presumed to be subtractive to the center, these cells should have a center-surround organization similar to that described in Chapter 6. The diffuse bipolar cells connect to parasol ganglion cells (labeled as "On MC-cell" and "Off MC-Cell" in the figure), whose axons leave the eye and connect with the magnocellular (large cell body) layers of the LGN. These cells in the LGN connect to specific layers of V1.

As described in Chapters 6 and 7, cells within the M pathway tend to have large receptive-center diameters in comparison to neurons in the other streams that project to the LGN, have poor spatial resolution (unable to respond to high spatial frequency stimuli), respond to rapid flicker, have high contrast gain (the slope of the contrast-response function is steep), and respond with excitation (increased firing rate of action potentials) or inhibition (decreased firing rate) to all wavelengths. In other words, they are spectrally nonopponent cells. They appear to play virtually no role in chromatic opponency but may be involved in providing information to the black-white luminance channel that was postulated by Hering.

The parvocellular visual pathway carries color-opponent information

The retinal neurons in the other stream, the **parvocellular (P) pathway**, include neurons that produce red-green color opponent information and blue-yellow opponent information. The current candidate for red-green opponency is the pathway through midget bipolar and midget ganglion cells. Within the central area of the retina, up to approximately 7° from the fovea, individual midget bipolar cells receive input from only a single cone and connect, in turn, to a single midget ganglion cell, as shown toward the right side of Color Plate 8.3. Therefore, the receptive-field center of the midget ganglion cell is cone specific (LWS or MWS but *not* SWS) and small (see Chapter 5, Figure 5.5). The midget ganglion cell's receptive-field surround is probably constructed from inputs drawn randomly from the LWS and MWS cone mosaic through the H1 horizontal cells. The midget ganglion cells are thus chromatically opponent and underlie color vision.

Another subdivision of the P pathway receives input from SWS cones. As shown at the right of Color Plate 8.3, there is a special cone bipolar cell type (labeled *S-Cone Bipolar*) that receives cone input only from the SWS cones. The SWS cone bipolar is an invaginating, wide-field, depolarizing (on) bipolar cell. It provides excitatory input to a small bistratified ganglion cell, and the axons of this ganglion cell type terminate in the interlaminar spaces within the parvocellular layers of the LGN. This SWS cone ganglion cell has been identified in humans as well as in macaque monkeys (Dacey 1993). LWS and MWS cone input to the blue-yellow opponent ganglion cell is probably directly inhibitory via a hyperpolarizing (off) bipolar cell. This scheme puts a potential candidate for blue-yellow opponency at the level of the inner plexiform layer of the retina.

Retinal ganglion cells and cells in the lateral geniculate nucleus of the brain show chromatic and spatial opponency

Psychophysical measures of both species have shown that macaque monkeys have similar color vision to humans. Electrical recordings that were made with microelectrodes from the visual pathway in macaques have shown that there are no essential differences in chromatic organization between the responses of retinal ganglion cells and cells in the LGN. Thus, data from the LGN can be taken as indicative of the responses of retinal ganglion cells. The color opponent nature of macaque monkey parvocellular LGN cells was demonstrated by DeValois et al. (1966). Using large stimuli that covered the entire receptive field (the center and the surround) of LGN cells, it was found that many cells respond by excitation (increased firing rate) to some wavelengths and by inhibition (decreased firing) to other wavelengths. The cells responded this way even when the luminances of the two lights were mismatched considerably, suggesting that the responses were truly wavelength specific. Figure 8.19 shows typical responses of LGN cells to large spectral lights. The term +R–G, for example, means that the cell was excited to lights that appeared red to the

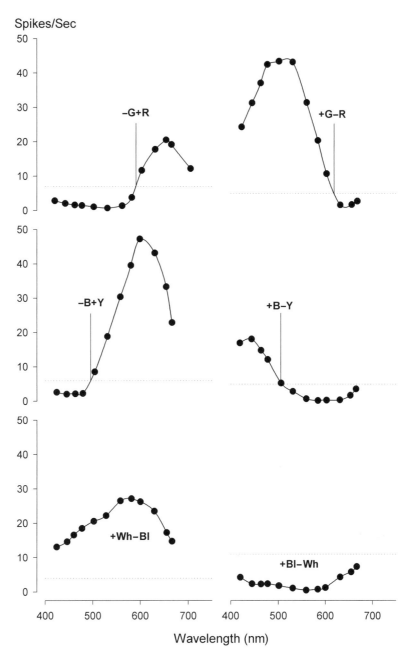

FIGURE 8.19 *Firing rates of six macaque monkey LGN cells in response to equal energy monochromatic stimuli that covered the entire receptive field. The horizontal line is the baseline firing rate of the cell when no stimulus is present. The four basic color opponent cells (+R–G, +G–R, +Y–B, +B–Y) increased their firing rates to some wavelengths and decreased their firing rates to others relative to their respective baseline rates. The two nonopponent cells (+Wh–Bl, +Bl–Wh) remained either above or below their respective baseline rates. (B = blue; Bl = black; G = green; R = red; Wh = white; Y = yellow.) (Modified from KK DeValois, RL DeValois. Spatial Vision. New York: Oxford University Press, 1988.)*

examiner, whereas lights appearing green inhibited it. Note that +R–G does not describe cone inputs. Rather, it refers to the fact that a cell increased its firing rate for long (red) wavelengths and decreased its firing rate for spectral wavelengths that appear as green.

DeValois et al. (1966) classified opponent cells into four groups based on the wavelength at which the response crossed from excitation to inhibition. The four groups were designated +R–G, +G–R, +Y–B, and +B–Y. This finding was thus suggestive that these cells constituted the physiological basis of Hering's opponent colors theory. In fact, DeValois et al. (1966) were able to show that the responses of these four cell groups plus a nonopponent cell type were able to account for psychophysical data on saturation discrimination, hue naming, and brightness perception. Thus, one has two physiologically based stages of color vision that can account for a great deal of psychophysical data. The first stage is at the level of the cones themselves; this stage accounts for trichromacy. The second stage is at the level of the retinal ganglion cells; this stage sees the first color opponent transformation.

The basic finding of color opponent LGN cells has been confirmed many times by others (DeMonasterio & Gouras 1975), but some important discrepancies between LGN cell responses and perceptual color opponency are now recognized. Today, more is known about cortical processing of color signals, and the transformations at the level of the ganglion cell and LGN are considered an early step in color processing.

By exploring the receptive fields of LGN cells with small white spots of light or gratings of various spatial frequencies, instead of large colored lights, such as those used in the previously mentioned DeValois study, it is found that cells are spatially opponent. They have a circular center-surround organization. This means that illuminating the entire receptive field with a large white light produces almost no response. Why, then, do LGN cells respond well to large colored lights but poorly to large white lights? The key to understanding this is to consider the cone inputs to the center and surround mechanisms. A +R–G cell (a cell excited by red and inhibited by green) might have, for example, a single LWS cone feeding the center mechanism and several MWS and LWS cones feeding the surround mechanism. Using a white light to which LWS and MWS cones are roughly equally sensitive, it is possible to map out the luminance receptive field that reflects the spatial antagonism rather than any spectral properties of the cell. A small white light that is the size of the receptive-field center mechanism produces an excitatory response. If the spot is enlarged to encroach on the surround, the inhibitory surround mechanism is stimulated and reduces the responses of the cell. When center and surround are fully covered, the cell's response is minimal. This is the same pattern of antagonistic center-surround organization that was described in Chapter 6.

If an isoluminant chromatic stimulus is used (i.e., no luminance modulation), the +R–G cell shows little center-surround spatial antagonism. When the entire receptive field is illuminated with white light, the cell responds little. If the wavelength of the light falling on just the center mechanism becomes 640 nm (red), LWS cones become more excited, and the LGN cell's response increases. As the 640 nm spot gets larger and starts to encroach on the surround, the MWS cones, which feed the surround, become less stimulated (because they are less sensitive to 640 nm than to white light of equal luminance); this reduces the surround antagonism, and the LGN cell's response continues to grow. Thus, one can see why large colored spots are effective at driving color opponent cells. In effect, each LGN cell has two superimposed receptive fields (DeValois & DeValois 1975). The luminance receptive field demonstrates spatial opponency, but the chromatic one does not. This accounts functionally for the lower spatial resolution that is observed when using stimuli that vary only in chromaticity versus luminance, and it accounts for the low pass rather than band pass shape of the spatial contrast sensitivity function to chromatic variations (DeValois & DeValois 1988) (see Chapter 6 for an explanation of these attributes of the contrast sensitivity function).

What happens to color signals after they leave the LGN? Signals are transmitted to V1 (also called *striate cortex*), where inputs from the P pathway terminate in layer 4cβ, and inputs from the M pathway terminate in layer 4cα of the cortex. The M pathway signals continue on to layer 4B, and from there to a different brain area, the middle temporal (MT) cortex. In the MT, there are many directionally selective neurons, and, as described in Chapter 7, it is generally believed that this is an important area for motion perception. It seems to be of little importance to color perception.

The P pathway signals from V1 layer 4cβ appear to connect to the superficial layers of V1, where they converge with a branch of the M pathway. Here, many cells are influenced by both the M and P pathways. The vast majority of the two major cell types encountered in V1, "simple" and "complex" cells, are chromatically opponent, although the opponency is often weaker than in the LGN (weaker opponency results when one cone type is weighted much more heavily than another). It has been shown that most cortical neurons are no more narrowly tuned to color variations than LGN cells (Lennie et al. 1990). Furthermore, the clear clustering of cells as red-green opponent or blue-yellow opponent that is seen in LGN cells is not found in V1. Rather, the cells appear to be tuned to many different colors (Thorell et al. 1984). The organization discovered in the LGN that was such a good match with the suggestions of psychophysical color opponent theory appears to be changed in V1.

A difficulty with detailing color processing in V1 and beyond is that one does not know precisely what one is looking for. In the vast majority of cells, some form of opponent cone inputs can be demonstrated, but it is not clear whether this means that all these cells are involved in color processing. Cortical cells transform signals in ways that more peripheral elements do not. A V1 cell might be color selective in the sense that it responds to a limited spectral region, but it no longer appears to carry an overtly opponent signal, and therefore it might not be considered to be involved in color processing. The relevance of the chromatic properties of cortical cells to color perception is not completely understood.

Cerebral achromatopsia suggests that there is a specialized cortical area for the perception of color

Cerebral achromatopsia is a condition that presents as a loss of color vision and is often permanent. The most frequent cause of cerebral achromatopsia is a stroke that damages two local areas of cortex in the inferior regions of both hemispheres near the **calcarine sulcus**. Cerebral achromats complain of loss of color in their world, but they often have excellent visual acuity, motion perception, stereopsis, and so on. However, the degree to which other visual functions are affected may be related to the extent of the cortical damage. Most cerebral achromats also experience *prosopagnosia*, or failure to recognize familiar faces, and this implies that the cortical mechanisms involved in face recognition and color vision lie in close proximity (Zeki 1990). The important implication of this rare and fascinating condition is that there is a specialized cortical area that is critically important for color perception. It has been suggested that cortical area V4 in the macaque monkey is the homologue of the human color area that is affected in cerebral achromatopsia. It also serves as a reminder that it is the brain that colors the world. Retinal mechanisms and afferent pathways organize the chromatic response, but cortical neurons are necessary for conscious color vision.

Deficient Color Vision

As described early in this chapter, the ability to precisely match all visible wavelengths by mixing three **primary colors**, trichromacy, is a logical extension of the presence of three different classes of photosensitive pigments (although it is not necessarily linked to just three). Although trichromacy is considered the normal condition of color vision, a substantial fraction of people have some degree of color deficiency.

Anomalous trichromats have an abnormal absorption spectrum for one cone photopigment while dichromats completely lack one of the cone photopigments

Approximately 6% of males and less than 0.4% of females are anomalous trichromats. One of their cone pigments has an action spectrum that is different from the normal action spectra that are shown in the top left panel of Figure 8.20 (Curcio & Allen 1990; Wassle et al. 1989). As a result, when presented with a color-matching task, these people use significantly different proportions of the three primaries to match some colors. Figure 8.20 shows, in addition to normals, the action spectra found in people with several types of color anomalies. On the left are **anomalous trichromats**, including conditions specifically known as **protanomaly** (1% of males) and **deuteranomaly** (5% of males).

In deuteranomaly, the anomalous photopigment occurs in the MWS cone. In protanomaly, it occurs in the LWS cone. In each condition, the effect is for the

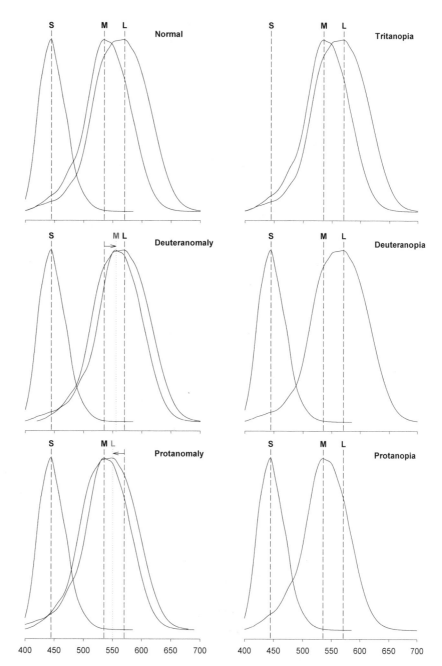

FIGURE 8.20 *Schematic representations of photopigment absorption spectra for the short-wavelength (S), middle-wavelength (M), and long-wavelength (L) sensitive cones in humans with normal color vision and with color deficiencies. The dashed vertical lines indicate the wavelengths of the peaks of the absorption spectra for the normal photopigments. The dotted lines indicate that in deuteranomaly the M peak is shifted toward longer wavelengths and in protanomaly the L peak is shifted toward shorter wavelengths. The dichromats shown in the right column are missing one cone photopigment.*

action spectrum of the anomalous photopigment to be shifted toward the action spectrum of the other, normal photopigment. Thus, in deuteranomaly, the anomalous MWS cone's action spectrum is shifted toward the LWS cone's action spectrum. In protanomaly, the LWS cone's action spectrum is shifted toward that of the normal MWS cones. These shifts in the action spectrum of one photopigment towards the other affect hue and saturation discriminations in the people who have these altered photopigments and also may affect the brightness of certain colors.

The right column in Figure 8.20 shows the color-matching situation for color-defective people who are known as *dichromats*; the conditions of dichromacy are **protanopia**, **deuteranopia**, and **tritanopia**. In **dichromacy**, one of the three classes of normal photopigments is missing. Two percent of males and less than 0.02% of females can match all colors with a mixture of only two primary colors, which is a direct result of having only two functional cone photopigments. In protanopia (1% of males), the observer lacks the LWS cone pigment. In deuteranopia (1% of males), the MWS cone pigment is missing. The genes that control the structure and expression of the MWS and LWS photopigments are found on the X chromosome, which explains the higher prevalence of these hereditary red-green color defects in males.

The SWS cone photopigment is controlled by a gene on chromosome 7. Tritanopia, the lack of functional SWS cones as an inherited condition, results from a small number of point mutations in the gene that codes the protein portion of the SWS cone photopigment. The defect follows a dominant inheritance pattern and the incidence is rare, estimated at 1 in 50,000 to 1 in 15,000. **Tritanomaly** might exist as a separate genetic activity.

Rod monochromats, individuals totally without cones or having only a few scattered cones, were mentioned earlier in this chapter. They constitute less than 1 in 30,000 of the population, and there are approximately equal numbers of males and females who have this condition. The genetic defect lies on chromosome 2, and, as with other types of inherited color defects and, indeed, with retinal dystrophies, there is genetic heterogeneity.

It should come as no surprise that having anomalous photopigments or having a photopigment totally absent produces characteristic differences between normal and color deficient individuals in psychophysical measurements of hue and saturation discrimination as well as the brightness of colors. These differences underlie the design and construction of clinical tests for the identification and classification of deficient color vision as discussed in greater detail throughout the remaining sections of this chapter.

Colors that a dichromat cannot distinguish fall on straight lines in the CIE (x, y) color space

Recall, in Figure 8.14, that if one starts with any color in the CIE 1931 (x, y) chromaticity diagram and changes its color in any direction, then when the x or y values change sufficiently, a normal trichromatic observer can distinguish that the color has changed. For protanopes, deuteranopes, and tritanopes, extensive color changes in certain directions cannot be discriminated. The colors that cannot be distinguished by dichromats lie along straight lines on the CIE 1931 (x, y) color space and are called **confusion lines**. Examples are shown in Figure 8.21. In the trichromatic observer, colors that lie along confusion lines produce changing quantal absorptions in just one of the three cone types, whereas the absorptions in the remaining two cone types remain constant.

The point on the CIE 1931 (x, y) chromaticity diagram at which all the confusion lines of one type of dichromacy intersect is called the **copunctal** or **convergence point**. This point theoretically represents the chromaticity coordinates of an imaginary light that would stimulate only the missing fundamental response function to which this chapter referred earlier. For protanopes, the copunctal point is close to 700 nm. For tritanopes, it is close to 400 nm. All three copunctal points actually lie outside the spectral locus, and the color at each copunctal point is therefore imaginary. The precise location of these copunctal points is extremely important in deriving the spectral sensitivities of the human cone photopigments.

One particular confusion line in Figure 8.21 deserves special mention: the one that passes through the center of the diagram where a white light (CIE Standard Illuminant C) is represented. It intersects the spectral locus at a point called the **neutral point**. Dichromats, when asked to match a monochromatic light to a specified white light, are able to do so for one wavelength. Its position on the spectral locus varies with the white chosen as a reference; the higher the color temperature, the shorter the wavelength of the matching light. A tritanope's neutral point is in the neighborhood of 570 nm, whereas those of a protanope and deuteranope are generally between 490 and 500 nm. The wavelength of the protanope's neutral point is consistently a few nanometers shorter than that of the deuteranope. Thus, a color vision test designed to assess a color-deficient person's neutral point could be used to classify these different types of dichromatic color defects.

Also to be noted in Figure 8.21 is that for both the protanope and deuteranope, there is a confusion line at the right of the CIE (x, y) color space that is essentially parallel to the most linear part of the spectral locus from approximately 540 to 700 nm. This indicates that these individuals cannot distinguish among monochromatic lights from the middle- to long-wavelength end of the spectrum, a fact that was also presented in Figure 8.12. All of these spectral colors collapse, effectively, into one color sensation. Notice, thus, that if a person reported that 700 nm and 540 nm lights match, their color vision must be dichromatic, but from this observation alone, it remains unclear whether their dichromacy is due to protanopia or deuteranopia.

Refer again to Figure 8.12, and compare the wavelength discrimination function for normal trichromats with that of protanopes and deuteranopes. Protanopes and deuteranopes have their best wavelength discrimination at wavelengths near their spectral neutral point (490–500 nm). Consistent with the notion of color opponency and the physiology of color opponent cells (see

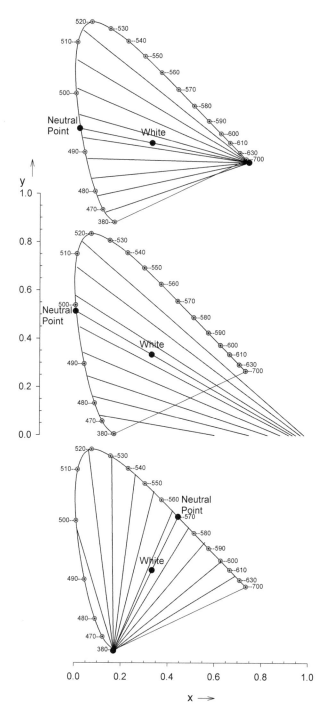

FIGURE 8.21   *Representative confusion lines of (**top**) protanopes, (**middle**) deuteran-opes, and (**bottom**) tritanopes are shown in the CIE 1931 (x, y) chromaticity diagram. A subset of all possible confusion lines is shown for each dichromatic condition. (Modified from G Wyszecki, WS Stiles. Color Science: Concepts and Methods, Quantitative Data and Formulae [2nd ed]. New York: Wiley, 1982.)*

Figure 8.19), the response of the blue-yellow opponent process changes most rapidly about the neutral points in protanopes and deuteranopes, and the response of their respective +B–Y (or –B+Y) LGN cell is at the baseline firing rate (neutral or no color response). For wavelengths longer than approximately 540 nm, light absorption by SWS cone photopigment is insignificant. Therefore, deuteranopes and protanopes are, respectively, LWS and MWS cone monochromats in this region of the spectrum. Consequently, the blue-yellow opponent process that is responsible for color discrimination should not be functional. This notion also is consistent with the existence of a confusion line that is collinear with the spectral locus from 540 to 700 nm for protanopes and deuteranopes, as described previously.

Tritanopes have their best wavelength discrimination at approximately 570 nm, and they are poor at discriminating lights in the region of 450 nm. The wavelength discrimination functions of protanomalous and deuteranomalous trichromats are quite variable and range from a flat W-shaped function, similar to normal, all the way to a nearly U-shaped function that is similar to that of protanopes and deuteranopes (see Figure 8.12).

Colorimetric purity discrimination thresholds are reduced in all color deficiencies

Saturation (colorimetric purity) discriminations for **deutans** (deuteranomalous trichromats and deuteranopes) and **protans** (protanomalous trichromats and protanopes) are shown in Figure 8.22. Remember, from Figure 8.13, that the task in this discrimination is to determine the amount of light at a given wavelength that must be added to a reference (4,800 K) white light for a subject to detect a jnd from the white light. When a small quantity of monochromatic light is added to white, the resulting mixture has low purity. If an observer can notice a change in saturation when a small quantity of monochromatic light is added, then the observer's purity discrimination is good. If, however, a lot of monochromatic light must be added to white for the observer to detect its presence, the purity of the light is higher, and the person's saturation discrimination is poor. Notice, in Figure 8.22, that for deuteranopes and protanopes, saturation discrimination falls to zero at one spectral point. This means that a pure monochromatic light of 495 nm (for the protanope) or 500 nm (for the deuteranope) is indistinguishable from the 4,800 K white light. These wavelengths correspond to the uniquely dichromatic neutral points that were described previously. Notice also that the minima for the saturation discrimination function are nearly where the wavelength discrimination of protanopes and deuteranopes is best (see Figure 8.12). Like normal trichromats, anomalous trichromats do not have neutral points. They are able to distinguish white from all spectral lights. Nearly everywhere in the visible spectrum, however, colors are more saturated for normal trichromats than for protan and deutan color defectives.

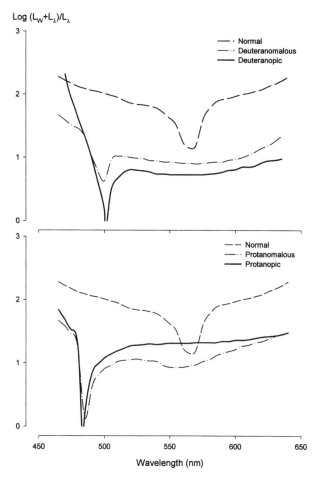

Log $(L_W+L_\lambda)/L_\lambda$

FIGURE 8.22 *Colorimetric purity (saturation discrimination) functions for X-linked dichromats and anomalous trichromats. The task was the same as for the subjects whose thresholds are shown in Figure 8.13. (L_λ = luminance of the monochromatic light that is added to the white; L_w = luminance of the white.) (Modified from J Pokorny, VC Smith, G Verriest, AJ Pinkers. Congenital and Acquired Color Vision Defects. New York: Grune & Stratton, 1979.)*

Protan color-defective observers perceive reds as dim or dark

As shown in the Appendix, Figure A.1, the normal photopic **luminosity** curve peaks at approximately 555 nm. It has this shape because there is a disproportionately large input (approximately 2 or 3 to 1) from LWS cones compared to MWS cones and little or no input from SWS cones. Consequently, compared to color normals, one would predict that protanopes, who lack LWS photopigment, and protanomalous trichromats, who have an LWS photopigment that is more like the normal MWS photopigment, would experience a severe reduction in the relative brightness of red lights. A number of practical examples show that this is, in fact, the case. First, protanopes and many protanomalous

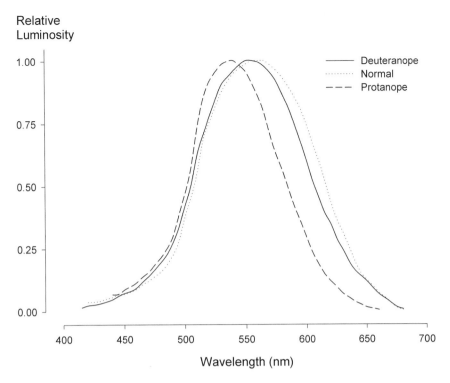

FIGURE 8.23 *Photopic luminosity (luminous efficiency) functions of protanopes, deuteranopes, and color normals. The normal curve is the same as that shown in the Appendix, Figure A.1. (Modified from G Wyszecki, WS Stiles. Color Science: Concepts and Methods, Quantitative Data and Formulae [2nd ed]. New York: Wiley, 1982.)*

individuals have difficulty seeing automobile brake lights under conditions in which it is easy for color normals to see them. This can lead to delayed reaction times, which has been linked to a higher incidence of rear-end automobile accidents in protans. Second, deep-red (long-wavelength) surface colors may look quite black to protanopic observers, and the red light–emitting diodes on consumer electronic devices can be difficult for protans to see. Deep-red laser pointers can be invisible to protans. Deutans have no significant relative loss of luminosity compared to normals, as Figure 8.23 clearly shows. This also is the case for deuteranomalous trichromats.

Significant color vision defects are acquired with eye disease

Any disorder or disease that affects the visual sensory pathways has the potential to affect color vision. The mechanisms by which color vision is affected by disease are largely unknown, and there are clearly many pathophysiologic causes for acquired color vision defects (Pokorny et al. 1979). For example, the cause of the color defect in **Stargardt's juvenile macular dystrophy** is different from that in **optic neuritis** because the disorders affect

Table 8.6 Distinctions between X-linked inherited and acquired color defects

Congenital X-linked inherited	Acquired
Symmetrical or equal for the two eyes	Eyes affected to different degrees
Rarely blue-yellow; almost always red-green	Often blue-yellow
Rarely misname colors	Frequent color naming errors
Stable throughout life	May vary with severity of underlying condition

different tissues. Patients with these disorders may make similar errors on color vision tests, however. There are important distinctions between inherited (congenital, X-linked recessive) and acquired color defects, as shown in Table 8.6.

Testing for Color Vision Defects

The anomaloscope is the gold standard for diagnosing vision defects

An **anomaloscope** is an instrument that is used to characterize color-matching behavior. The **Rayleigh equation** is the gold standard for diagnosing the four major X-linked color defects. The anomaloscope uses an additive mixture of 670 nm (spectral red light) plus 546 nm (spectral green light) combined in one hemifield of a bipartite field, and a 589 nm (spectral orange-yellow light) in the other hemifield. The task of the observer is to adjust the relative energies of the 670 and 546 nm primaries until their mixture appears identical to the reference 589 nm light (a metameric match).

Color vision testing is based on knowledge of confusion lines

It is the existence of highly predictable confusion lines that allows for clever diagnostic distinction between color defective types. For protanopes and deuteranopes, the spectrum above 540 nm is detected essentially by one photopigment: the MWS (for protanopes) or LWS (for deuteranopes) photopigment. Consequently, for these dichromats, any anomaloscope mixture of 546 nm plus 670 nm matches the 589 nm light, including the match extremes, that is, the 546 or 670 nm primaries alone. If a dichromat now needs to reduce the intensity of the 589 nm light when matching a pure (non-mixture) 670 nm light, then he identifies himself as a protanope. The yellow-intensity setting of a deuteranope is virtually the same as the one he or she uses to match the 546 nm light alone.

Anomalous trichromats characterize themselves by requiring more (deuteranomalous) or less (protanomalous) 546 nm light (green) in the mixture to match 589 nm light than color normal people. Like color normal people, and unlike dichromats, many anomalous trichromats accept a specific mixture of 670 nm plus 546 nm; other anomalous trichromats may accept a wide range of mixtures but never the entire range. This different anomaloscope mixture-match behavior of anomalous trichromats is consistent with the notion that their color confusions are less extensive than those of dichromats.

Book or plate tests have been remarkably successful in detecting color defective vision. The colors of the figure and background are carefully chosen to lie close to confusion lines (see Figure 8.21). For example, many figures on the **Ishihara Color Plate Test** use reddish, orange, and yellow dots in a background within which is embedded a green number made up of dots with the same brightness range (so that the number cannot be detected by brightness difference alone). Color defectives may be unable to discriminate the green number from the background, because both color sets lie close together and are close to one of their confusion lines. Therefore, the number is hidden for color defectives but not for normal trichromats. Ishihara's book tests have one or more diagnostic plates on which the color normal sees a red and a purple number on a gray background. These plates help distinguish protan from deutan observers.

Color Plate 8.4 shows the rationale behind similarly designed diagnostic plates of the **Hardy-Rand-Rittler (HRR) Color Plate Test**. The colored figures represented in this test (a circle and a triangle) have chromaticities in the greenish and bluish-green regions of the CIE diagram (Figure 8.24). Other colored figures are along the same protan and deutan confusion lines, but in the red and red-purple regions of the CIE diagram. By locating these colors at different distances from the gray background along the two confusion lines, the type and degree of severity (extent of confusion) of a color defect may be distinguished. A dichromat would fail to see colors most distant from the gray background, whereas anomalous trichromats would rarely miss such saturated (for them) colors.

Perhaps the most clinically useful test is the **Farnsworth D-15 Color Test** and its related desaturated versions of the test. The locations of the 15 colors plus a fixed reference color in the CIE 1931 (x, y) diagram are plotted in Figure 8.25, along with confusion lines for protanopes and deuteranopes (see also Figure 8.21). The test colors are Munsell papers.

The Farnsworth D-15 Color Test was designed to classify patients into those who are likely to experience difficulties with their color vision and those who are not. A patient arranges 15 colored caps in a tray with a fixed reference cap at one end. Each successive cap is the closest match to the one that preceded it. The spacing of colors along confusion lines makes it a relatively easy test to pass for normal trichromats and many anomalous trichromats, but almost all dichromats fail. A protanope, for example, places cap No. 15 next to the reference cap, cap No. 1 next to cap No. 15, cap No. 14 next to cap No. 1, and so on, consistent with protanopic confusions.

A common clinical situation is for a young male to fail the Ishihara Color Plate Test but pass the Farnsworth D-15 arrangement test. This almost certainly

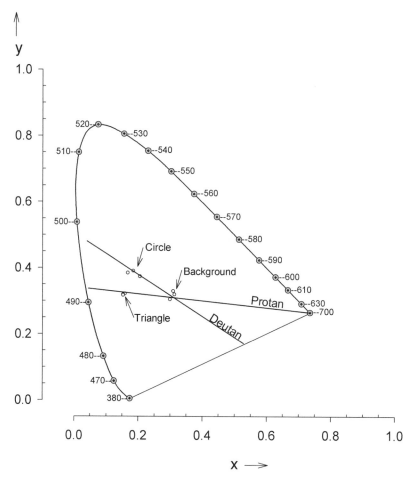

FIGURE 8.24   *The chromaticities of the circle and triangle figures of plate 13 on the Hardy-Rand-Rittler Color Plate Test are shown in the CIE 1931 (x, y) chromaticity diagram, along with the chromaticities of the neutral (gray) background. The protanope is unable to see the triangle but sees the circle; the deuteranope sees the triangle but not the circle. For clarity, the chromaticities of the figures are exaggerated. (Modified from Committee on Vision. Procedures for testing color vision—report of Working Group 41. Washington: National Academy Press, 1981.)*

indicates anomalous trichromacy, but if there are no errors on the Farnsworth D-15 test, there is no indication whether the protan or deutan variety is present. Protanopes and deuteranopes, as well as extreme anomalous trichromats (who are nearly dichromatic), fail both the Ishihara and Farnsworth D-15 tests, and their error axes are diagnostic of these conditions.

The **Farnsworth-Munsell 100-hue test**, consisting of 85 caps taken from the 100 possible hues of the Munsell color ordering system (described in an earlier section), allows a normal observer to arrange color caps within a single quadrant of the color circle. Because of this division of the color circle, the observer is never allowed to make confusions across the hue circle. Again, the color

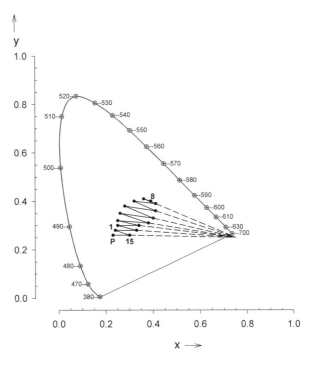

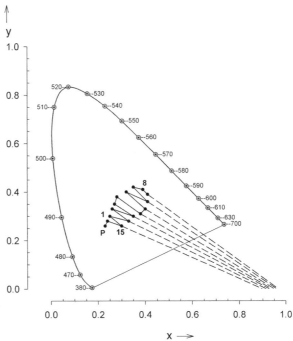

FIGURE 8.25 *Chromaticity coordinates of the 16 caps of the Farnsworth D-15 test are plotted with the confusion lines of protanopes (**top**) and deuteranopes (**bottom**) to show the expected cap arrangement of each color defective. The task is to order the colors from P, the reference cap, to cap 15 in a logical sequence. (Modified from Committee on Vision. Procedures for testing color vision—report of Working Group 41. Washington: National Academy Press, 1981.)*

confusion lines and their empirical separation in color space account for the poor performance by the color defective.

Color testing may need to be performed monocularly

Clinicians need to be aware that testing color vision binocularly simply tests the better eye. If ocular dysfunction is a concern, monocular testing is necessary (see Table 8.6). However, most vocational color standards require binocular testing.

Few color vision tests were designed for acquired color vision defects that are associated with eye disease

Many forms of eye disease that alter the sensory retina, preretinal filtering, or any part of the visual sensory pathways can produce disturbance of vision. The processing of the signals from the three cone photoreceptor types in the retina before the signals leave the eye perhaps makes it inevitable that disturbances of sensory retina will reflect color vision alterations. The association of retinal and visual pathway disease with color vision defects has been reported for over a century and is most popularly characterized by Kollner's rule. Although an oversimplification, the rule has sufficient validity to assist clinicians in complex diagnoses of retinal and visual pathway disorders. The rule is that lesions at the level of the photoreceptors or in the preretinal media are more commonly associated with blue-yellow (better termed as **tritan**) disorders of color vision. Lesions in the postreceptoral layers (inner retina, ganglion cells) are more likely to exhibit red-green color disorders.

Short Wavelength Automated Perimetry detects early visual sensitivity loss in glaucoma

As was discussed in Chapter 3, new strategies have recently been developed for use in visual field testing to detect early changes due to glaucoma. In Short Wavelength Automated Perimetry (SWAP), which is used for early glaucoma testing, blue test targets are flashed on a bright yellow background. Through selective adaptation of the MWS and LWS cones by the yellow light, their sensitivity relative to SWS cones is decreased while the adaptive background is present (see Figure 8.2). This forces detection of the blue test light by the SWS cone pathway, which is believed to be selectively damaged in the earliest stages of glaucoma. It has been shown that characteristic glaucomatous visual field changes can be identified with SWAP in eyes that, several years later, develop field defects that are demonstrable by standard increment threshold perimetry. Note that glaucoma is one of the diseases that does not follow Kollner's rule. In early diabetes, the SWS cone system not only has a selective sensitivity loss, but its sensitivity appears to be correlated with changes in blood glucose levels. This offers hope for a sensitive vision test of a diabetic's glucose control.

e of most color defects is an altered or absent photopig-
g the world through colored lenses does not correct this
s little reason to believe that colored filters improve the
nations of a color defective. If one eye receives a different
ther, then there is the theoretical possibility that the brain
: could learn to interpret this differential information in a
ncrease in color discrimination abilities overall. This does
. however.

l, it is clear that the color defective has well-defined and
; with specific colors. It is relatively straightforward to
ilter that can exaggerate the brightness differences of two
if a color defective observer is unable to distinguish a red
bject, viewing through a red filter creates a lightness or
, with the red object becoming relatively brighter and
le. Selective filtering of the most desaturated colors for
Figure 8.22) may enhance the appearance of an other-
, colors that fall on the confusion lines of dichromats can
lowever, it should always be assumed that the discrimina-
lors has been reduced by adding this filter. Nonetheless,
workplace in which a limited number of important col-
shed from each other, there is a good application of filters

luding tinted spectacle or contact lenses) should never be
r tests. Use of colored filters to help an individual pass an
example, is like allowing an individual to stand closer to
hat he can read the 6/6 line (see Chapter 5, Figure 5.9).
ng. Also, a monocularly worn, tinted contact lens (such as
the X chrom lens) should never be worn for driving because of possible impairment of depth perception.

Study Guide

1. How have the spectral sensitivities of human cones been studied by means of psychophysics?
2. Why are individual cones and, therefore, persons with only one type of cone present in their retina, totally color blind?
3. What is meant by the term *primaries*, as used in color-matching studies? Distinguish between real and imaginary primaries.
4. How is it possible to represent colors that are seen by a normal trichromatic observer in a two-dimensional diagram?
5. What are complementary colors? How are they located on the CIE (x, y) color diagram?
6. Given the chromaticity coordinates of a color, how are the dominant wavelength and excitation purity of the color determined?

7. What are the physical correlates of the hue, saturation, and brightness of a color? Describe how such a color would be specified using the Munsell Color System.

8. What are the spectral locations of best wavelength and purity discrimination in normal trichromats?

9. What are MacAdam discrimination ellipses, and what are their consequences for specifying color appearance using the CIE 1931 (x, y) color diagram?

10. What lines of psychophysical and electrophysiological evidence support color opponency?

11. How does the luminance of a color affect its hue and saturation? What are the wavelengths of invariant hues for normal trichromats?

12. Compare and contrast the functional color aspects of the M and P visual pathways.

13. In what way is the circuitry of the SWS cone pathway distinct from the MWS and LWS cone pathways?

14. Sketch the wavelength discrimination functions of protanopes and deuteranopes. What feature of each curve is related to the minimum of the respective purity discrimination function?

15. Sketch a CIE 1931 (x, y) chromaticity diagram, and show at least three confusion lines and the location of the convergence point of a protanope and a deuteranope. Draw an additional confusion line to show how to locate their spectral neutral points.

16. Why is anomalous trichromacy considered to be deficient color vision? Why is it not possible to distinguish anomalous trichromats from dichromats using common clinical tests?

17. List at least three distinguishing characteristics of hereditary and acquired color deficiencies.

18. What is Kollner's rule? What are its implications for clinical color vision tests?

19. What is SWAP? How is selective chromatic adaptation used to isolate SWS cone pathways that are damaged in eye disease?

Glossary

Abney effect: the change in hue of a color that accompanies a change in its purity or saturation.

Achromatic color: sensation or perception that is characterized by brightness without hue; neutral color.

Action spectrum: a plot of the radiant energy at various wavelengths that is required for a constant biological effect, such as rate of nerve discharge or number of activated molecules of photopigment.

Anomaloscope: an instrument for testing color vision by means of mixing colors, usually a red plus a green to match a yellow. Significant deviation from the normal mixture match characterizes the type and degree of severity of the color vision deficiency present.

Anomalous trichromat: a person who has anomalous trichromatic color vision, specified as protanomaly, deuteranomaly, or tritanomaly.

Bezold-Brücke effect: the change in hue of most spectral colors that accompanies a change in their intensity.

Blackbody radiator: a thermal radiator whose spectral power distribution is determined solely by its temperature.

Brightness: the subjective correlate of photometric luminance or luminous intensity.

Calcarine sulcus: calcarine fissure. A deep cleft on the medial aspect of the occipital lobe of the brain adjacent to V1.

Cerebral achromatopsia: total color blindness due to lesions in the brain cortex near the calcarine sulcus.

Chroma: the designation of saturation in the Munsell Color System.

Chromatic adaptation: prolonged, continuous viewing of a color that is chosen to depress the sensitivity of one or two classes of cones, thereby partially isolating a remaining class of cones to concurrently measure its spectral sensitivity.

Chromatic valence functions: curves that describe the extent to which a spectral stimulus excites yellow-blue and green-red pairs of opponent colors.

Chromaticity: the color quality of a stimulus that refers to its hue and saturation.

Chromaticity diagram: a two-dimensional graphic representation of the gamut of color stimuli; the rectilinear coordinates differ depending on the selected primaries.

Chromophore: the light-absorbing portion of photopigment.

CIE 1931 RGB color-matching functions: tristimulus values of real primary colors (red, green, and blue) standardized by the International Commission on Illumination and subsequently used by the same group to create a set of color-matching functions by mathematic transformation for a set of imaginary primaries, X, Y, and Z.

CIE 1931 XYZ system: a means for specifying color based on the tristimulus values of imaginary color primaries—X, Y, and Z—that were standardized by the International Commission on Illumination.

CIE 1931 (x, y) chromaticity diagram: a two-dimensional graphic representation of color stimuli; the rectilinear coordinates (x, y) are the ratios of each tristimulus value of the color stimulus to their sum.

CIE 1976 (u', v') uniform color space diagram: a transformation of the CIE 1931 (x, y) chromaticity diagram such that equal distances between the coordinates (u', v') represent approximately equal perceptual differences between the corresponding color stimuli.

Color blindness: defective color vision regardless of degree of severity. Because true, total color blindness is extremely rare, color deficiency is a better term.

Color constancy: stability of color perception of objects in spite of changes in the wavelength composition of incident light.

Color discrimination: the judgment of just noticeable differences in hue, saturation, or brightness or a combination of these attributes of color as compared with a reference stimulus.

Color matching: the act of mixing colors to achieve the same hue, saturation, and brightness as a sample color.

Color specification: a numeric or alphanumeric description of a color based on measurement of its objective or subjective attributes.

Color temperature: the temperature of a blackbody radiator at which its color matches a given color sample.

Color vision: the attribute of sight that provides appreciation of differences in the physical composition of wavelengths of light.

Colorimeter: a device used to specify a color.

Colorimetric purity: the proportional amount of a spectral light in a mixture of the spectral light and a white light.

Complementary colors: pairs of colors that match a specified white light when mixed in proper proportions.

Cone opsins: various proteins that combine with the chromophore 11-*cis*-retinaldehyde to synthesize molecules of photopigment in cones; the variation of the protein moiety determines the differences in the cones' spectral absorption properties.

Confusion lines: the loci of colors in a chromaticity diagram that appear identical to a dichromat.

Convergence point: one of three locations at which the confusion lines of dichromatic color vision intersect in a chromaticity diagram. Theoretically, the point represents the CIE specification of lights that would stimulate each of the fundamentals.

Copunctal point: convergence point

Correlated color temperature: specification of a light source in terms of the temperature of a blackbody radiator that is a colorimetric match.

Deutans: deuteranopes and deuteranomalous individuals.

Deuteranomaly: anomalous trichromatic color vision due to alteration of the normal MWS cone photopigment.

Deuteranopia: dichromatic color vision due to an absence of the MWS cone pigment.

Dichromacy: dichromatic color vision.

Dichromat: a person who has dichromatic color vision, specifically, protanopia, deuteranopia, or tritanopia.

Dominant wavelength: the physical correlate of hue. When properly mixed with a specified white light, the mixture matches a given sample color.

Excitation purity: the extent to which a color stimulus differs from white or its dominant wavelength, as gauged by its location between them on a chromaticity diagram.

Farnsworth-Munsell 100-hue test: a test of color discrimination that involves the arrangement of 85 of the 100 possible hues in the Munsell Color System at constant chroma (saturation) and value (brightness) that can be scored quantitatively for classification of a color defect by type and degree of severity.

Farnsworth D-15 Color Test: arrangement color test of only 15 hues that progress uniformly around the color circle from a reference hue. It is useful for dichotomizing mild and severe color defects, and if the defect is severe, it may be classified according to type.

Fundamental response function: the one particular set of color-matching functions that corresponds to the actual spectral sensitivities of the three response systems that are present in the normal trichromatic retina (i.e., the spectral sensitivity of each of the cone photopigments).

Hardy-Rand-Rittler (HRR) Color Plate Test: a test that was designed for screening and classification, if necessary, of deficient color vision. The colors of geometric figures to be identified on a series of plates lie along dichromatic confusion lines that pass through a neutral gray that is used as the background of each plate, making the test one of saturation discrimination.

Hue: the perceptual correlate of the dominant wavelength of a color, to be distinguished from its other perceptual attributes, namely saturation and brightness, which are designated respectively as chroma and value in the Munsell Color System.

Imaginary primaries: mathematically transformed real primaries (an unreal color) that serve to locate primary reference points in a CIE chromaticity diagram.

Ishihara Color Plate Test: a test primarily designed for screening of red-green deficient color vision. The colors of digits to be identified on the majority of plates differ from the surrounding background, but figure and background lie on or near a confusion line that is separated by no more than a near-threshold distance for persons with normal color vision.

Isomer: one of a pair of color stimuli that have identical color appearance and wavelength composition.

Luminosity: the luminous effect of radiant energy that is dependent on wavelength, as described in relative values by the photopic luminous efficiency coefficient, the symbol V_λ.

Magnocellular (M) pathway: magnocellular channel. One of two retinocortical pathways that carries no information about color or high spatial resolution but otherwise all other information that is not transmitted by the parallel P pathway.

Metamer: one of a set of color stimuli, all of which have identical color appearance but different spectral composition.

Monochromatic: light or electromagnetic radiation that is emitted over a narrow band of wavelengths.

Neutral point: a spectral wavelength that a dichromat selects to match a specified white light.

Nonspectral colors: any color that is not on the spectral locus. Colors that cannot be matched by a single spectral light.

Optic neuritis: inflammation of the optic nerve that may be intraocular and observable or extraocular and usually not visible to a clinician and that is marked by sudden vision loss, which often affects color perception.

Parvocellular (P) pathway: parvocellular channel. One of two retinocortical pathways that carries information about color and high spatial resolution but is not capable of high contrast sensitivity or any other characteristics of the parallel M pathway.

Planckian locus: a collection of points on a chromaticity diagram that represent blackbody radiation of various temperatures.

Primary colors: color stimuli by whose mixture all other color stimuli can be matched.

Protanomaly: anomalous trichromatic color vision due to alteration of the normal LWS cone photopigment.

Protanopia: dichromatic color vision due to absence of the LWS cone type.

Protans: protanopes and protanomalous individuals.

Rayleigh equation: the proportional amounts of spectral red and green lights in a mixture that matches a spectral yellow light, usually derived from color vision testing with an anomaloscope to characterize deficient color vision.

Saturation: the perceptual correlate of colorimetric purity that refers to the difference between chromatic (colored) and achromatic (gray or white) visual stimuli of the same brightness.

Simultaneous color contrast: color in an area that surrounds an object tends to induce in the object a hue in the direction of the surround's complement.

Spectral color: light that is composed of a single wavelength; monochromatic light.

Spectral composition: the set of wavelengths that constitute a color.

Spectral light: spectral color.

Spectral locus: the location of points on a chromaticity diagram that represent color stimuli across the entire visible spectrum.

Spectral sensitivity: a plot of the reciprocal of the radiometric energy at various wavelengths necessary to elicit a constant visual response, such as equality of brightness in reference to a fixed standard light.

Standard Illuminant C: a light source with color temperature 6,774 K that was adopted by the CIE as a standard for colorimetry.

Stargardt's juvenile macular dystrophy: an autosomal recessive disorder that usually occurs at puberty and affects the function of the pigment epithelium and photoreceptor layers within the maculas of both eyes.

Successive color contrast: a colored stimulus induces a hue in a subsequently viewed stimulus close to the complement of the inducing color; the duration of the effect is dependent on the strength and viewing time of the original stimulus.

Transmittance: the ratio of radiant energy that is transmitted by a medium to that which is incident on it.

Tristimulus values: the actual amounts of each of three primary colors that are needed in a mixture to match a sample color.

Tritanomaly: a rare and poorly understood type of anomalous trichromatic color vision due to presumed alteration of the normal SWS cone photopigment.

Tritanopia (tritanopic): dichromatic color vision due to absence of the SWS pigment.

Tritans: tritanopes and tritanomalous individuals.

Trichromacy (trichromatic vision): color vision that requires mixtures of not fewer than three primary colors (usually red, green, and blue) to match all perceived hues.

Value: the designation of brightness in the Munsell Color System.

Wavelength discrimination: color discrimination of spectral (monochromatic) light.

Wavelength discrimination threshold: the threshold for determining the test wavelength differs from a reference wavelength.

9 Postnatal Human Vision Development

Deborah Orel-Bixler

Overview

Although age has not been considered as a variable to be controlled or tested in the visual functions discussed in the previous chapters of this book, it has dramatic effects on vision in infancy and early childhood. This chapter describes the infant visual system and its development. It also introduces a new psychophysical method that can be used in situations in which a subject or patient cannot respond verbally to a stimulus.

The human visual system has been found to be surprisingly mature at birth. Nevertheless, there is continued rapid maturation of the eye, visual pathways, and visual behavior during the first days, weeks, and months of life. Because standard psychophysical methods do not work in infants, new psychophysical methods had to be devised specifically for infants and young children. Two-alternative forced-choice preferential looking (FPL) is based on the fact that infants prefer to look at patterned targets rather than plain ones. In FPL, an observer judges which stimulus the infant appears to fixate. Combined with the Method of Constant Stimuli, FPL provides measures of thresholds. Visual evoked potentials (VEPs) are used to measure visual thresholds objectively.

Absolute threshold is initially over 1 log unit higher in infants than adults, but decreases to adult levels by 6 months of age. Ricco's law holds for infants for stimuli that are larger than in adults. Increment thresholds are higher than adults, but follow a function resembling Weber's law. Visual acuity is poor at birth and improves rapidly during the first 6 months. VEP measures indicate better acuity than FPL measures. Vernier acuity also improves rapidly during the first 6 months. By 2–3 months of age the spatial contrast sensitivity function is band pass, but the peak sensitivity is lower than in adults and occurs at a much lower spatial frequency. Critical flicker frequency (CFF) develops rapidly in infants. The temporal contrast sensitivity function is band pass by 4 months, but the sensitivity remains low. Dichromatic (tritanopic) color vision is present by 2 months and trichromacy is present by 3 months of age. The photopic and scotopic luminosity functions in infants resemble those of adults. These measures provide baseline values that permit early detection of vision disorders in infants.

The human visual system is surprisingly mature at birth

Over a century ago, the psychologist William James (1899) said that the infant's world must be "a blooming, buzzing confusion, a blank slate to be written on by his world." Perhaps this impression was influenced by observations of infant facial expressions, like the one shown in Figure 9.1. It was generally believed that vision in infants was extremely poor, and that they could do little more than see light and dark (Restak 1986). Fifty years later, the popular pediatrician Benjamin Spock (1957) stated that infants could feel discomfort and pain, but were "just a bundle of organs and nerves during the first month." Textbooks for pediatricians and ophthalmologists in the 1960s stated that infants could see light and dark, but could not see patterns.

This impression has changed considerably over the past 35 years as infant vision and visual development has been more extensively studied by develop-

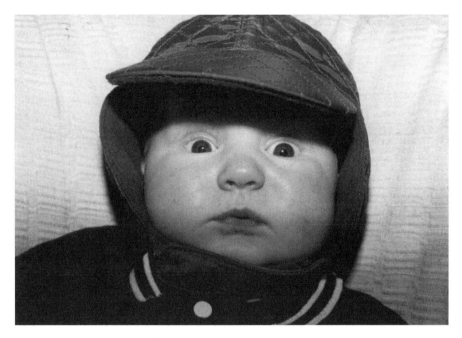

FIGURE 9.1   *The blooming, buzzing confusion of infancy.*

mental psychologists, vision scientists, and vision care practitioners. For instance, it has been learned that newborn infants can imitate their parents' facial expressions immediately after birth (Figure 9.2). As reviewed by Teller (1997), it has been found that vision is more mature at birth than was previously thought, and undergoes rapid development in the early postnatal weeks and months. Indeed, most aspects of visual function examined in this chapter reach adult levels during the first year after birth. Restak (1986) wrote

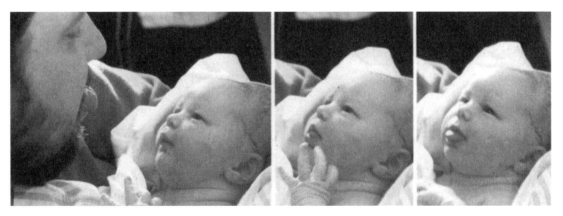

FIGURE 9.2   *Within hours after birth, this infant imitates his father's facial expression. (Reprinted with permission from L Nilsson, L Hamberger. A Child is Born. New York: Delacorte Press, 1990.)*

When one considers that people have been having babies since Adam and Eve, the question arises: Why only in the past twenty-five years has the neonate been appreciated as a psychological being capable of learning, influencing parents and being influenced? . . . If an infant is studied with sufficient sensitivity to its mood, wakefulness, inclination, and brain development, truly marvelous performance can be achieved.

Part of the problem was that the psychophysical methods used for the study of adult vision must be modified for use with infants.

Development of the visual system is rapid during the first year of life

The eye of the newborn is approximately two-thirds of its adult size. It undergoes its most rapid growth during the first year of life and finally reaches the adult length and size by adolescence. At birth, the anterior structures of the eye, the cornea, lens, and iris, are more developed than the retinal structures in the posterior eye. Yuodelis and Hendrickson (1986) showed that both rods and cones are present at birth but are immature in size and spacing. After birth, the inner layers of the retina differentiate further. The specializations of the fovea, however, lag behind the development of the peripheral retina. Foveal maturation is not complete until approximately 6 months of age. The optic nerve, which conveys information from the eye to the brain, is relatively full size at birth, but myelination, which speeds the neural conduction rate, is not complete until age 2 years. The next stage of the pathway to the visual cortex, the lateral geniculate nucleus, has the full complement of neurons present at birth, but they enlarge and establish more connections to other neurons with age. The visual cortex has the adult number of neurons present at birth, but these are still migrating to the superficial layers of the cortex and forming their neural connections (Hickey & Peduzzi 1987). This anatomical and physiological development of the visual system is accompanied by a rapid improvement in visual abilities.

New psychophysical techniques had to be devised for studying visual function in infants

The standard psychophysical methods, described in Chapter 1 and used in the other chapters of this book to measure various visual functions, do not work with infants. Part of the problem is in the presentation of stimuli to infants. They cannot sit in front of a stimulus display by themselves. They need both physical support, so that they can look at visual displays, and emotional support, because they can easily become upset. A crying infant does not pay attention to visual stimuli. In addition, when making psychophysical measures on preverbal children, detecting whether the child sees a stimulus can be very difficult. Even older children who can talk may have difficulty either performing a psychophysical task or communicating their responses. Indeed, many of the clinical tests that use standard psychophysical tasks are unreliable in children as old as 5–6 years of age. As a consequence, accurate information on the visual capabilities of infants had to await the development of clever new ways of measuring infant vision.

An extremely useful psychophysical test, called **forced-choice preferential looking (FPL)** has been developed in recent years. It is based on the fact that visual fixation is evident in the newborn and accurate fixation is achieved by 6–9 weeks. This chapter examines the results obtained with this technique and with another technique, the **visual evoked potential (VEP)**. The latter is an objective technique that complements the psychophysical technique. Both have been used to quantify spatial, temporal, and color visual function in infants and young children.

The fact that infants prefer to look at patterned targets rather than unpatterned ones is the basis for the preferential looking technique

In early work by Fantz (1958), infants were shown a series of pairs of stimuli. In each pair, one stimulus was more complex than the other. A bold patterned stimulus, such as a checkerboard, a bull's-eye, or any of several geometric shapes was paired with a plain stimulus, or one with less visual complexity. Various aspects of the infant's behavior to these stimuli were observed by an investigator, who watched the infant through a peephole so the presence of the investigator did not distract the infant. The investigator recorded the direction of the infant's first look when the stimuli were revealed, the amount of time that was spent looking at each object, and the number of fixations on each object. From this work with a variety of stimulus comparisons, it became clear that infants prefer to look at patterned targets rather than unpatterned ones or targets of intermediate complexity rather than very simple ones. The quantitative measurement of this looking behavior is called the *preferential looking technique*.

In forced-choice preferential looking, an observer judges at which of two stimuli an infant looks

Davida Teller and her coworkers at the University of Washington modified the investigator's task into making a two-alternative forced-choice judgment and named it *forced-choice preferential looking*. In FPL, the infant is held by a parent or other comforting person. The stimulus, which may be, for example, a grating of black and white stripes, is presented to the infant's right or left. The mean luminance of the grating is equal to the luminance of the gray background to eliminate luminance differences as a cue if the grating cannot be resolved by the infant. The left or right location of the grating target is varied randomly with each presentation. When the stimulus is presented, the observer views the infant through a peephole located between the left and right stimulus positions. The observer does not know whether the stimulus is on the left or right, and must judge the location of the grating based on the infant's looking behavior. This is a forced-choice task (see Chapter 1)

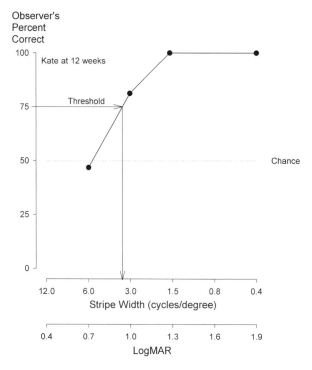

FIGURE 9.3   *Two-alternative forced-choice preferential looking (FPL) data for infant grating acuity. The observer's percent correct ranged from near chance (50%) for the grating with the smallest stripe width (highest spatial frequency) to 100% for the gratings with the two largest stripe widths (lowest spatial frequency). Visual resolution acuity was estimated to be approximately 10' (1 [logMAR] = 1.0) at the level of 75% correct. Each data point is based on at least 20 trials. (Modified from V Dobson. Behavioral tests of visual acuity in infants. Int Ophthalmol Clin 1980;20:233–250.)*

because the observer must say that the infant appeared to look to the left or to the right, even if it is difficult to discern. The observer's judgment of the location of the grating is compared with the actual stimulus location. If the observer is correct more frequently than expected by chance, then the infant must be detecting the grating target. This technique has been used extensively to measure visual thresholds in infants and, with modifications, in older children.

An example of a study of visual resolution acuity is shown in Figure 9.3. In this study, the spatial frequency of a high-contrast square-wave grating was varied. The smallest stripe width that the infant reliably fixated was judged to be the estimate of visual resolution (grating) acuity. The Method of Constant Stimuli (see Chapter 1) was used. Four gratings that ranged from 6 cycles per degree to 0.4 cycles per degree were each presented at least 20 times in random order. A plot of the percent of trials in which the observer correctly identified the grating location versus the grating spatial frequency produces a standard, forced-choice psychometric function with chance performance at 50%. The infant's visual acuity is defined as the spatial frequency at which the observer's judgment of the location of the grating was correct 75% of the time.

Absolute thresholds reach adult levels approximately 6 months after birth

The absolute threshold (see Chapter 2) has been measured in infants using modified two-alternative FPL procedures. A dark-adapted infant is shown large stimuli of durations of less than 1 second that are presented to either the left or right side of the infant's center of gaze. The observer reports the stimulus position based on the infant's eye and head movements. The results showed that absolute threshold decreases rapidly with age. There is reasonable agreement between studies that the threshold for completely dark adapted 4 week–old infants is approximately 1.4 log units higher than the adult absolute threshold. In 10 week–old infants, it is approximately 1 log unit higher, and in 18 week–olds, it is two-thirds of a log unit higher (Hansen & Fulton 1993). Extrapolations from these suggest that absolute threshold reaches adult levels approximately 6 months after birth.

Spatial summation areas are larger in infants than in adults

In both infants and adults, the absolute threshold is constant over a range of stimulus areas as shown by the flat regions of the curves in Figure 9.4. For smaller stimulus areas, threshold is inversely proportional to stimulus area, that is, Ricco's law

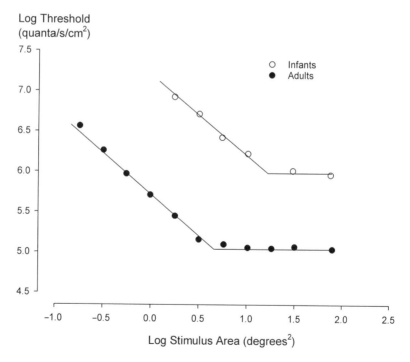

FIGURE 9.4   *Log threshold versus log stimulus area for infants and adults. The critical area occurs at the intersection of the sloping line with the horizontal line. (Modified from RM Hansen, RD Hamer, AB Fulton. The effect of light adaptation on scotopic spatial summation in 10-week-old infants. Vision Res 1992;32:387–392.)*

holds (see Chapter 2). Studies with infants 4–11 weeks of age have shown that these relations between threshold and area are shifted toward larger areas and higher thresholds in infants relative to those observed for adults. This means that the critical area, the area beyond which Ricco's law does not hold, is larger in infants than in adults. As discussed in Chapter 2, spatial summation occurs from the convergence of photoreceptors onto bipolar cells. This determines the size of the receptive-field center and, therefore, the region over which spatial summation occurs. The decrease in the critical area between infants and adult may occur because the receptive-field–center size decreases with postnatal age, as has been shown to occur in various animal species.

Increment threshold functions are similar to those of adults and obey Weber's law by 2–4 months of age

In Chapter 3, the effect of a background luminance on the threshold ΔL in adults was described. Figure 9.5 shows increment threshold versus background intensity functions (also known as *threshold versus intensity* or *TVI curves*) for adults and 4, 10, and 18 week–old infants measured at scotopic levels of background luminance. Figure 9.5 shows that the rod-mediated increment threshold functions of infants are similar in shape to those of adults,

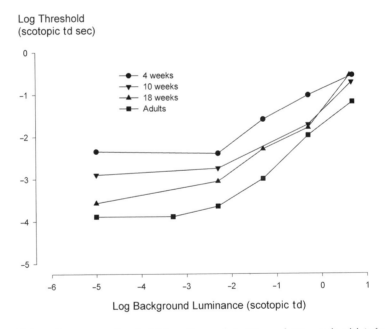

FIGURE 9.5   *Increment threshold functions of 4, 10, and 18 week–old infants and adults versus background luminance. Stimuli were 10°, 1 second, blue (wavelength shorter than 510 nm) flashes presented 20° from fixation. Each point is the mean of five threshold determinations at that level of background adaptation. (Modified from R Hansen, A Fulton. Development of Scotopic Retinal Sensitivity. In K Simons [ed], Early Visual Development, Normal and Abnormal. New York: Oxford University Press, 1993;130–142.)*

but that the threshold ΔL is highest in 4 week–old infants and decreases with age at each background luminance level.

As described in Chapter 3, the Weber fraction is the ratio of the threshold luminance (ΔL) to the luminance of an adapting field (L), or $\Delta L/L$. Numerous infant studies indicate that the Weber fraction for infant rod vision decreases at the same rate as the absolute threshold over the first 6 months of life. Recall that where Weber's law holds, $\Delta L/L$ is a constant. On the log-log axes of Figure 9.5, a slope of 1 indicates that Weber's law holds. For adults, this occurs for a background luminance above –2 log scotopic trolands. In infants, there also is a linear relationship, but the slope is less than 1. The slope is approximately 0.5 for 4 to 6 week–olds, which suggests that they follow the deVries-Rose law (see Chapter 3). The slope is 0.83 for 10 week–old infants. Linearity holds over approximately the same range of adapting luminances in 2 month–old infants as in adults. Thus, if the stimuli are large and of long duration, the increment threshold function slope increases to reach adult-like slopes (0.8–1.0) by 2–4 months of age. According to Hansen and Fulton (1993), immaturity or absence of rod-cone interactions may account for the shallow slope of the increment threshold versus background intensity functions of young infants.

Up to 6 months postnatal, grating acuity in cycles per degree equals age in months

There is general agreement across studies that grating acuity, when measured with FPL, develops from approximately 1 cycle per degree (1.5 logMAR) at 1 month of age to 6 cycles per degree (0.7 logMAR) by 6 months of age with little measurable improvement from 6 to 12 months. According to Mayer et al. (1995), grating acuity does not reach adult levels (30 cycles per degree, 0 logMAR) until approximately 3 years of age.

A better way to report an infant's visual acuity with PL techniques is to reference it to age-matched norms. Getz et al. (1992) found that acuity development in premature infants is predictable from post-term (corrected) age rather than from postnatal age. For example, if an infant is born 4 weeks prematurely and is tested at 20 weeks postnatal, his or her acuity data should be compared to the normative data of a 16 week–old infant rather than the 20 week–old infant, at least during the first year of life.

Infant visual acuity also can be measured with visual evoked potentials

The VEP is an electrical signal that is generated by neurons in the occipital region of the cortex (where the visual cortical areas are located) in response to visual stimulation (Sokol 1976). The visual stimulus is usually a patterned stimulus, such as a checkerboard or a grating that produces a pattern VEP. The cortical response is produced by *counterphasing* the contrast of the stimulus, so that dark areas become light and light areas become dark. After a delay (latency) that involves phototransduction, processing in the retina, and trans-

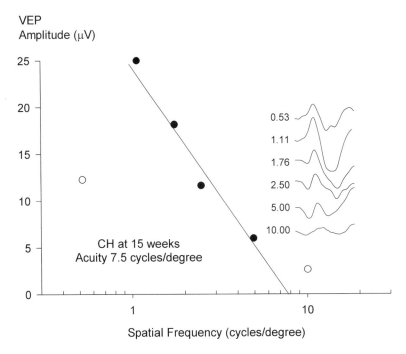

FIGURE 9.6 *Inset. Visual evoked potential (VEP) produced by a counterphased grating in a 15 week–old infant. The stimulus contrast was reversed at the left end of each line, producing, after a delay, the evoked response in the cortex. The spatial frequency of the stimulus is next to each VEP line.* **Main graph**. *The amplitude of the major positive (upward-going) component of each trace in the inset is plotted (circles) versus the spatial frequency of the grating. The visual acuity threshold is determined from a linear extrapolation of the VEP amplitude to 0 μV. Filled circles indicate the data points that were used in the extrapolation, with spatial frequencies ranging from 1.11 to 5.00 cycles per degree. The visual evoked potential acuity estimate is 7.5 cycles per degree (0.6 logMAR). (Modified from D Orel-Bixler. Electrodiagnostics, neuroimaging, ultrasound and photorefraction. In B Moore [ed], Eye Care for Infants and Young Children. Boston: Butterworth–Heinemann, 1997;89–122.)*

mission through the visual pathways, the VEP appears as a small change in electrical activity in the cortex. This is measured by placing electrodes on the scalp that are connected to amplifiers that magnify the evoked potentials. A computerized system calculates the average VEP produced by a large number of contrast reversals, displays the VEPs on a monitor or print-out, and stores them for further analysis. The latency and amplitude of the pattern VEP is sensitive to changes in contour and edge features of the stimulus.

To measure visual acuity, the amplitude of the VEP response is recorded for a series of gratings of different spatial frequencies. A large response indicates that the grating is visible. As the spatial frequency is increased, the amplitude of the VEP declines, as shown in the inset of Figure 9.6. The assumption is that when a grating does not produce a response, it is not visible. To determine the acuity threshold, the VEP amplitude is plotted versus spatial frequency, as shown in Figure 9.6. A straight line is fit to the data and is extrapolated to 0 μV (i.e., no response) to yield the acuity estimate in cycles per degree.

A more rapid measure of visual acuity in infants can be obtained using the **swept spatial frequency VEP** (Norcia & Tyler 1985). This technique is more rapid because it presents many spatial frequencies quickly. As with standard VEP measures of acuity, a high-contrast grating is counterphased several times per second to produce a VEP. During a 10 second period, the spatial frequency is increased 1 cycle per degree every 0.5 seconds while the VEP is recorded (see Figure 9.7A,B). Thus, the infant is presented with a range of spatial frequencies (e.g., 1 to 20 cycles per degree) in a very brief time. A computer program calculates the VEP amplitude at each spatial frequency (see Figure 9.7C). As expected, the VEP amplitude decreases as the spatial frequency increases. The acuity is calculated to be the point at which a straight line fit to the decline in VEP amplitude reaches 0. In normal adults, thresholds that are determined with the swept VEP technique agree with psychophysical measures of grating acuity.

The rate of acuity development measured with the visual evoked potential is more rapid than that measured with preferential looking techniques

Elwin Marg and colleagues (1976) demonstrated that visual acuity, when measured with VEPs, approaches 20 cycles per degree (approximately 0.2 logMAR) as early as 6 months of age. This rapid phase of acuity development is followed by a long, slow second phase that lasts until at least 5–11 years of age when the highest spatial frequency level (60 cycles per degree, –0.3 logMAR) is reached (Orel-Bixler 1989).

Psychophysical studies that used FPL generally have found a slower rate of acuity development before 3 years of age, as shown in Table 9.1. The differences in results have not been resolved. They cannot be explained solely by investigative technique, such as differences in scoring criteria or stimuli, and illustrate the difficulties inherent in measuring thresholds in infants and young children. VEPs measure visual responses in early cortical processing, whereas FPL techniques rely on the whole infant. The later stages of visual processing, attention, and motor control that are needed to produce looking behavior may influence the results. It is possible that the information is available in primary visual cortex, but for some reason the infant, as a whole being, is unable to use the information to guide his or her looking behavior.

Although the results obtained with these techniques differ in details, both show an initially rapid improvement in acuity with age that parallels anatomical changes. Hickey and Peduzzi (1987) showed that postreceptor development limits visual acuity during early postnatal life. Also, there is significant postnatal development of the macular area, which includes an increase in foveal receptor density and cone outer segment length. In addition, foveal cones become thinner, and ganglion cells and cells in the inner nuclear layers migrate away from the center of the foveal region. Cones migrate towards the center of the developing fovea continuously during development, from the time they first differentiate at 13 weeks of gestation.

Predictions of cone-mediated MAR can be derived from actual cone dimensions and cone spacing, as discussed in Chapters 5 and 6. Changes in cone spacing between 15 months of age and adulthood are of the same relative

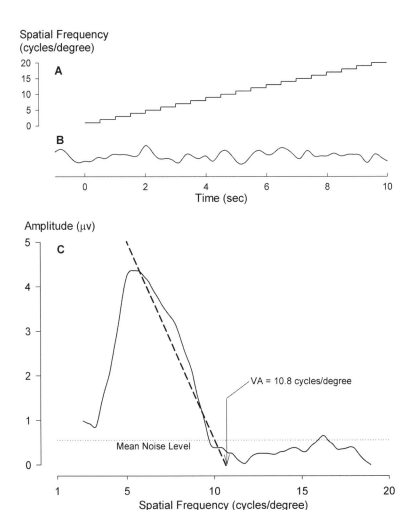

FIGURE 9.7   *Estimate of the visual acuity of a 29 week–old infant using the swept spatial frequency VEP paradigm.* **A.** *During a 10 second period, the spatial frequency of a counterphased grating was increased in steps from 1 to 20 Hz.* **B.** *The activity recorded through the electrodes located over the visual cortical areas during the presentation of the grating.* **C.** *The amplitude of the VEP as a function of the spatial frequency of the grating. The largest response occurred when the spatial frequency was approximately 5 cycles per degree. As the spatial frequency was increased, the amplitude of the VEP declined. The acuity was estimated to be 10.8 cycles per degree—the point at which a line fit to the declining portion of the VEP amplitude function reached 0 mV. (Modified from AM Norcia, CW Tyler. Spatial frequency sweep VEP: visual acuity during the first year of life. Vision Res 1985;25:1399–1408.)*

magnitude as the improvement in grating acuity over these ages. Early in life, however, grating acuity is less than predicted by cone spacing, which suggests a postreceptor limitation on acuity in normal eyes. Rapid development of retinal surface area and morphological changes in the lateral geniculate nucleus and cortex probably determine the rapid phase of acuity development in the first 8 months of age in normal children.

TABLE 9.1 Visual evoked potential grating acuity data and monocular grating acuity with the acuity card procedure

Age (mos)	VEP (cycles/degree)	FPL (cycles/degree)	VEP (mins of arc)	FPL (mins of arc)	VEP (6/6 notation)	FPL (6/6 notation)
1	5	0.94	6	31.9	6/36	6/191
2.5	7.8	2.16	3.85	13.9	6/23	6/83
4	12	2.68	2.5	11.2	6/15	6/67
6	18	5.65	1.65	5.3	6/10	6/32
9	23	6.79	1.3	4.4	6/8	6/26
12	25	6.42	1.2	4.6	6/7	6/28
18	—	8.59	—	3.5	—	6/21
24	—	9.57	—	3.1	—	6/19

FPL = forced-choice preferential looking; VEP = visual evoked potential.
SOURCE: *Modified from AM Norcia, CW Tyler. Spatial frequency sweep VEP: visual acuity during the first year of life. Vision Res 1985;25:1399–1408; and DL Mayer, AS Beiser, AF Warner, et al. Monocular acuity norms for the Teller Acuity Cards between ages one month and four years. Invest Ophthalmol Vis Sci 1995;36:671–685.*

Between birth and 6–8 months of age, Vernier acuity reaches a level that is twice that of grating acuity

Localization acuity, also known as *Vernier acuity* or *hyperacuity* (see Chapter 5), has a different developmental time course than grating acuity. Most FPL studies agree that Vernier acuity is not reliably measurable before approximately 10 weeks of age. In infancy, one study (Brown 1997) found that Vernier acuity is initially equal to or worse than grating acuity and then dramatically improves relative to grating acuity between approximately 2 and 8 months of age (Figure 9.8). The different rates of development of grating and Vernier acuity result in a crossover at approximately 4–8 months of age, when Vernier acuity becomes better than grating acuity. Other investigators (Manny & Klein 1984) reported that Vernier acuity was twice as good as grating acuity across all ages. Although these studies seem at odds with each other in terms of the rate of Vernier acuity development, the actual Vernier acuity values were similar in the two studies. Carkeet et al. (1997) demonstrated that although Vernier acuity shows a faster improvement than grating acuity initially, Vernier acuity has a longer time course to reach adult levels. They speculate that cortical immaturity may play a role in children's relative Vernier acuity deficits.

Abbreviated preferential looking techniques have a clinical application for measurement of grating acuity

In laboratory studies, a single acuity estimate requires an average of approximately 60 trials over 15 minutes of test time. This makes the procedure impractical for the clinical setting. A more rapid procedure, the **acuity card procedure**, was developed by McDonald et al. (1986) specifically for use in

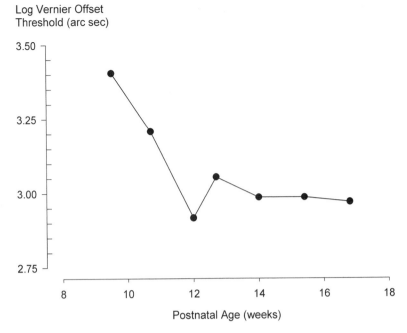

Log Vernier Offset
Threshold (arc sec)

FIGURE 9.8   *Vernier acuity as a function of postnatal age. (Modified from AM Brown. Vernier acuity in human infants: rapid emergence shown in a longitudinal study. Optom Vis Sci 1997;74:732–740.)*

clinical settings. In the acuity card procedure, the examiner's task on each trial is to judge whether the infant can resolve that grating based on the quality and consistency of the infant's looking behavior. When the stripes are wide and easily seen, and the infant's looking behavior is clearly in the direction of the grating, then only two presentations of the grating are needed. As the infant's acuity limit is approached, the looking behavior becomes less consistent, and the tester may need to show the grating cards several times to determine whether the infant is consistently looking at the grating. Thus, the tester uses the overall looking behavior of the infant on a small number of presentations to judge whether the grating was visible to the infant. However, with the many possible distractions in a clinical setting, one cannot conclude that a grating that is not preferentially fixated is not resolvable to an infant. Thus, acuity may be better than is measured with this technique.

Adult-like band pass spatial filtering appears by 2–3 months postnatal

As described in Chapter 6, the spatial CSF describes the amount of contrast that is needed to detect gratings of different spatial frequencies. The development of the spatial CSF has been studied both with FPL and VEP techniques.

Several studies have used FPL to examine the development of spatial CSF during the first 8 postnatal months. Over the course of the first 1–3 months of

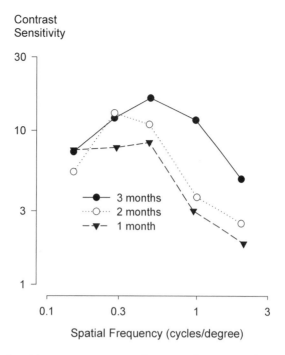

Contrast
Sensitivity

- 3 months
- 2 months
- 1 month

Spatial Frequency (cycles/degree)

FIGURE 9.9 *Spatial contrast sensitivity functions for 1, 2, and 3 month–old infants. (Modified from MS Banks, P Salapatek. Acuity and contrast sensitivity in 1-, 2-, and 3-month-old human infants. Invest Ophthalmol Vis Sci 1978;17:361–365.)*

age (Figure 9.9), there is an increase in overall contrast sensitivity across all spatial frequencies. The first appearance of a low spatial frequency rolloff (see Chapter 6) is at approximately 2–3 months of age. By 6 months of age, infants show a band pass spatial CSF, but compared with adults, the cutoff high spatial frequency is quite low.

Sensitivity to high spatial frequencies continues to develop beyond 6 months of age

VEP measurements of contrast sensitivity at 6 months of age indicate that the infant has the same contrast sensitivity as the adult for spatial frequencies of less than 2 cycles per degree. For spatial frequencies greater than 2 cycles per degree, sensitivity is higher in adults than in infants (see Chapter 6, Figure 6.15). Swept VEP measurements indicate that contrast sensitivity for low spatial frequency grating targets (less than 1 cycle per degree) develops rapidly between birth and 10–12 weeks of age. According to Norcia et al. (1990), the contrast sensitivity for coarse targets of 10 week–old infants is only a factor of two lower than for adults. However, contrast sensitivity at high spatial frequencies continues to develop long after 10 weeks of age. At 32 weeks of age, the contrast sensitivity for a fine target (16 cycles per degree) was a factor of 20 lower than for adults.

Photoreceptor maturation may explain the rise in contrast sensitivity with age; cone packing density and image size may explain the shift toward higher spatial frequencies

Once the spatial CSF develops its band pass shape, the primary changes with age are a rise in contrast sensitivity and a shift in the peak contrast sensitivity toward higher spatial frequencies. As may be seen by comparing the 3 month–old data with the 2 month–old data in Figure 9.9, the entire spatial CSF moves upward, to higher contrast sensitivity, and rightward, to high spatial frequencies (Peterzell & Kelly 1997).

The initially low contrast sensitivity in young infants may be due to reduced quantal absorption by the relatively short, immature cone outer segments, although immaturity of central visual structures may also play a role. The shift of the spatial CSF toward higher spatial frequencies may be due to two factors. One is the decrease in cone diameter with development of the fovea. This causes there to be a higher packing density of cones, decreases the size of the receptive-field center in the midget bipolar cells, and (see Chapter 5) allows the detection of higher spatial frequencies. A second factor is that the enlargement of the eye with age causes the size of images on the retina to change such that one cycle of any spatial frequency covers a larger retinal area. This, also, could contribute to an increase in the cutoff high spatial frequency.

The temporal contrast sensitivity function matures more rapidly than the spatial contrast sensitivity function

The maturation of temporal vision has been studied by measurement of the CFF and the temporal CSF. Infants prefer to look at rapidly flickering stimuli instead of a steady light. FPL measures have found that the CFF is 40 Hz by 1 month of age and 50 Hz by 2–3 months of age.

As shown in Chapter 7, the adult temporal CSF has a peak contrast sensitivity at intermediate temporal frequencies (approximately 20 Hz at high luminance levels), a low temporal frequency rolloff, and a cutoff high temporal frequency (DeLange 1958). The cutoff high temporal frequency is approximately the same as the CFF. Compared to adults, infants have an overall reduction in temporal contrast sensitivity (Figure 9.10). Temporal contrast sensitivity increases with age with a shift in the peak frequency toward higher temporal frequencies: 2 Hz at 2 months of age, 4 Hz at 3 months of age, and 8 Hz at 4 months of age. The shape of the temporal CSF changes from a low-pass function having no attenuation of low relative to intermediate frequencies at 2 months of age to band pass (low frequency rolloff present) at 3 months of age (see Figure 9.10). By 3 months of age, the shapes of the temporal CSF of the infant and the adult are nearly identical, but infants require greater contrast across all temporal frequencies and cannot detect high frequencies (see Chapter 6, Figure 6.15). Compared with adults, their sensitivity is approximately 1.5 log units lower. The temporal CSF shows the same shift toward higher sensitivity and higher cutoff frequency as does the spatial CSF. At 4 months of age, the infant CSF is still reduced by more than 1 log unit

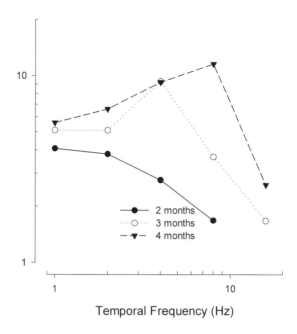

FIGURE 9.10   *Temporal contrast sensitivity function at three ages. (Modified from TA Rasengane, D Allen, RE Manny. Development of temporal contrast sensitivity in human infants. Vision Res 1997;37:1747–1754.)*

compared to adults. The low infant CFF and the low cutoff high frequency of the temporal CSF may be explained by reduced quantum absorption by immature infant foveal cone outer segments. This reduces the effective luminance of stimuli, and following the Ferry-Porter law, lowers the CFF (see Chapter 7). Thus, as characterized by the CFF and temporal CSF, temporal vision develops more rapidly than spatial vision.

Visual evoked potential measures indicate that short-wavelength sensitive (SWS) cones develop later than middle- and long-wavelength sensitive (MWS, LWS) cones

Using VEP measures, Allen et al. (1993) showed that infants as young as 2 weeks of age have functional MWS and LWS cones and the postreceptor circuits that are needed to relay color information to the visual cortex. A similar VEP study by Volbrecht and Werner (1987) demonstrated that infants as young as 5 weeks of age have functional SWS cones. Although the color processes that were sampled by evoked potentials imply that neonates have mature color vision, behavioral measures indicate that color discrimination develops at a later age.

By 8–10 weeks, infants demonstrate dichromatic (tritanopic) color vision; trichromatic vision is present by 3 months of age

Early FPL studies of infant color vision were fraught with the difficulty of ensuring that the infants were responding to wavelength differences in the stimulus rather than luminance differences (Teller 1997). A successful strategy for testing infant color vision with FPL techniques has been to measure color discrimination in the presence of luminance difference. In this situation, the test stimulus at a particular wavelength can have a variety of luminance levels. The underlying premise is that an infant without color vision performs at chance discrimination when there is no luminance difference, whereas an infant with color vision fixates the target when the luminance is equal to the background, but the color is different. Therefore, using a range of luminance differences that includes the equiluminance condition makes luminance an unreliable cue and allows the determination of whether color vision is present.

Color discrimination by 3 to 4 week–old infants is poor, but by 8–10 weeks of age, it has reached a level consistent with the notion that infants have at least two functional classes of cones. However, at this age, chromatic discriminations fail in the yellow-greens (540–560 nm) and middle nonspectral purple zones, which indicate a tritan-type color defect (Figure 9.11; see also Chapter 8).

The age at which color vision becomes adult-like is not yet known. The anatomical limitation of infant color vision does not appear to be photoreceptor immaturity; rather, it is thought to be limited by postreceptor processing that may involve the formation of chromatically opponent channels.

Infant luminous efficiency is derived from the measurement of the minimally discriminable luminance of a test wavelength and a standard light

FPL techniques have been used to measure V_λ, the photopic luminous efficiency function (see Appendix, Figure A.1), in infants. The task that is required is somewhat like a side-by-side heterochromatic brightness matching using a bipartite field used to produce V_λ. Here, however, the background, which fills the field of view, is the reference light. The monochromatic test light is presented on top of the background, either on the right or left. A "dummy" light that matches the background light closely in both luminance and spectral composition is presented on the other side. Using the Method of Constant Stimuli, the investigator varies the luminance of the test light from trial to trial over a large range of closely spaced luminances. The luminance range is assumed to include the luminance levels that are high enough to be detected and low enough to be indistinguishable from the background. The FPL procedure yields a psychometric function that plots discrimination versus luminance. At the infant's match point, the infant performs at a chance level. Discrimination-versus-luminance difference functions with a variety of test stimulus wavelengths are used to generate a spectral luminous efficiency curve. The photopic spectral sensitivity function resembles that of adults tested under similar conditions. The scotopic spectral sensitivity curve (V'_λ) in 1

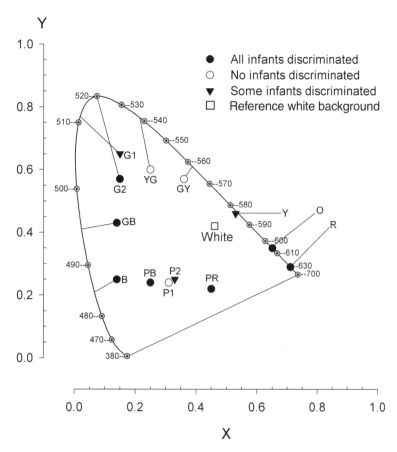

FIGURE 9.11   *Location on the CIE 1931 (x,y) chromaticity diagram of the color stimuli that were used in forced-choice preferential looking studies to examine the maturation of color discrimination in 2 month–old infants. The color of the various wavelengths is indicated by the abbreviations. Colors that are reliably discriminated from the white reference background are indicated by filled circles. Colors that were not discriminated are indicated by open circles. Triangles indicate colors that were discriminated by some infants. The lines connect the chromaticity coordinates to the spatial color that matched the stimulus in hue. See Color Plate 2 for the appearance of the stimuli at the chromaticity coordinates. (B = blue; G = green; O = orange; P = purple; R = red; Y = yellow.) (Modified from DY Teller, DR Peeples, M Sekel. Discrimination of chromatic from white light by two-month-old human infants. Vision Res 1978;18:41–48.)*

month–old infants also has been measured and is well fit by the adult standard scotopic curve over most of the spectrum.

The infant photopic and scotopic spectral luminous efficiency curves are evidence that rods and at least one cone type are functional by the first postnatal month. Possible explanations for any difference between infant and adult luminous efficiency functions include the optical density of screening pigments in the lens and macula, as well as rod and cone photopigment densities. Infant spectral sensitivity also may depend on different combinations of cone and rod responses than adults.

Knowledge of the normal developmental pattern is necessary for clinical detection of vision disorders

According to Gerali et al. (1990), vision disorders are the fourth most common disability of children in the United States and the leading cause of handicapping conditions in childhood. From studies of the postnatal development using FPL and VEP, the time course of normal development has been determined for many different visual functions. Using modified FPL techniques, and the more objective VEP, it is possible to quantify many of the visual functions (e.g., visual acuity, contrast sensitivity, and color vision) of infants in a clinical setting. Having norms against which an individual child's vision can be compared is useful in determining whether that child has a vision problem.

Study Guide

1. What behavior of infants allowed the development of the FPL technique?
2. Describe the task of the observer in FPL.
3. Describe the development of absolute threshold.
4. Describe the development of spatial summation (Ricco's law).
5. What is the time course of development of the Weber fraction?
6. How different are the estimates of grating acuity as determined by VEP and FPL measures?
7. Describe the development of Vernier acuity.
8. When does the spatial CSF become band pass?
9. By what age is the infant CFF 50 Hz?
10. Which cone class appears to develop more slowly than the other two?
11. When is trichromatic vision present?
12. Describe the procedure for measuring the photopic luminous efficiency (V_λ) curve.
13. How does knowledge of normal vision development help the clinician?

Glossary

Acuity card procedure: a clinical adaptation of FPL in which the examiner uses fewer stimulus presentations.

Forced-choice preferential looking (FPL): a technique in which an observer judges the location (left or right) of a stimulus based on watching an infant's looking behavior when the stimulus is presented.

Swept spatial frequency VEP: a technique for measuring grating acuity in which the VEP is recorded while the spatial frequency of a counterphased grating is rapidly increased (swept).

Visual evoked potential (VEP): electrical responses that are recorded from visual cortex in response to changes in a visual stimulus, such as a grating.

10   The Aging Visual System

Karlene K. Ball

Overview

Although the normal developmental changes that occur in the eye and visual system during infancy and childhood rapidly enhance visual functions, those that occur throughout adulthood slowly degrade some aspects of visual function. It is important to establish normative data on these changes so that the effects of pathology can be distinguished from the normal effects of aging. It is also important to understand the effects of changes in visual function on the ability of the elderly to perform the tasks of daily living.

There are numerous physical changes that occur in the eye and visual system over time. Increased light scatter, increased absorption by the ocular media, and decreased pupil diameter (miosis) reduce contrast and retinal illuminance. The lens becomes thicker and eventually hardens such that accommodation is no longer possible. In addition, the lens yellows and may develop opacities. At the retinal level, there is a gradual loss of photoreceptors and a decrease in the optical density of photopigments. Foveal cone density decreases. Changes occur in the electrical properties of the photoreceptors so they become less responsive to light. There may be cell loss and changes in neurotransmitters in the visual pathways and cortex.

These physical changes lead to a measurable decline in numerous visual functions with advancing age. There is an increase in the absolute threshold and a decrease in the rate of dark adaptation. Resolution acuity decreases, especially after 60 years of age. The spatial CSF decreases at intermediate and high spatial frequencies. The CFF decreases with age. Temporal contrast sensitivity does not seem to decrease, but visual stimuli appear to persist longer in the elderly. Visual fields become smaller with age.

In addition to real changes in visual function, elderly patients may appear to have greater losses than they actually have because they tend to adopt more conservative response criteria on psychophysical tests. It is sometimes necessary to alter a standard psychophysical measurement in a clinical setting to account for this response bias.

The decline in visual function can affect the ability of the elderly to perform the routine tasks of daily living. Visual acuity losses may be less important in everyday activities than the changes in the spatial CSF. A new measure, the useful field of view, is a better predictor of automobile accidents than other psychophysical measures.

Normal aging can lead to degraded visual function that must be distinguished from the effects of pathology

The fastest growing segment of the U.S. population is comprised of adults aged 85 years and older. This is largely due to the combined effects of general population growth and increases in longevity. The large age shift affects all institutions, from universities to the workplace. According to Crews (1994), there were approximately 860,000 older adults in the United States in 1950 who experienced vision impairment, defined in functional terms as the inability to read newsprint with best correction. By the year 2030, this number is likely to rise to nearly 6 million. There are many normal anatomical and physiological changes in the eye that occur gradually throughout life and that eventually can lead to observed impairment in visual performance. In addition, ocular diseases and their associated vision losses are much more prevalent in older adults.

One of the challenges for vision science, as well as for clinical practice, is to better understand the often subtle distinctions between normal aging and early pathology. Such distinctions are made more difficult by the fact that measurement variability increases with age, partly because people age at different rates. The result is that the distinction between normal aging changes in the eye and the early stages of eye disease is somewhat arbitrary. Any anatomical and physiological change observed in an older eye, if minor, may be considered to be due to normal aging. The same observed change may be designated as a disease process in other cases. For example, the presence of some pigmentary mottling and the presence of a few drusen are common in the retina of older individuals and could be considered a result of normal aging. However, when these changes are more pronounced, and accompanied with acuity loss, they are considered to be age-related macular degeneration.

Another challenge is to understand how specific visual impairments impact the performance of everyday activities. Many older adults never experience any significant visual impairment and the subtle age-related changes that occur naturally do not interfere with their everyday visual activities. In other instances, however, older persons have difficulty in their everyday activities but have no demonstrable evidence of ocular pathology. Thus, it is important to understand the complex interrelationships between vision and visual information processing skills.

The ocular media become less clear with age, thereby increasing light scatter and reducing contrast

Although there may be a loss of clarity in the cornea and an increase in debris (floaters) in the vitreous humor, the most dramatic age-related changes occur in the crystalline lens. As it ages, the lens increases in diameter and thickness, hardens, increases in optical density, and accumulates more light-absorbing pigmentation. Ultimately, the lens may undergo some noticeable opacification that is an early sign of cataract.

As pigmentation in the crystalline lens increases, the absorption of light by the lens becomes wavelength dependent. The lens of the neonate's eye is transparent to all visible wavelengths. In the older eye, absorption is greater for short-wavelength light (violet and blue) than for intermediate and long wavelengths (yellow, orange, and red). This selectivity produces progressive yellowing of the crystalline lens throughout life. By the third decade of life, yellowing is noticeable. It continues to increase thereafter, although to varying degrees in different individuals.

Johnson et al. (1988) used chromatic adaptation to determine the course of age-related loss of sensitivity to short wavelengths. They estimated that approximately 40% of the loss could be accounted for by increased absorption of the shorter wavelengths by the lens. Loss of short-wavelength sensitivity can have a dramatic impact on color vision. Vivid blue-green and green colors may be confused, as are other colors that are characteristic of a tritan type of color vision deficiency (see Chapter 8). Reliance on color coding, as may be used on medication labels, therefore is potentially confusing for an elderly person unless care is taken in selecting the colors to be used.

Retinal illuminance decreases with age as pupil size decreases

By age 60 years, retinal illuminance is approximately one-third of what it was at age 20 years. One optical contribution to this change is a decrease in resting pupil size (*miosis*) with age until it becomes essentially fixed at 2–3 mm by age 80. In combination with the increased lens absorption, miosis exacerbates the problems of seeing at lower light levels and exerts additional influences on visual function. As less light reaches the retina, there is a decline in acuity and loss of contrast sensitivity (see Chapter 5, Figure 5.14 and Chapter 6, Figure 6.15).

Although smaller pupil size reduces the retinal illuminance, there are, perhaps, two advantages: reduced optical aberrations and increased depth of focus. These help maintain a degree of image sharpness even when an object may be out of focus owing to **presbyopia**.

Age-related anatomical and physiological changes can occur in the eye and central pathways

At the level of photoreceptors, there can be an age-related loss of photoreceptors (both rods and cones) and reduction in photopigment density (see Chapter 8). Misalignment or improper orientation of the cone photoreceptor outer segments may develop. The resting membrane potential of the photoreceptors may decrease (become more hyperpolarized). This, in turn, can produce a decline in photoreceptor response amplitude. There may also be a decrease in the levels of neurotransmitters. All of these factors can contribute to reduced visual sensitivity (Sturr & Hannon 1991). Possible postreceptor mechanisms for age-related loss include reduced receptor pooling due to reduced convergence onto bipolar cells, ganglion cell loss, decreased response amplitude of the neurons, decreased levels of retinal neurotransmitters, cortical cell loss, and a decrease in the levels of cortical neurotransmitters. All of these factors can and do occur as a function of age but not always at the same rate in different individuals. The variability of the extent of these changes contributes to the variable results obtained in psychophysical measures of vision.

The elderly tend to adopt a more conservative response criterion in psychophysical measurements than younger observers

Visual function is typically evaluated clinically with a variety of tests that use psychophysical methods. In Chapter 9, it was shown that a new technique (two-alternative forced-choice preferential looking) was needed in order to assess the visual capabilities of infants. Although most elderly people do not need such specialized procedures, clinicians and others who test vision in the elderly need to understand that they may not respond the same way on psychophysical tests (e.g., acuity, visual field testing) as do younger adults. These methods rely on the observer's subjective report of what is or is not seen. There can be the appearance of visual impairment in older individuals relative to younger ones, not because of any vision loss, but simply because many elderly are reluctant to say that they detect a target unless they are very sure. In other words, older persons tend to adopt a more stringent, conservative criterion and do not report that an object is seen or read farther down a letter chart, unless the sensory evidence is extremely strong. Younger observers, on the other hand, are much more likely to guess and therefore may appear to have a lower sensory threshold or better visual function.

Because older patients may tend to adopt a more conservative response criterion when standard clinical testing methods are used, it is critical that they be encouraged to continue to read a letter chart or to respond to another type of stimulus even when they are not sure what they see. In addition, a forced-choice procedure can be used in which the individual must respond even if she or he is not certain that she or he can see the stimulus. This can be done, for example, by having the patient identify a light's position or orientation rather than simply its presence. Using this testing approach, it is typically found that stimuli can be detected or discriminated at levels far lower than the thresholds determined by methods in which the subject can choose to not respond. Thus, many early studies that reported an age-related decline in vision may have overestimated the amount of sensory loss due to age.

There is a decrease in the rate of dark adaptation and an increase in absolute threshold with increasing age

The elderly tend to experience more visual difficulties with dark adaptation than with light adaptation. Figure 10.1 clearly shows the effect of age on the

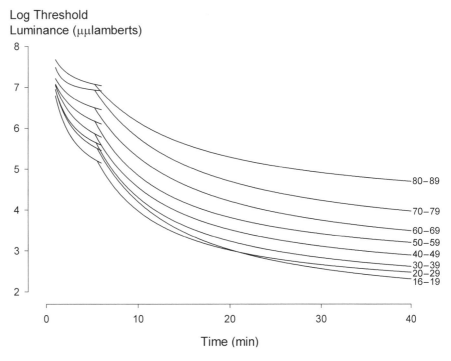

FIGURE 10.1   *Dark-adaptation curves for different age groups. (Modified from RA McFarland, RG Domey, AB Warren, DC Ward. Dark adaptation as a function of age: I. A statistical analysis. J Gerontol 1960;15:149–154.)*

standard dark-adaptation curve. Thresholds are increasingly higher with age throughout the entire time course of dark adaptation as well as at the end of the dark-adaptation period. In the oldest group tested, thresholds were elevated 1–2 log units.

There may be two factors at work to cause these effects on the dark-adaptation curve. One is that the absolute threshold of the visual system increases with age, as shown at the end of the dark-adaptation period. Another is that the rate of dark adaptation is slowed, producing the flattening of the curves observed in Figure 10.1.

The higher absolute threshold may have several causes. One potential cause is rod photoreceptor loss. The number of rods in histologic sections within 4° of the foveal center decreases with age. It appears, however, that rod outer segments enlarge with age, which may at least partially compensate for the decreased number of rods and the resultant reduction in quantal absorptions.

The slowed rate of dark adaptation may be due to a slowed rate of rhodopsin regeneration with age that results in an increase in the rhodopsin regeneration time constant (see Chapter 4, Figure 4.12). Such a change may be linked to changes observed in the photoreceptor mosaic or to an increased thickness of *Bruch's membrane*, the outermost layer of the retina through which nutrients from the blood supply must diffuse from the choroid.

Finally, optical factors, such as a decrease in pupil diameter and an increase in the optical density of the lens, also probably contribute to normal age-related changes in dark adaptation. Such changes should produce an upward displacement of the curves in Figure 10.1. Nearly the same result can be obtained in a young eye by placing a light absorbing filter in front of it and adjusting the filter transmittance. In this way, it is possible to produce the thresholds observed at any age in a single individual. Duplication of results does not, of course, prove that all of the change in threshold is due to optical factors. In addition, the change in the rate of dark adaptation is best accounted for by a slowing of the photopigment regeneration kinetics. Researchers are actively seeking a comprehensive model to explain the relative contributions of all possible mechanisms to the difficulties that older adults experience because of slower dark adaptation and higher absolute threshold. One such difficulty is the increased possibility of injury that is caused by falling while walking at night, even in familiar surroundings.

Visual acuity decreases with normal aging

Weymouth (1960) reported that 93.5% of patients 40–44 years of age had a corrected resolution acuity of 1' (0.0 logMAR) or better. 41.9% of patients in the 70–74 year–old bracket had that acuity. In this group, 14.5% of the patients whose corrected visual acuity was poorer than 1.25' (0.1 logMAR) had no apparent degenerative or disease conditions. Visual acuity in those patients apparently declined, although the eyes were normal clinically. Figure 10.2 illustrates the relationship between visual resolution acuity and age.

A number of clinical studies have reported a better than standard normal acuity of 1' (0.0 logMAR) from ages 20 to 60 years, with an average decline to

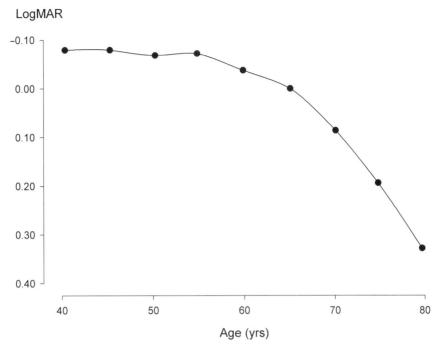

LogMAR

FIGURE 10.2 *Relation between median logMAR acuity and age. (Modified from FW Weymouth. Effect of age on visual acuity. In MJ Hirsch, RE Wick [eds], Vision of the Aging Patient. Philadelphia: Chilton Co., 1960; 37–62.)*

2' (0.3 logMAR) by 80 years of age. This is a loss of slightly more than one line of letters per decade (0.15 logMAR; see Chapter 5) above age 60 years. As described in Chapter 5, resolution acuity is typically measured by having a patient read a high-luminance, high-contrast letter chart at a standardized viewing distance. Many visual acuity tests are based on the standard normal value of 1' (0.0 logMAR or Snellen 6/6). Although this may be acceptable for screening purposes, younger adults, on average, have acuities that are better than 1' (see Chapter 5). Therefore, using 1' as a reference point for resolution acuity may have the effect of underestimating the onset and rate of acuity decline with age. An advantage of the logMAR system is that it allows a more precise measure of acuity that can provide more accurate comparisons of changes in a patient's acuity with age.

Several factors in the acuity testing situation, including luminance level, amount of contrast, and letter spacing, have, in general, a much more significant impact on the acuity values that are measured in older adults than those measured in younger persons. In Chapter 5, Figure 5.14 showed that acuity decreases with luminance, and Figure 5.15 showed that it decreases as contrast is reduced. If acuity testing is done under conditions of reduced luminance or contrast, or both, the results from young adults may not be affected. However, because of reduced pupil size, increased absorption by the ocular media, and increased light scatter, older adults may produce results that indicate reduced acuity. If the luminance or contrast, or both, were increased, their measured acuity might then become normal. Any real, age-related acuity differences would be amplified because the decreased retinal illuminance and contrast place older adults at a disadvantage relative to younger individuals. In addition, the spacing of the letters on an acuity chart, which is known to affect acuity because of contour interactions, may affect older adults' acuity performances if contour interactions extend over a larger spatial area for older individuals. Thus, some of the reported age-related decline in acuity may, in fact, be due to the testing conditions.

As was suggested in Chapter 5, the spacing of cones in the fovea should affect resolution acuity. Histologic studies carried out by Curcio et al. (1987) showed that there is as much as a threefold difference in maximum foveal cone density in young adults. This variation may contribute to individual differences in visual acuity. Although it seems reasonable that changes in the foveal mosaic would play a role in acuity during aging, the variability that occurs across individuals makes it difficult to detect whether the age-related foveal cone loss actually affects visual acuity. As of yet, there are no quantitative data that show that a significant loss of foveal cones is correlated with a similar loss of acuity. Indeed, recent work by Curcio (Curcio et al. 1990; Curcio & Owsley 2000) showed that rods rather than cones are more vulnerable to the effects of aging.

Spatial contrast sensitivity is stable in young adults and declines with age at intermediate and high spatial frequencies

When measured with foveally fixated targets, spatial contrast sensitivity has been found to decline in the intermediate and higher spatial frequencies but not at low spatial frequencies (Figure 10.3). The loss in sensitivity at high spatial frequencies, which is, in effect, a measure of resolution acuity, can be accounted for by the same optical factors (miosis, absorption, and light scattering) that were suggested to account for decreased acuity. As expected from Figure 6.15 in Chapter 6 and the reduced retinal illuminance with increasing age, the amount of the age-related contrast sensitivity reduction at high and middle spatial frequencies is greatly magnified if testing occurs under conditions of reduced luminance. As a result, the decline in contrast sensitivity can be offset partially by increasing the luminance level used in testing.

The loss of contrast sensitivity under scotopic and mesopic conditions occurs only at intermediate and high spatial frequencies and therefore points to a neural basis other than general cell loss. A deficit in the parvocellular visual pathway is likely because damage to this pathway has been shown to selectively reduce contrast sensitivity to middle and high spatial frequencies.

An alternative approach to measuring contrast sensitivity is to bypass the eye's optics by creating interference fringe patterns with a variety of spatial frequencies directly on the retina with two laser beams imaged in the pupil. In spite of the advantages of this technique, a number of studies have been unable to clarify the relative role of optical and neural factors in the age-related loss of spatial contrast sensitivity.

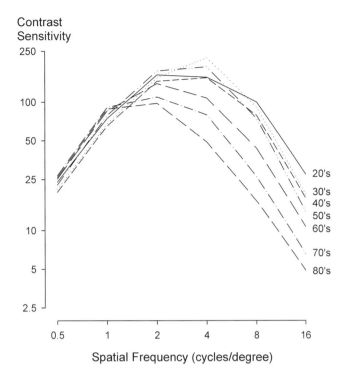

FIGURE 10.3   *Spatial contrast sensitivity function as a function of age for 100 subjects, aged 19–87 years, who had no ocular pathology or cataract. The display subtended 4.2° × 5.5° and had a mean luminance of 103 candelas per square meter. (Modified from C Owsley, R Sekuler, D Siemsen. Contrast sensitivity throughout adulthood. Vision Res 1983;23:689–699.)*

Sensitivity to temporally modulated stimuli declines with age

One way to evaluate the temporal resolving ability of the visual system is to measure the CFF (see Chapter 7). Older adults tend to have lower CFFs than do younger adults. Although the loss may have some neural basis, the CFF depends on mean retinal illuminance (the Ferry-Porter law), and mean retinal illuminance declines with age.

Measurements of the temporal CSF in older adults generally show reduced sensitivity primarily at intermediate and high temporal frequencies. Although reduced pupil size does play a role, it cannot fully explain the reduction. Using a methodology that was designed to minimize and control for optical factors, Tyler (1989) gathered flicker sensitivity data from approximately 1,000 visitors to the Exploratorium Science Museum in San Francisco; the sample ranged in age from 5 to 75 years. Analysis showed that, although sensitivity to flicker does not decrease from age 15 to 75 years, there is an increase in the persistence of visual stimuli with increasing age. The extent and cause of loss of temporal resolving power of the visual system is not yet clear, but may be due to changes in the functioning of the magnocellular pathway.

Ball and Sekuler (1986) found that older adults are less accurate than young adults in judging the direction of motion. This study followed earlier work by Owsley et al. (1983), who demonstrated decreased spatial contrast sensitivity for moving targets in older adults compared to younger adults. This can have important implications in everyday life because the elderly are more heavily dependent on visual information for maintaining their balance and preventing falls. These aging-related deficits cannot fully be explained by optical factors, such as reduced retinal illuminance, or by cognitive factors, thus implying that they have a neural basis.

Visual fields become smaller and peripheral sensitivity decreases with age

Much of the visual information that is critical for everyday activities comes from outside of the foveal region. Peripheral vision serves many important functions. It is critical for visual attention, the guidance of eye movements to important visual events, postural stability, and mobility. Visual sensitivity throughout the field of view is adversely affected by age, both in terms of the size of the visual field and the thresholds to detect a peripheral luminance target, as shown in Figure 10-4. The visual field isopters (see Chapter 3) are constricted—the limits

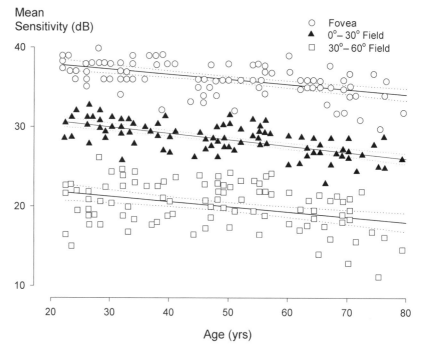

FIGURE 10.4   *Visual field sensitivity as a function of age for the fovea, 0°–30° field and the 30°–60° field in a Humphrey perimeter. (Modified from RS Brenton, CD Phelps. The normal visual field on the Humphrey field analyzer. Ophthalmologica 1986; 193: 56–74.)*

move closer to the point of fixation—in older adults, and by age 70 years, the binocular visual field declines from approximately 180° to 140°.

Figure 10.4 shows that the visual field sensitivity declines at a constant rate from ages 20 to 80 years. In addition, although the sensitivities are different for the 0°–30° and the 30°–60° fields, the rate of decline is essentially the same. Consistent with other age-related reductions in vision, these changes in the visual field cannot be accounted for completely by changes in the optics of the older eye, thus implying a role in neural factors as well.

The useful field of view is a psychophysical assessment of visual fields designed to test functional vision

Assessing the **useful field of view** involves testing the ability of a subject to localize and identify complex visual stimuli in the periphery. Standard visual field testing (see Chapter 3) seeks to minimize the presence of environmental factors that are typical of everyday situations. Assessing the useful field of view (Figure 10.5) includes features that are designed to mimic everyday visual activities. It uses complex visual scenes with distracting stimuli and requires simultaneous use of both central and peripheral vision. The limits of the useful field of view are affected by many factors, such as the presence of a secondary task and distracting stimuli.

The impact of these variables is much greater for older adults. Numerous studies have demonstrated that aging is associated with a reduced useful field of view. An older adult's useful field of view can be many times smaller than that of younger adults (Ball et al. 1988). Although Ball and Sekuler (1986) showed that the size of the useful field of view declines, on average, with age, more recent work by Ball et al. (1988) has established the contribution of three factors to this reduction: (1) reduced speed of visual processing, (2) reduced ability to divide attention, and (3) reduced salience of the target against its background. These factors operate independently. Some individuals experience a decline in only one of the factors (e.g., divided attention), whereas others experience decline in multiple factors. The effects of multiple causes, when they occur, are additive. As a group, individuals with all three factors have a loss of 85% of the useful field of view relative to the group that experiences none or fewer of the problems.

Visual field loss, as tested with perimetry, is not a necessary condition for a constricted useful field of view. Many older adults who have impairments in the useful field of view have normal visual fields when measured using standard methods. Thus, visual attention ability depends not only on the integrity of visual sensory information, but also on the attentional factors noted previously. In this sense, measurement of the useful field of view complements traditional measures.

The age-related decline in vision observed in the laboratory or clinic does not necessarily affect everyday visual activities

The preceding discussion has dealt primarily with the results of psychophysical measures of vision using clinical or laboratory tests. There is, however, a

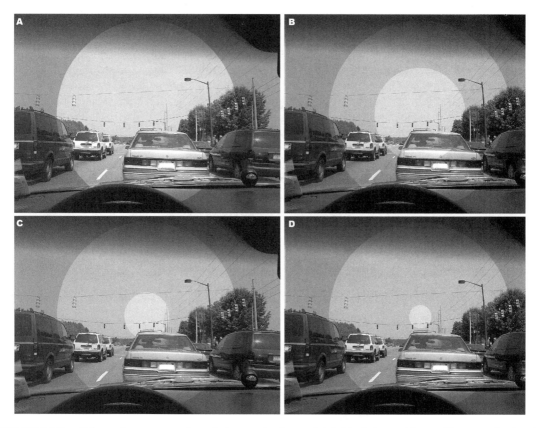

FIGURE 10.5   *Schematic representation of changes in the useful field of view with age. The areas in the circles do not represent the actual size of the visual field but are scaled to represent relative reductions in the size of the useful field of view.* **A.** *The circle represents the size of the attentional window for individuals with no restriction in the useful field of view.* **B.** *The smaller, lighter circle represents the window of individuals who have experienced a significant decline in the speed of visual information processing.* **C.** *Further reduction in the window size is due to both a slowing and an extreme sensitivity to distraction.* **D.** *Individuals with an attentional window of the smallest size have reduced processing time, increased sensitivity to distraction, and the inability to divide attention between central and peripheral tasks. If a person with this size window were concentrating only on the traffic lights, she or he would be unaware of the actions of the surrounding vehicles. (Modified from K Ball and C Owsley. The useful field of view test: a new technique for evaluating age-related declines in visual function. J Am Opt Assoc 1993;64:71–79.)*

considerable difference between someone's ability to perform, for example, a visual acuity test in a laboratory under optimal conditions and her or his ability to walk without falling, drive a vehicle, or recognize a friend in a crowd. Thus, the effects of aging on vision should also be evaluated in an environmental context in which the visual demands may be very different from the laboratory.

There has been increasing interest in the relationship between visual impairment and functional dependence among older adults. Several large population-based studies have demonstrated that visual impairment is associated with difficulty in performing both on the Activities of Daily Living measure and the more cognitive Instrumental Activities of Daily Living. These activities rely not only on sensory abilities but also on cognitive abilities, so there has been much interest in exploring the inter-relationships between vision and cognition among older adults.

Visual acuity is less important in everyday activities than contrast sensitivity

Older adults are at a disadvantage in recognizing faces at low ambient light levels. They typically need approximately twice as much contrast to detect and discriminate between faces as younger adults. The decline in the ability to recognize faces cannot fully be explained by poor acuity or a stricter threshold criterion, as noted earlier in this chapter. Rather, the best visual correlate of face perception is spatial contrast sensitivity (see Chapter 6, Figure 6.21), a more sensitive index of the ability to discriminate larger details.

Declining vision may also play a role in the increased prevalence of falls in the elderly. Reduced spatial contrast sensitivity is also associated with mobility problems, as described in Chapter 6. In addition, deficits in temporal processing and motion perception may also contribute to walking difficulty. Attention to the different lighting and contrast highlighting needs of the elderly can offset some of the increased risk of falls.

Older drivers have disproportionately more accidents and citations than middle-aged drivers

The accident profiles that describe the causes of automobile accidents that involve older drivers include failures to heed signs, yield the right of way, and turn safely, as well as an increased prevalence of intersection accidents. Impaired vision is typically thought to be responsible for these types of accidents. Most of the evidence linking visual sensory decline to driving problems is weak, however. For example, studies by Burg (1971) found static visual acuity to have extremely weak or nonexistent relationships to traffic accidents.

There are several reasons why one might not expect to find strong relationships between standard visual acuity test results and driving. Good acuity may be helpful in instances in which the vehicle is stopped or moving slowly, but is of less benefit while driving at normal speeds. Dynamic visual acuity (see Chapter 5), however, is also only weakly related to measures of driving performance. Furthermore, unlike real visual scenes, which vary in complexity, contrast, and illumination, the stimuli used to measure visual acuity are small, high contrast, and of low complexity. Spatial contrast sensitivity is a slightly better predictor of driving ability than visual acuity, but the strength of the relationship is relatively weak, and there is not a significant relationship between spatial contrast sensitivity and crash rates.

Visual field sensitivity has also been evaluated as a possible basis for poor driving among older adults. Although most studies have found only very weak relationships, one exception is a large sample study (n = 10,000) by Johnson and Keltner (1986) who found that the small subset of older drivers with severe binocular field loss had crash and conviction rates that were twice as high as those with normal visual fields.

Driver inattention and deficiencies in visual information processing have also been proposed as factors in accident causation. In fact, hazard recognition errors have been interpreted by some investigators more as attention failures than as sensory deficiencies. Consistent with this interpretation, the useful field of view has been found to be a better predictor of crash involvement than all other visual sensory function measures combined. For example, useful field of view reductions of 22.5–40.0%, 41–60%, and more than 60% have been associated with a 5.2-, 16.5-, and 21.5-fold increased risk of an injurious crash, respectively, compared to those with reductions of less than 22.5% (Owsley et al. 1998). In addition, driving performance on a closed course is related to performance on the useful field of view, as is performance on simulated driving tasks. Thus, there is converging evidence from investigators using different measures of driving outcome that visual search skills are strongly related to driving performance among older adults.

Study Guide

1. Why is it important to distinguish normal aging from visual pathology?
2. What are the optical effects of aging-related ocular media changes?
3. List five age-related anatomical or physiological changes that can affect vision.
4. How can a more conservative response criterion lead a clinician to believe incorrectly that an elderly patient has a loss of visual function?
5. What ways can a clinician use to counteract any tendency of an elderly patient to use a conservative criterion?
6. Describe the two primary age-related changes in the dark-adaptation curve.
7. What physiological or anatomical changes, or both, may account for these two changes in the dark-adaptation curve?
8. What is the effect of aging on acuity, and when does it occur?
9. What is the effect of aging on the spatial CSF, and when does it occur?
10. What is the effect of aging on sensitivity to temporally modulated stimuli, and when does it occur?
11. What happens to visual fields as a function of age, and when does it occur?
12. What is the useful field of view?
13. How is the useful field of view useful clinically?
14. What psychophysical measures of visual function correlate best with mobility difficulties in the elderly?

Glossary

Presbyopia: the inability of a person to change the shape of the crystalline lens to accommodate to nearby objects.

Useful field of view: the portion of the visual field that is useful for activities of daily living, including driving.

Appendix

Measuring Light

Where vision is concerned, light is generally specified in photometric units not in quanta and energy

When measuring the absolute threshold for detecting light (see Chapter 2), Hecht, Shlaer, and Pirenne (1942) determined the minimum number of quanta necessary to elicit a visual response. This number could, in turn, be converted to energy equivalents. It would be convenient to continue to deal with quanta and energy units, but, unfortunately, it is necessary to delve into the world of photometric units. This is a quagmire of units populated by such denizens as trolands, stilbs, apostilbs, nits, phots, lux, lamberts, footlamberts, foot-candles, and lumens, to name a few. This confusing array of terms results partly from the fact that photometry was developed in several countries as an independent practice associated with the lighting industry. There is thus a mixture of metric and English systems of measurements. It is, however, possible to survive with just a few units in one's photometric vocabulary, as long as one has a basic understanding of the meaning of several key concepts. A more detailed description is available in Chapter 1 of Graham (1965b).

Radiometry is the measure of radiant energy in the electromagnetic spectrum

The light that stimulates the eye is electromagnetic radiation. There are, however, many wavelengths of electromagnetic radiation (e.g., ultraviolet, infrared) that are not visible to the human eye. For radiant energy to be "luminous," it must be absorbed by the photoreceptors and be effective for vision. Ultraviolet or infrared radiation is not luminous because the eye can not detect any of it.

Photometry is the measure of the luminous effect of radiant energy

Even within the visible spectrum (wavelengths of approximately 400–700 nm), equal amounts of radiant energy at different wavelengths usually have unequal luminous effects. Thus, in photometry, radiometric units are weighted by the relative sensitivity of the eye or the visual system, or both, to various wavelengths of light, and (usually, properly) the wavelength of the light is specified.

Figure A.1 is a plot of the luminous efficiency of radiant energy as a function of wavelength for photopic (cone-mediated) and scotopic (rod-mediated) vision. For simplicity, each function has been normalized to a value of 1 at its maximum. It should be noted, however, that the amount of radiant energy that is required to stimulate the eye under scotopic conditions is much less than that under photopic conditions, except at the long-wavelength end of the spectrum (Riggs 1965). Also, the effectiveness of radiant energy differs somewhat from one observer to another.

The curves in Figure A.1 represent the relative sensitivity of a "standard observer" as designated by the CIE. The luminosity coefficient is called V_λ (pronounced "V lambda") for photopic vision.* At a wavelength of 555 nm, the value of V_λ is 1, which indicates that a given level of radiant energy at this wavelength has the maximum effect on the eye owing to absorption by the cones. All other wavelengths have V_λ values that are less than 1. For example, at the two wavelengths at which V_λ is 0.5 (510 and 610 nm), the amount of radiant energy must be twice what it is at 555 nm to have the same luminous effect. Therefore, V_λ is the relative luminous efficiency of radiant energy: the luminous efficiency relative to the maximum at 555 nm.

For reasons discussed in Chapter 8, the V_λ curve does not have a simple relationship to the absorption spectrum of the three cone pigments. It plots the overall effectiveness of light of different wavelengths on vision under photopic conditions. The scotopic (rod-mediated) luminous efficiency function, V'_λ (pronounced "V prime lambda") is similar in shape to the photopic curve but

---

*As described in Chapter 8, this curve was selected by the CIE to also be the $\bar{y}_\lambda$ color-matching function.

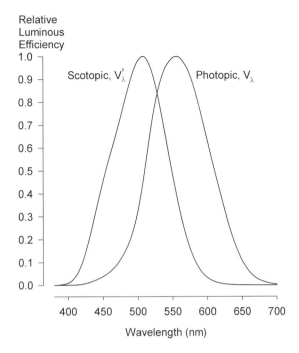

FIGURE A.1   *The photopic (V_λ) and scotopic (V'_λ) curves of relative spectral luminosity as standardized by the CIE. (Modified from WD Wright. The Measurement of Colour. New York: Macmillan, 1958.)*

has a peak at a shorter wavelength, 507 nm. This curve resembles the absorption spectrum for rhodopsin but differs, in part, from that spectrum because of filtering of wavelengths by the crystalline lens in the eye of a standard observer.

A note of caution is needed regarding the use of both the V_λ and the V'_λ curves. Luminous efficiency is *not* brightness. A light that is one-half as efficient as another is not one-half as bright. The primary utility of the V_λ and the V'_λ curves is to allow one to provide lights of different wavelengths that are photometrically equal and therefore have equal luminosity.

Photometric terminology describes what is emitted from a point source of light, what falls on a surface, and what is reflected or emitted from a surface

Figure A.2 is a simplified version of the most important photometric concepts. It begins on the left with a point source of light that ideally emits radiant energy in all directions equally. In photometric terms, the output of a point source is called *luminous flux*, and the unit of measure is the *lumen*. At a wavelength of 555 nm, one lumen is equal to approximately 4.07×10^{15} quanta per second emitted from the point source. In energy terms, this is 1.46×10^4 ergs or 1/685 W.

Note that these units are specified at 555 nm, the peak of the phototopic luminous efficiency function. As shown in Figure A.1, the luminous efficiency function of rod-mediated scotopic vision (V'_λ) is different from that of cone-mediated

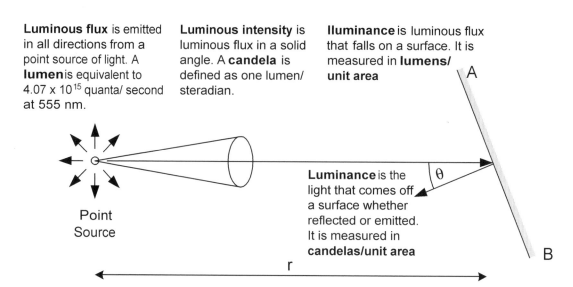

Luminous flux is emitted in all directions from a point source of light. A **lumen** is equivalent to 4.07×10^{15} quanta/ second at 555 nm.

Luminous intensity is luminous flux in a solid angle. A **candela** is defined as one lumen/ steradian.

Iluminance is luminous flux that falls on a surface. It is measured in **lumens/ unit area**

A

Luminance is the light that comes off a surface whether reflected or emitted. It is measured in **candelas/unit area**

θ

B

Point Source

r

FIGURE A.2 *Basic photometric concepts. (θ = the angle of tilt of the surface; r = perpendicular distance from the point source.)*

photopic vision. The V'_λ function may be used to evaluate the luminous flux of a stimulus under scotopic conditions (e.g., to measure *scotopic lumens*). One may, however, make photometric measurements based on the V_λ function at low light levels, and most measures are specified in photopic lumens.

If the light source in Figure A.2 were surrounded by a spherical surface, and one measured only the light that passed through a circular opening in the surface, the luminous flux that passed through that opening would be the luminous intensity. Thus, luminous intensity is luminous flux per unit solid angle. A solid angle, measured in steradians, is represented by the cone in Figure A.2. If one lumen is emitted per steradian, then by definition, the luminous intensity is equal to one *candela*. This term is derived from the early days of photometry (1860–1877) when the "standard candle" was made of whale oil. Thus, although formally defined previously, one candela is approximately the intensity of a candle. Table A.1 gives the luminous intensity values for some familiar sources.

TABLE A.1 Luminous intensity of various sources

Source	Approximate luminous intensity (candela)
Sun	10^{27}
Electric arc	10^{3}
40 W light bulb	10^{2}
Candle flame	10^{0}

Target/source	Illuminance (lux)
On the earth from the sun at noon	10^5
On an eye chart from room lights	$10^{2.5}$
On walls of a typical room interior from incident lighting	10^2
On the earth from a full moon	10^{-1}

*Illuminance** is a measure of the amount of light falling on a surface. It is expressed in lumens per unit area. One lumen per square meter is a *lux*. One lumen per square foot is a *foot-candle*, which is equal to approximately 10.8 lux. Table A.2 gives the illuminance values of some familiar situations.

Illuminance decreases in proportion to the square of the distance from the light source

If *F* is the total luminous flux (in lumens) that is emitted by a point source at the center of a sphere of radius *r*, then the illuminance (in lux) on the surface of the sphere is given by

$$\text{Illuminance} = \frac{F}{4\pi r^2} \qquad \text{Eq. A.1}$$

Because the denominator of the equation is the square of the radius of the sphere, the illuminance decreases in proportion to the square of the distance from the light source. This is the famous *Inverse Square Law*. Thus, if a light is a certain distance from a surface and one moves it twice as far away, the illuminance on the surface decreases to one-fourth of the original illuminance.

Illuminance changes with surface orientation relative to the source

The illuminance on a surface is also affected by the orientation of the surface relative to the source. For instance, in Figure A.2, surface AB is tilted at an angle, θ, to the incident light. The illuminance decreases in proportion to the cosine of the angle of tilt of the surface away from normal incidence. This is the *Cosine Law of Illuminance*. The basis for this effect is that the projected

---

*There is a convention in terminology that should be mentioned here. Words that end with the suffix "-tion" refer to a process, whereas words that end with the suffix "-ance" refer to the quantitative aspects of the process. Thus, "illumination" refers to light falling on a surface, whereas "illuminance" is the *amount* of light that falls on that surface. The quantitative measure of "reflection" is "reflectance," the ratio of the amount of light that is reflected to the amount of light that is incident.

TABLE A.3 Luminance of various sources

Source	Luminance (cd/m²)
Surface of sun at noon (clear day)	10^9
Tungsten filament	10^6
Upper limit of visual tolerance	$10^{4.7}$
White paper in sunlight (clear day)	10^4
Candle flame	10^4
Clear blue sky	$10^{3.8}$
Surface of moon (clear night)	$10^{3.3}$
Upper limit for rods (approximate)	10^2
White page in good reading light	$10^{1.7}$
Cone threshold (approximate)	10^{-2}
White paper in moonlight (clear night)	10^{-2}
White paper in starlight (clear night)	10^{-4}
Absolute threshold	10^{-6}

cd = candela.
SOURCE: *Modified from LA Riggs. Light as a Stimulus for Vision. In CH Graham (ed), Vision and Visual Perception. New York: Wiley, 1965;1–38; RM Boynton. Vision. In JB Sidowski (ed), Experimental Methods and Instrumentation in Psychology. New York: McGraw-Hill, 1966;273–330; and SH Bartley. The Psychophysiology of Vision. In SS Stevens (ed), Handbook of Experimental Psychology. New York: Wiley, 1951;921–984.*

area of a surface becomes smaller as it is rotated away from normal incidence. Combining the Inverse Square Law and the cosine law gives

$$\text{Illuminance} = \left(\frac{I}{r^2}\right)\cos\theta \qquad \text{Eq. A.2}$$

where r is the perpendicular distance from the source of luminous intensity, I, to the surface, and θ is the angle of tilt of the surface.

Luminance is a measure of the light emitted from a surface

Light can be reflected from a surface, as from the AB surface in Figure A.2, or it can be directly emitted, as in the case of a frosted light bulb, a fluorescent light, or a computer monitor. The intensity of the reflected or emitted light is expressed in *candelas per unit area* of the emitting surface, usually as candelas per square meter (cd/m²). Table A.3 shows some representative values of luminance for familiar light sources.

For reference
If one has to deal with stimulus luminance values in the real world, the following list of additional equivalencies from Riggs (1965) may be of use:

$$1 \text{ lumen/m}^2 = 0.0929 \text{ lumen/ft}^2 \text{ (e.g., foot candles)}$$
$$1 \text{ cd/m}^2 = 3.1416 \text{ apostilbs}$$
$$= 0.2919 \text{ footlamberts}$$
$$= 0.3142 \text{ millilamberts}$$

A troland is a measure of retinal illuminance

There is a final photometric unit that is not shown in the figure. The troland (td), a unit of retinal illuminance, is defined as L, the luminance of a surface (in the direction of viewing), multiplied by the area of the eye's pupil, S, in square millimeters. Thus,

$$td = L \times S \qquad \text{Eq. A.3}$$

For example, a stimulus with a luminance of 1 cd/m^2 that is viewed through a pupil with an area of 10 mm^2 (3.6 mm diameter) provides 10 trolands of retinal illuminance.

The utility of the troland is that if someone measures the luminance of a surface and fixes the pupil size by having a subject view the source through an artificial pupil, then anyone can reproduce the retinal illuminance conditions of the study later. Notice that the troland is not a true measure of retinal illuminance because it does not take into account differences in transmittance of the ocular media. Also, for large pupil diameters at photopic luminance levels, the troland somewhat overestimates the effectiveness of a light. It is nevertheless a very commonly used (and very useful) unit.

The reflectance of a surface is the ratio of reflected to incident light

Reflectance is not a photometric term, but is one that is useful to consider here. Obviously, both the incident and reflected light have to be in the same units. If the illuminance is given in lux, the reflected value should be in lux. However, for a diffusely reflecting (matte) surface, like the moon or nonglossy paper, if the illuminance is given in lux, the luminance in candelas per square meter can be calculated by multiplying the illuminance by the reflectance of the surface and dividing by π.

Contrast is an expression of the luminance or color difference between two surfaces

Contrast also is not a photometric term, but one that is extremely important. The difference may be one of luminance or color, or both. Any one of these differences may also occur over time (temporal contrast) in the same part of the visual field. The standard quantitative definition of contrast is

$$\frac{(L_T - L_B)}{L_B} \qquad \text{Eq. A.4}$$

where L_B is the luminance of the reference, or background, surface, and L_T is the luminance of the second, or test, surface. If L_T is greater than L_B, then the contrast is positive; otherwise, it is negative. For instance, the dark letters on an eye chart have negative contrast. If the illuminance is equal on any two surfaces, one can substitute the reflectances of the surfaces into the equation without changing the value of the contrast.

Grating contrast is calculated from the highest and lowest luminances

In Chapters 5, 6, and 7, another contrast calculation is used (Michelson contrast) for static stimuli composed of alternating bars of high luminance (L_{max}) and low luminance (L_{min}) (gratings) and as well as for lights that flicker between a high and low luminance over time. Michelson contrast is calculated as

$$\text{Contrast} = \frac{(L_{max} - L_{min})}{(L_{max} + L_{min})} \qquad \text{Eq. A.5}$$

Michelson contrast can have a value between 0 and 1 and is independent of the luminance values in the grating.

Specifying and Using Visual Angle

Stimulus size is often expressed in terms of visual angle

In psychophysical studies, rather than specifying stimulus size in terms of its width or height and distance from the eye, it is generally expressed as an angle. This has two advantages. First, it provides a measure of the size of the stimulus on the retina. This, in turn, enables one to approximate, for example, how many photoreceptors would be stimulated by a particular target. Second, it enables investigators to duplicate stimulus size in different experiments without having to construct an exact duplicate of the experimental apparatus. Figure A.3A shows how stimulus size and distance determine the angular extent of stimuli on the retina.

Figure A.3A shows three objects, A, B, and C, represented by vertical arrows at distances d_1, d_2, and d_3 from the corneal apex. A and B are the same physical size (x). C is half the size (y) of A and B, but is closer to the cornea. The principal ray connecting the bottom of the objects and the principal rays from the tip of the objects pass through a point inside the eye, called the *nodal point* (N), and intersect the retina in an arc. These principal lines create similar triangles. Thus, the visual angle, α, is the same outside and inside that eye, as is angle β.

Objects are said to *subtend* an angle at the eye. Even though objects A and B are the same size, they subtend different angles on the retina because they are at different distances from the cornea. On the other hand, since objects A and C have common principal rays, they subtend the same angle on the retina despite being different sizes and different distances from the eye. This means that they cover retinal areas of identical size, and, in the case shown in the figure, identical positions on the retina. As far as the retina

A

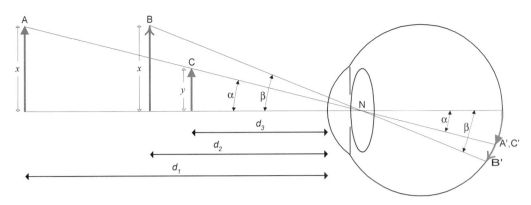

B

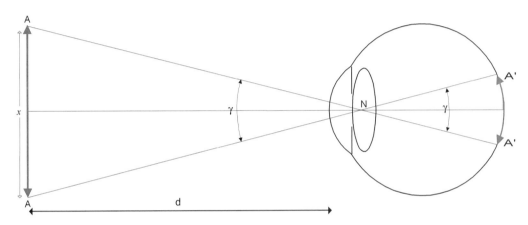

FIGURE A.3   *Geometric relationships used for defining visual angle. See text for details.*

is concerned these two stimuli would be indistinguishable on the basis of size and retinal position alone.

In Figure A.3A it is a straightforward matter to calculate the visual angles of the three stimuli:

$$\alpha = \tan^{-1}\left(\frac{x}{d_1}\right)$$ Eq. A.6

$$\beta = \tan^{-1}\left(\frac{x}{d_2}\right)$$ Eq. A.7

$$\alpha = \tan^{-1}\left(\frac{y}{d_3}\right)$$ Eq. A.8

Note that the distance between the corneal apex and the nodal point is not added to the distances because, at approximately 7 mm, it is generally negligible when compared to the distances of objects from the eye. As a rule of thumb, it is safe to ignore the 7 mm for stimuli larger than 0.5 cm and distances larger than 50 cm.

Figure A.3B shows a more general case where the object AA extends on either side of the perpendicular principal ray. The object in this case subtends the visual angle, which can be calculated as

$$\gamma = 2 \times \tan^{-1}\left(\frac{x/2}{d}\right)$$

Eq. A.9

For ratios of object size to distance of 0.1 or less, it is not necessary to use half the object length and multiply the resulting angle by 2. This holds for visual angles of 6° or smaller.

Visual angles are expressed in degrees, minutes, or seconds

Large stimuli generally subtend visual angles expressed in degrees (°). Smaller stimuli have units of minutes of arc ('). There are 60' in a degree. This is an important unit in visual acuity, for example, where resolution acuity is standardized to 1'. Finally, even smaller stimuli are expressed in seconds of arc ("). There are 60" in 1' of arc. Vernier acuity has a threshold measured in seconds, for example.

Visual angle can be used to determine the retinal dimensions of a stimulus

Suppose, for example, that angle α in Figure A.3A is 1°. The tangent of 1° is 0.017. Because this is the ratio of retinal image size to the distance of the retina from the nodal point (approximately 17 mm), it is a simple matter to calculate that a stimulus subtending a visual angle of 1° will cover approximately 0.3 mm or 300 μm. Knowing that the center-to-center spacing of cones in the fovea is in the range of 20" to 40" (see Chapter 5) it is possible to calculate that the spacing is approximately 0.002 mm or 2 μm, assuming the middle of the range.

Study Guide

1. What does photometry measure?
2. What are V_λ and V'_λ?
3. Define lumen, candela, illuminance, luminance, troland, reflectance, and contrast.
4. Write the Inverse Square Law.
5. Write the Cosine Law of Illuminance.
6. Be able to calculate visual angle given stimulus size and distance from the cornea.
7. Be able to convert between degree, minutes of arc, and seconds of arc.
8. Be able to calculate the retinal dimensions of a stimulus given the visual angle.
9. Given the dimensions of an anatomical feature on the retina, be able to calculate its visual angle.

References

Abadi R, Pascal E. Visual resolution limits in human albinism. Vision Res 1991; 31:1445–1447.

Ahnelt P, Kolb H. Horizontal cells and cone photoreceptors in primate retina: a Golgi-light microscopic study of spectral connectivity. J Comp Neurol 1994;343:387–405.

Aiba TS, Stevens SS. Relation of brightness to duration and luminance under light- and dark-adaptation. Vision Res 1964;4:391–401.

Alexander KR, Fishman GA. Rod-cone interaction in flicker perimetry. Br J Ophthalmol 1984;68:303–309.

Alexander KR, Fishman GA. Rod-cone interaction in flicker perimetry: evidence for a distal retinal locus. Doc Ophthalmol 1985;60:3–36.

Alexander KR, Xie W, Derlacki D. The effect of contrast polarity on letter identification. Vision Res 1993;33:2491–2497.

Allen D, Banks MS, Norcia AM. Does chromatic sensitivity develop more slowly than luminance sensitivity? Vision Res 1993;33:2553–2562.

Alpern M. Metacontrast. J Opt Soc Am 1953;43:648–657.

Anderson DR. Perimetry with and without Automation. St. Louis: Mosby, 1987.

Appelle S. Perception and discrimination as a function of stimulus orientation: the "oblique effect" in man and animals. Psychol Bull 1972;78:266–278.

Arden GB, Hogg CR. A new cause for difficulty in seeing at night. Doc Ophthalmol 1985;60:121–125.

Arden GB, Jacobson JJ. A simple grating test for contrast sensitivity: preliminary results indicate value in screening for glaucoma. Invest Ophthalmol Vis Sci 1978;17:23–25.

Ariyasu R, Lee P, Linton K, et al. Sensitivity, specificity, and predictive values of screening tests for eye conditions in a clinic-based population [See comments]. Ophthalmology 1996;103:1751–1760.

Bailey IL, Bullimore M, Raasch T, Taylor H. Clinical grading and the effects of scaling. Invest Ophthalmol Vis Sci 1991;32:422–432.

Bailey IL, Lovie JE. New design principles for visual acuity letter charts. Am J Optom Physiol Opt 1976;53:740–745.

Baker HD. The instantaneous threshold and early dark adaptation. J Opt Soc Am 1953;43:798–803.

Barlow HB, Hill RM. Selective sensitivity to direction of motion in ganglion cells in the rabbits' retina. Science 1963;139:412–414.

Bartley SH. Subjective brightness in relation to flash rate and the light-dark ratio. J Exp Psychol 1938;23:313–319.

Ball K, Owsley C. The useful field of view test: a new technique for evaluating age-related declines in visual function. J Am Optom Assoc 1993;64:71–79.

Ball K, Sekuler R. Improving visual perception in older observers. J Gerontol 1986;41:176–182.

Ball KK, Beard BL, Roenker DL, et al. Age and visual search: expanding the useful field of view. J Opt Soc Am A 1988;5:2210–2219.

Banister H. Block capital letters as tests of visual acuity. Br J Ophthalmol 1927;11:49–61.

Banks MS, Geisler WS, Bennett PJ. The physical limits of grating visibility. Vision Res 1987;27:1915–1924.

Banks MS, Salapatek P. Acuity and contrast sensitivity in 1-, 2-, and 3-month-old human infants. Invest Ophthalmol Vis Sci 1978;17:361–365.

Banks MS, Sekuler AB, Anderson SJ. Peripheral spatial vision: limits imposed by optics, photoreceptors, and receptor pooling. J Opt Soc Am A 1991;8:1775–1787.

Barlow H. Temporal and spatial summation in human vision at different background intensities. J Physiol (Lond) 1958;178:477–504.

Barlow HB. Single units and sensation: a neuron doctrine for perceptual psychology? Perception 1972;1:371–394.

Barlow HB, Fitzhugh R, Kuffler SW. Change of organization in the receptive fields of the cat's retina during dark adaptation. J Physiol 1957;137:338–354.

Baron W, Westheimer G. Visual acuity as a function of exposure duration. J Opt Soc Am 1973;63:212–219.

Bartley SH. The Psychophysiology of Vision. In SS Stevens (ed), Handbook of Experimental Psychology. New York: Wiley, 1951;921–984.

Baylor D. How photons start vision. Proc Natl Acad Sci U S A 1996;93:560–565.

Baylor DA, Lamb TD, Yau KW. Responses of retinal rods to single photons. J Physiol (Lond) 1979;288:613–634.

Baylor DA, Nunn BJ, Schnapf JL. Spectral sensitivity of cones of the monkey macaca fascicularis. J Physiol (Lond) 1987;390:145–160.

Békésy G. A new audiometer. Acta Otolaryngol (Stockh) 1947;35:411–422.

Berlin B, Kay P. Basic color terms; their universality and evolution. Berkeley, CA: University of California Press, 1969;178.

Bennett AG. Ophthalmic test types. A review of previous work and discussions on some controversial questions. Br J Physiol Opt 1965;22:238–271.

Blackwell HR. Contrast thresholds of the human eye. J Opt Soc Am 1946;36:624–643.

Blackwell HR. Psychophysical thresholds: experimental studies of methods of measurement. Bulletin of the Engineering Research Institute 1953;36:1–227.

Blakemore C, Campbell FW. On the existence of neurons in the human visual system selectively sensitive to the orientation and size of retinal images. J Physiol (Lond) 1969;203:237–260.

Blakemore C, Rushton W. The rod increment threshold during dark adaptation in normal and rod monochromat. J Physiol (Lond) 1965;181:629–640.

Bodis-Wollner I. Visual acuity and contrast sensitivity in patients with cerebral lesions. Science 1972;178:769–771.

Boynton RM. Vision. In JB Sidowski (ed), Experimental Methods and Instrumentation in Psychology. New York: McGraw-Hill, 1966;273–330.

Boynton RM, Gordon J. Bezold Brücke hue shift measured by color naming technique. J Opt Soc Am 1977;55:78–86.

Boynton RM, Olson CX. Salience of chromatic basic color terms confirmed by three measures. Vision Res 1990;30:1311–1317.

Bradley A, Thibos L, Wang Y, et al. Imaging FWC. Ophthalmic Physiol Opt 1992; 12:128.

Brenton RS, Phelps CD. The normal visual field on the Humphrey field analyzer. Ophthalmologica 1986;193:56–74.

Broca A, Sulzer D. La sensations luminen en function des temps. J Physiol Paris 1902;4:632–640.

Brown AM. Vernier acuity in human infants: rapid emergence shown in a longitudinal study. Optom Vis Sci 1997;74:732–740.

Brown B. Dynamic visual acuity, eye movements and peripheral acuity for moving targets. Vision Res 1972;12:305–321.

Brown JL, Graham CH, Leibowitz H, Ranken HB. Luminance thresholds for the resolution of visual detail during dark adaptation. J Opt Soc Am 1953;43:197–202.

Burg A. Vision and driving: a report on research. Hum Factors 1971;13:79–87.

Burr DC, Holt J, Johnstone JR, Ross J. Selective depression of motion sensitivity during saccades. J Physiol 1982;333:1–15.

Burr DC, Morrone MC, Ross J. Selective suppression of the magnocellular visual pathway during saccadic eye movements. Nature 1994;371:511–513.

Burr D, Ross J. Contrast sensitivity at high velocities. Vision Res 1982;22:479–484.

Campbell F, Green D. Optical and retinal factors affecting visual resolution. J Physiol (Lond) 1965;181:576–593.

Campbell F, Gubish R. Optical quality of the human eye. J Physiol 1966;186:558–578.

Campbell F, Robson J. Application of Fourier analysis to the visibility of gratings. J Physiol (Lond) 1968;197:551–566.

Campbell FW, Wurtz RH. Saccadic omission: why we do not see a grey-out during a saccadic eye movement. Vision Res 1978;18:1297–1303.

Carkeet A, Levi DM, Manny RE. Development of Vernier acuity in childhood. Optom Vis Sci 1997;74:741–750.

Casagrande VA. A third parallel visual pathway to primate area V1. Trends Neurosci 1994;17:305–310.

Chapanis A. The dark adaptation of the color anomalous measured with lights of different hues. J Gen Physiol 1947;30:423–437.

Chung ST, Bedell HE. Effect of retinal image motion on visual acuity and contour interaction in congenital nystagmus. Vision Res 1995;35:3071–3082.

Chung ST, Levi DM, Bedell HE. Vernier in motion: what accounts for the threshold elevation? Vision Res 1996;36:2395–2410.

Coletta NJ, Adams AJ. Rod-cone interaction in flicker detection. Vision Res 1984;24:1333–1340.

Committee on Vision. Recommended standard procedures for the clinical measurement and specification of visual acuity. Report of working group 39. Committee on vision. Assembly of Behavioral and Social Sciences, National Research Council, National Academy of Sciences, Washington, D.C. Adv Ophthalmol 1980;41:103–148.

Committee on Vision. Procedures for testing color vision—report of Working Group 41. Washington: National Academy Press, 1981.

Conner JD, MacLeod DIA. Rod photoreceptors detect rapid flicker. Science 1977;195:698–699.

Corliss DA. A comprehensive model of clinical decision making. J Am Optom Assoc 1995;66(6):362–371.

Cornsweet TN. Visual Perception. New York: Academic, 1970.

Crawford BH. Visual adaptation in relation to brief conditioning stimuli. Proc R Soc Lond B Biol Sci 1947;128:283–302.

Crews J. The demographic, social, and conceptual contexts of aging and vision loss. J Am Optom Assoc 1994;65:63–68.

Curcio CA, Allen KA. Topography of ganglion cells in human retina. J Comp Neurol 1990;300:5–25.

Curcio CA, Owsley C, Jackson GR. Spare the rods, save the cones in aging and age-related maculopathy. Invest Ophthalmol Vis Sci 2000;41(8): 2015–2018.

Curcio CA, Sloan KR, Kalina RE, Hendrickson AE. Human photoreceptor topography. J Comp Neurol 1990;292:497–523.

Curcio CA, Sloan KR Jr, Packer O, et al. Distribution of cones in human and monkey retina: individual variability and radial asymmetry. Science 1987;236: 579–582.

Dacey DM. Morphology of a small-field bistratified ganglion cell type in the macaque and human retina. Vis Neurosci 1993;10:1081–1098.

Dacey DM. Circuitry for color coding in the primate retina. Proc Natl Acad Sci U S A 1996;93:582–588.

Dacey DM, Lee BB, Stafford DK, et al. Horizontal cells of the primate retina: cone specificity without spectral opponency. Science 1996;271:656–659.

Davson H. The Physiology of the Eye (3rd ed). New York: Academic, 1976.

DeLange HD. Research into the dynamic nature of the human fovea-cortex systems with intermittent and modulated light: attenuation characteristics with white and colored lights. J Opt Soc Am 1958;48:777–784.

Demer JL, Amjadi F. Dynamic visual acuity of normal subjects during vertical optotype and head motion. Invest Ophthalmol Vis Sci 1993;34:1894–1906.

De Monasterio FM, Gouras P. Functional properties of ganglion cells of the rhesus monkey retina. J Physiol 1975;251:167–195.

Derrington AM, Lennie P. Spatial and temporal contrast sensitivities of neurones in lateral geniculate nucleus of macaque. J Physiol 1984;357:219–240.

DeValois KK, DeValois RL. Spatial Vision. New York: Oxford University Press, 1988.

DeValois RL, Abramov I, Jacobs GH. Analysis of response patterns of LGN cells. J Opt Soc Am 1966;56:966–977.

DeValois RL, DeValois KK. Neural Coding of Color. In EC Carterette, MP Friedman (eds), Handbook of Perception: Seeing. New York: Academic, 1975;117–166.

DeValois RL, Morgan H, Snodderly DM. Psychophysical studies of monkey vision. 3. Spatial luminance contrast sensitivity tests of macaque and human observers. Vision Res 1974;14:75–81.

deVries HL. The quantum nature of light and its bearing upon the threshold of vision, the differential sensitivity and visual acuity of the eye. Physica 1943;10:553–564.

Dobson V. Behavioral tests of visual acuity in infants. Int Ophthalmol Clin 1980; 20:233–250.

Donner K, Hemila S. Modelling the spatio-temporal modulation response of ganglion cells with difference-of-Gaussians receptive fields: relation to photoreceptor response kinetics. Vis Neurosci 1996;13:173–86.

Dowling JE. The Retina: An Approachable Part of the Brain. Cambridge, MA: Belknap Press of Harvard University Press, 1987.

Drum B. Hue signals from short- and middle-wavelength-sensitive cones. J Opt Soc Am A 1989;6:153–157.

D'Zmura M, Lennie P. Shared pathways for rod and cone vision. Vision Res 1986;26:1273–1280.

Enroth-Cugell C, Lennie P. The control of retinal ganglion cell discharge by receptive field surrounds. J Physiol 1975;247:551–578.

Falcao-Reis FM, Hogg CR, Frumkes TE, Arden GB. Nyctalopia with normal rod function: a suppression of cones by rods. Eye 1991;5(1):138–144.

Fantz R. Pattern vision in young infants. Psychol Rev 1958;8:43–47.

Ferris FL III, Kassoff A, Bresnick GH, Bailey I. New visual acuity charts for clinical research. Am J Ophthalmol 1982;94:91–96.

Field DJ. Relations between the statistics of natural images and the response properties of cortical cells. J Opt Soc Am A 1987;4:2379–2394.

Flom MC. New concepts on visual acuity. Optometric Weekly 1966;57:63–68.

Flom MC. Contour interaction and the crowding effect. Probl Optom 1991;3:237–257.

Flom MC, Heath GG, Takahashi E. Contour interaction and visual resolution: contralateral effects. Science 1963;142:979–980.

Frumkes TE, Eysteinsson T. The cellular basis for suppressive rod-cone interaction. Vis Neurosci 1988;1:263–273.

Geisler WS. Sequential ideal-observer analysis of visual discriminations. Psychol Rev 1989;96:267–314.

Gerali P, Flom MC, Raab EL. Report of Children's Vision Screening Task Force. National Society to Prevent Blindness, Schaumburg, IL 1990.

Gervais MJ, Harvey LO Jr, Roberts JO. Identification confusions among letters of the alphabet. J Exp Psychol Hum Percept Perform 1984;10:655–666.

Gescheider GA. Psychophysics, Method, Theory and Application. Hillsdale, NJ: Erlbaum Associates, 1985.

Getz L, Dobson V, Luna B. Grating acuity development in 2-week to 3-year-old children born prior to term. Clin Vis Sci 1992;7:251–256.

Glaser J, Goodwin J. Neuro-Ophthalmologic Examination: The Visual System. In J Glaser (ed), Neuro-Ophthalmology (2nd ed). Philadelphia: Lippincott, 1990;9–36.

Goldberg SH, Frumkes TE, Nygaard RW. Inhibitory influence of unstimulated rods in the human retina: evidence provided by examining cone flicker. Science 1983;221(4606):180–182.

Goldmann H. Examination of the fundus of the cataractous eye. Am J Ophthalmol 1972;73:309–320.

Gordon J, Abramov I. Color vision in the peripheral retina. II. Hue and saturation. J Opt Soc Am 1977;67:202–207.

Graham CH. Vision and Visual Perception. New York: Wiley, 1965b.

Graham CH, Margaria R. Area and the intensity-time relation in the peripheral retina. Am J Physiol 1935;113:299–305.

Granit R, Harper P. Comparative studies on the peripheral and central retina: II. Synaptic reactions in the eye. Amer J Physiol 1930;95:211–227.

Green DG, Dowling JE, Siegal IM, Ripps H. Retinal mechanisms of visual adaptation in the skate. J Gen Physiol 1975;65:483–502.

Gregg JB, Heath GG. The Eye and Sight. Boston: Heath, 1964.

Guild J. The colorimetric properties of the spectrum. Philos Trans R Soc Lond A 1931;230:149–187.

Haegerstrom-Portnoy G, Schneck ME, Verdon WA, Hewlett SE. Clinical vision characteristics of the congenital achromatopsias. I. Visual acuity, refractive error, and binocular status. Optom Vis Sci 1996;73:446–456.

Haley MJ. The Field Analyzer Primer. San Leandro, CA: Allergan Humphrey, 1986.

Hallett PE, Marriott FH, Rodger FC. The relationship of visual threshold to retinal position and area. J Physiol (Lond) 1962;160:364–373.

Hansen R, Fulton A. Development of Scotopic Retinal Sensitivity. In K Simons (ed), Early Visual Development, Normal and Abnormal. New York: Oxford University Press, 1993;130–142.

Hansen RM, Hamer RD, Fulton AB. The effect of light adaptation on scotopic spatial summation in 10-week-old infants. Vision Res 1992;32:387–392.

Harmon LD. The recognition of faces. Sci Am 1973;229:71–82.

Harris MJ, Robins D, Dieter JM Jr, et al. Eccentric visual acuity in patients with macular disease. Ophthalmology 1985;92:1550–1553.

Hart JW. Visual Adaptation. In RA Moses, JW Hart (eds), Adler's Physiology of the Eye (8th ed). St. Louis: Mosby, 1987;389–414.

Hart PM, Chakravarthy U, Stevenson MR. Questionnaire-based survey on the importance of quality of life measures in ophthalmic practice. Eye 1998;12:124–126.

Harwerth RS, Smith EL III, DeSantis L. Mechanisms mediating visual detection in static perimetry. Invest Ophthalmol Vis Sci 1993;34:3011–3023.

Hecht S. Vision II. The Nature of the Photoreceptor Process. In C Murchison (ed), Handbook of General Experimental Psychology. Worcester, MA: Clark University Press, 1934;704–828.

Hecht S. The chemistry of visual substances. Annu Rev Biochem 1942;11:465–496.

Hecht S, Haig C, Chase AM. The influence of light adaptation on subsequent dark adaptation of the eye. J Gen Physiol 1937;20:831–850.

Hecht S, Haig C, Wald G. Dark adaptation of retinal fields of different size and location. J Gen Physiol 1935;19:321–337.

Hecht S, Hsia Y. Dark adaptation following light adaptation to red and white lights. J Opt Soc Am 1945;35:261–267.

Hecht S, Ross S, Mueller CG. The visibility of lines and squares at high brightnesses. J Opt Soc Am 1947;37:500–507.

Hecht S, Shlaer S. Intermittent stimulation by light. V. The relation between intensity and critical frequency for different parts of the spectrum. J Gen Physiol 1936;19:965–979.

Hecht S, Shlaer S, Pirenne MH. Energy, quanta and vision. J Gen Physiol 1942; 25:819–840.

Hecht S, Williams RE. The visibility of monochromatic radiation and the absorption spectrum of visual purple. J Gen Physiol 1922;5:1–33.

Hedin A, Olsson K. Letter legibility and the construction of a new visual acuity chart. Ophthalmologica 1984;189:147–156.

Herse PR, Bedell HE. Contrast sensitivity for letter and grating targets under various stimulus conditions. Optom Vis Sci 1989;66:774–781.

Hess RF, Nordby K. Spatial and temporal limits of vision in the achromat. J Physiol (Lond) 1986;371:365–385.

Hess RF, Sharpe LT, Nordby K. Night Vision: Basic, Clinical and Applied Aspects. Cambridge, UK: Cambridge University Press, 1990.

Hickey T, Peduzzi J. Structure and Development of the Visual System. In P Salapatek, LB Cohen (eds), Handbook of Infant Perception. New York: Academic, 1987;1–42.

Hoffstetter HW, Griffin JR, Berman MS, Everson RW. Dictionary of Visual Science (5th ed). Boston: Butterworth–Heinemann, 2000.

Horner DG, Paul AD, Katz B, Bedell HE. Variations in the slope of the psychometric acuity function with acuity threshold and scale. Am J Optom Physiol Opt 1985;62:895–900.

Hurvich LM. Color Vision. Sunderland, MA: Sinauer, 1981.

Hurvich LM, Jameson D. Some quantitative aspects of an opponent-colors theory. II. Brightness, saturation, and hue in normal and dichromatic vision. J Opt Soc Am 1955;45:602–616.

Ivers RQ, Cumming RG, Mitchell P, Attebo K. Visual impairment and falls in older adults: the Blue Mountains Eye Study. J Am Geriatr Soc 1998;46:58–64.

Jacobs RJ. Visual resolution and contour interaction in the fovea and periphery. Vision Res 1979;19:1187–1195.

James W. Principles of Psychology. New York: H Holt and Company, 1899.

Johnson CA, Adams AJ, Casson EJ, Brandt JD. Blue-on-yellow perimetry can predict the development of glaucomatous visual field loss. Arch Ophthalmol 1993;111:645–650.

Johnson CA, Adams AJ, Twelker JD, Quigg JM. Age-related changes in the central visual field for short-wavelength sensitive pathways. J Opt Soc Am A 1988;5:2131–2139.

Johnson CA, Casson EJ. Effects of luminance, contrast, and blur on visual acuity. Optom Vis Sci 1995;72:864–869.

Johnson CA, Keltner JL. Incidence of visual field loss in 20,000 eyes and its relationship to driving performance. Arch Opthamol 1986;101:371–375.

Johnson CA, Samuels SJ. Screening for glaucomatous visual field loss with frequency-doubling perimetry. Invest Ophthalmol Vis Sci 1997;38:413–425.

Kaiser PK, Boynton RM. Human Color Vision. Washington: Optical Society of America, 1996.

Kelly DH. Motion and vision I. Stabilized images of stationary gratings. J Opt Soc Am 1979a;69:1266–1274.

Kelly DH. Motion and vision II. Stabilized spatio-temporal threshold surface. J Opt Soc Am 1979b;69:1340–1349.

Kelly DH. Visual responses to time-dependent stimuli. I. Amplitude sensitivity measurements. J Opt Soc Am 1961;51:422–429.

Kirschen DG, Rosenbaum AL, Ballard EA. The dot visual acuity test—a new acuity test for children. J Am Optom Assoc 1983;54:1055–1059.

Kling JW, Riggs LA. Woodworth & Schlosberg's Experimental Psychology (3rd ed). New York: Holt, Reinhart and Winston, 1971.

König A, Brodhun E. Experimentelle Untersuchungen über die psychophysische Fundamentalformel in Bezug auf den Gesichtssinn. Sitzungsber, Berlin: Preuss Akad. Wiss., 1889;27:641–644.

Kraft TW, Schneeweis DM, Schnapf JL. Visual transduction in human rod photoreceptors. J Physiol 1993;464:747–765.

Kuyk T, Elliott JL. Visual factors and mobility in persons with age-related macular degeneration. J Rehabil Res Dev 1999;36:303–312.

Lakshminarayanan V, Lang AJ, Portney V. The "Expected Visual Outcome" (EVO) model: methodology and clinical validation. Optom Vis Sci 1995;72:511–521.

Laming D. On the Limits of Visual Detection. In JJ Kulikowski, V Walsh, IJ Murray (eds), Vision and Visual Dysfunction: Limits of Vision (vol 5). Boca Raton, FL: CRC Press, 1991;6–14.

Lange G, Frumkes TE. Influence of rod adaptation upon cone responses to light offset in humans: II. Results in an observer with exaggerated suppressive rod-cone interaction. Vis Neurosci 1992;8:91–95.

Lee BB, Dacey DM. Structure and Function in Primate Retina. In C Cavonius, AJ Adams (eds), Colour Vision Deficiencies XIII: Proceedings of the Thirteenth Symposium of the International Research Group on Colour Vision Deficiencies held in Pau, France, July 27–30, 1995. Boston: Kluwer Academic Publishers, 1997;107–117.

Lee BB, Martin PR, Valberg A. Sensitivity of macaque retinal ganglion cless to chromatic and luminance flicker. J Physiol 1989;414:223–243.

Legge GE, Rubin GS, Luebker A. Psychophysics of reading—V. The role of contrast in normal vision. Vision Res 1987;27:1165–1177.

Lennie P, Krauskopf J, Sclar G. Chromatic mechanisms in striate cortex of macaque. J Neurosci 1990;10:649–669.

Levi DM, Klein SA. Differences in vernier discrimination for grating between strabismic and anisometropic amblyopes. Invest Ophthalmol Vis Sci 1982;23:398–407.

Levi DM, Klein SA. Equivalent intrinsic blur in amblyopia. Vision Res 1990;30:1995–2022.

Levi DM, Klein SA, Aitsebaomo AP. Vernier acuity, crowding and cortical magnification. Vision Res 1985;25:963–977.

Logothetis NK, Schall JD. Neuronal correlates of subjective visual perception. Science 1989;245(4919):761–763.

Ludvigh EJ. Visual acuity while one is viewing a moving object. Arch Ophthalmol 1949;42:14–22.

Ludvigh E, McCarthy EF. Absorption of visible light by the refractive media of the human eye. Arch Ophthalmol 1938;20:37–51.

Lynn JR, Felman RL, Starita RJ. Principles of Perimetry. In R Ritch, MB Shields, T Krupin (eds), The Glaucomas. St Louis: Mosby, 1996;491–521.

Lythgoe RJ, Tansley K. The relation of the critical frequency of flicker to the adaptation of the eye. Proc Roy Soc (Lond) 1929;105B:60–92.

MacAdam DL. Visual sensitivities to color differences in daylight. J Opt Soc Am 1942;32:247–274.

Maddess T, Hemmi JM, James AC. Evidence for spatial aliasing effects in the Y-like cells of the magnocellular visual pathway. Vis Res 1998;1843–1859.

Maffei L. Spatial Frequency Channels: Neural Mechanisms. In R Held, H Leibowitz, M Teuber (eds), Handbook of Sensory Physiology: Perception (vol 8). Berlin: Springer-Verlag, 1978;39–66.

Mandelbaum J, Sloan LL. Peripheral visual acuity. Am J Ophthalmol 1947;30:581–588.

Manny RE, Klein SA. The development of vernier acuity in infants. Curr Eye Res 1984;3:453–462.

Marg E, Freeman D, Peltzman P, Goldstein P. Visual acuity in human infants: evoked potential measurements. Invest Ophthalmol 1976;15:150–152.

Maxwell JC. Experiments on colour, as perceived by the eye, with remarks on colour blindness. Trans R Soc (Edinburgh) 1855;21:275–298.

Mayer DL, Beiser AS, Warner AF, et al. Monocular acuity norms for the Teller Acuity Cards between ages one month and four years. Invest Ophthalmol Vis Sci 1995;36:671–685.

Mayer MJ, Spiegler SJ, Ward B, et al. Foveal flicker sensitivity discriminates ARM-risk from healthy eyes. Invest Ophthalmol Vis Sci 1992;33:3143–3149.

Mayer MJ, Ward B, Klein R, et al. Flicker sensitivity and fundus appearance in pre-exudative age-related maculopathy. Invest Ophthalmol Vis Sci 1994;35:1138–1149.

McDonald M, Sebris SL, Mohn G, et al. Monocular acuity in normal infants: the acuity card procedure. Am J Optom Physiol Opt 1986;63:127–134.

McFarland RA, Domey RG, Warren AB, Ward DC. Dark adaptation as a function of age: I. A statistical analysis. J Gerontol 1960;15:149–154.

Merigan WH, Katz LM, Maunsell JH. The effects of parvocellular lateral geniculate lesions on the acuity and contrast sensitivity of macaque monkeys. J Neurosci 1991;11:994–1001.

Merigan WH, Maunsell JHR. How parallel are the primate visual pathways? Annu Rev Neurosci 1993;16:369–402.

Miller DM. Optics and Refraction: A User Friendly Guide. In SM Podos, M Yanoff (eds), Textbook of Ophthalmology. New York: Gower, 1991.

Movshon JA, Adelson EH, Gizzi MS, Newsom WT. The analysis of moving visual patterns. In Chagas C, Gattass R, Gross C (eds). Pattern Recognition Mechanisms. Exp Brain Res Suppl 11. New York: Springer-Verlag, 1985;117–185.

Nakayama K. Biological image motion processing: a review. Vision Res 1985;25:625–660.

Newacheck JS, Haegerstrom-Portnoy G, Adams AJ. Predicting visual acuity from detection thresholds. Optom Vis Sci 1990;67:184–191.

Newsome WT, Britten KH, Movshon JA. Neuronal correlates of a perceptual decision. Nature 1989;341:52–54.

Newsome WT, Mikami A, Wurtz RH. Motion selectivity in macaque visual cortex. III. Psychophysics and physiology of apparent motion. J Neurophysiol 1986;55:1340–1351.

Nilsson L, Hamberger L. A Child Is Born. New York: Delacorte Press, 1990.

Norcia AM, Tyler CW. Spatial frequency sweep VEP: visual acuity during the first year of life. Vision Res 1985;25:1399–1408.

Norcia AM, Tyler CW, Hamer RD. Development of contrast sensitivity in the human infant. Vision Res 1990;30:1475–1486.

Norton TT, Godwin DW. Inhibitory GABAergic control of visual signals at the lateral geniculate nucleus [Review]. Prog Brain Res 1992;90:193–217.

Nye PW, Naka KI. The dynamics of inhibitory interaction in a frog receptive field: a paradigm of paracontrast. Vision Res 1971;11:377–392.

Omoruyi GI, Leat SJ. Selection of potential image processing algorithms for improving the visibility of images for low vision observers. Invest Ophthalmol Vis Sci 2000;38:S431(abst).

Ophthalmic Standards Committee. Specification for test charts for determining distance visual acuity. British Standard 4274. London, British Standards Institution 1968;1–14.

Orel-Bixler D. Subjective and visual evoked potential measures of acuity in normal and amblyopic adults and children. Doctoral dissertation, University of California, Berkeley CA 1989;47–60.

Orel-Bixler D. Electrodiagnostics, Neuroimaging, Ultrasound and Photorefraction. In B Moore (eds), Eye Care for Infants and Young Children. Boston: Butterworth–Heinemann, 1997;89–122.

Østerberg G. Topography of the layer of rods and ones in the human retina. Acta Ophthalmol Scand Suppl 1935;6:1–106.

Owsley C, Sekuler R, Siemsen D. Contrast sensitivity throughout adulthood. Vision Res 1983;23:689–699.

Owsley C, Sloane ME. Contrast sensitivity, acuity, and the perception of 'real-world' targets. Br J Ophthalmol 1987;71:791–796.

Oyster CW. The Human Eye. Sunderland, MA: Sinauer Associates, 1999.

Palmer GA. Theory of Colours and Vision. London: S. Leacroft, 1777.

Pantle A. Motion after-effect magnitude as a measure of the spatio-temporal response properties of direction sensitive analyzers. Vision Res 1974;14:1229–1236.

Patorgis CJ. Contrast Sensitivity. In JB Eskridge, JF Amos, JD Bartlett (eds), Clinical Procedures in Optometry. Philadelphia: Lippincott, 1991;498–504.

Peli E. Limitations of image enhancement for the visually impaired. Optom Vis Sci 1992;69:15–24.

Peli E, Lee E, Trempe CL, Buzney S. Image enhancement for the visually impaired: the effects of enhancement on face recognition. J Opt Soc Am A 1994;11:1929–1939.

Pelli DG, Robson JG, Wilkins AJ. The design of a new letter chart for measuring contrast sensitivity. Clinical Vision Sciences 1988;2:187–199.

Peterzell DH, Kelly JP. Development of spatial frequency tuned "covariance" channels: individual differences in the electrophysiological (VEP) contrast sensitivity function. Optom Vis Sci 1997;74:800–807.

Pflug R, Nelson R, Ahnelt PK. Background-induced flicker enhancement in cat retinal horizontal cells. I. Temporal and spectral properties. J Neurophysiol 1990;64:313–325.

Pirenne MH. Absolute Thresholds and Quantum Effects. In Davson H (eds), The Eye. New York: Academic, 1962;125–130.

Pitts DG, Kleinstein RN. Environmental Vision: Interactions of the Eye, Vision and the Environment. Boston: Butterworth–Heinemann, 1993.

Pokorny J, Smith VC, Verriest G, Pinkers AJ. Congenital and Acquired Color Vision Defects. New York: Grune & Stratton, 1979.

Prager TC. Essential Factors in Testing for Glare. In MP Nadler, D Miller, DJ Nadler (eds), Glare and Contrast Sensitivity for Clinicians. New York: Springer-Verlag, 1990;33–44.

Prince JH, Fry GA. The effect of errors of refraction on visual acuity. Am J Optom Arch Am Acad Optom 1956;33:353–373.

Quigley HA, Dunkelberger GR, Green WR. Retinal ganglion cell atrophy correlated with automated perimetry in human eyes with glaucoma. Am J Ophthalmol 1989;107:453–464.

Quigley HA, Sanchez RM, Dunkelberger GR, et al. Chronic glaucoma selectively damages large optic nerve fibers. Invest Ophthalmol Vis Sci 1987;28:913–920.

Rasengane TA, Allen D, Manny RE. Development of temporal contrast sensitivity in human infants. Vision Res 1997;37:1747–1754.

Regan D. Spatiotemporal Abnormalities of Vision in Patients with Multiple Sclerosis. In D Regan (ed), Spatial Vision. Boca Raton, FL: CRC Press, 1991;239–249.

Regan D, Neima D. Low-contrast letter charts as a test of visual function. Ophthalmology 1983;90:1192–1200.

Restak R. The Infant Mind. Garden City, NY: Doubleday, 1986.

Riggs LA. Light as a Stimulus for Vision. In CH Graham (ed), Vision and Visual Perception. New York: Wiley, 1965;1–38.

Riggs LA, Ratliff F, Cornsweet JC, Cornsweet TN. The disappearance of steadily fixated visual test objects. J Opt Soc Am 1953;43:495–501.

Robson JG. Spatial and temporal contrast-sensitvity functions of the visual system. J Opt Soc Am 1966;56:1141–1142.

Rodieck RW. The First Steps in Seeing. Sunderland, MA: Sinauer Associates, 1998.

Rose A. The sensitivity performance of the eye on an absolute scale. J Opt Soc Am 1948;38:196–208.

Roufs JA. Dynamic properties of vision. I. Experimental relationships between flicker and flash thresholds. Vision Res 1972;12:261–278.

Roufs JAJ, Meulenbrugge HJ. The quantitative relation between flash threshold and the flicker fusion boundary for centrally fixated fields. Institute for Perception Research, Eindhoven, The Netherlands 1967;Annual Progess Report 2:133–139.

Rovamo J, Virsu V, Nasanen R. Cortical magnification factor predicts the photopic contrast sensitivity of peripheral vision. Nature 1978;271:54–56.

Rubin GS, Legge GE. Psychophysics of reading. VI—The role of contrast in low vision. Vision Res 1989;29:79–91.

Rushton WAH. The Ferrier lecture. Visual adaptation. Proc R Soc Lond B Biol Sci 1965;162:20–46.

Rushton WAH, Powell DS. The rhodopsin content and the visual threshold of human rods. Vision Res 1972;12:1073–1081.

Salzman CD, Britten KH, Newsome WT. Cortical microstimulation influences perceptual judgements of motion direction [Published erratum appears in Nature 1990;346(6284):589.] [See comments]. Nature 1990;346:174–177.

Salzman CD, Murasugi CM, Britten KH, Newsome WT. Microstimulation in visual area MT: effects on direction discrimination performance. J Neurosci 1992;12:2331–2355.

Savage GL, Haegerstrom-Portnoy G, Adams AJ, Hewlett SE. Age changes in the optical density of human ocular media. Clin Vis Sci 1993;8:97–108.

Schnapf JL, Nunn BJ, Meister M, Baylor DA. Visual transduction in cones of the monkey Macaca Fascicularis. J Physiol 1990;427:681–713.

Schultz M. Zur anatomie und physiologie der retina. Archiv fur Mikroscopische Anatomische Entwicklungsmechanie 1866;2:175–286.

Sekuler R, Pantle A. A model for after-effects of seen movement. Vision Res 1967; 7:427–439.

Sergent J. Microgenesis of Face Perception. In HD Ellis (ed), Aspects of Face Processing. Boston: Martinus Nijhoff, 1986;17–33.

Shapley R. Neural Mechanisms of Contrast Sensitivity. In D Regan (ed), Spatial Vision. Boca Raton, FL: CRC Press, 1991;290–305.

Shapley R, Reid RC. Contrast and assimilation in the perception of brightness. Proc Natl Acad Sci U S A 1985;82:5983–5986.

Shlaer S. The relation between visual acuity and illumination. J Gen Physiol 1938; 21:165–188.

Sloan LL. New test charts for the measurement of visual acuity at far and near distances. Am J Ophthalmol 1959;48:807–813.

Smith G. Ocular defocus, spurious resolution and contrast reversal. Ophthalmic Physiol Opt 1982;2:5–23.

Sokol S. Visually evoked potentials: theory, techniques and clinical applications. Surv Ophthalmol 1976;21:18–44.

Southall JPC, trans-ed. Helmholtz's Treatise on Physiological Optics. New York: Dover, 1962.

Sperling G. Temporal and spatial visual masking. I. Masking by impulse flashes. J Opt Soc Am 1965;55:541–559.

Steinman RM, Levinson JZ. The Role of Eye Movement in the Detection of Contrast and Spatial Detail. In E Kowler (ed), Eye Movements and Their Role in Visual and Cognitive Processes. New York: Elsevier, 1990;115–212.

Sterling P, Freed M, Smith RG. Microcircuitry and functional architecture of the cat retina. Trends Neurosci 1986;9:186–192.

Stevens SS. A scale for the measurement for a psychological magnitude: loudness. Psychol Rev 1936;43:405–416.

Stevens SS. Problems and methods of psychophysics. Psychol Bull 1958;55:177–196.

Stevens SS. The Psychophysics of Sensory Function. In WA Rosenblith (ed), Sensory Communication. Cambridge, MA: M.I.T. Press, 1961;1–33.

Stevens SS. Psychophysics. New York: Wiley, 1975.

Stockman A, Sharpe LT, Zrenner E, Nordby K. Slow and fast pathways in the human rod visual system: electrophysiology and psychophysics. J Opt Soc Am A 1991;8:1657–1665.

Sturr J, Hannon D. Methods and Models for Specifying Sites and Mechanisms of Sensitivity Regulation in the Aging Visual System. In P Bagnoli, W Hodos (eds), The Changing Visual System. New York: Plenum, 1991.

Tanner JW, Swets JA. The human use of information: I Signal detection for the case of the signal known exactly. Transactions of the IRE Professional Group on Information Theory 1954;4:213–221.

Teller DY. First glances: the vision of infants. The Friedenwald lecture. Invest Ophthalmol Vis Sci 1997;38:2183–2203.

Teller DY, Peeples DR, Sekel M. Discrimination of chromatic from white light by two-month-old human infants. Vision Res 1978;18:41–48.

Thorell LG, De Valois RL, Albrecht DG. Spatial mapping of monkey V1 cells with pure color and luminance stimuli. Vision Res 1984;24:751–769.

Thorn F, Schwartz F. Effects of dioptric blur on Snellen and grating acuity. Optom Vis Sci 1990;67:3–7.

Traquair HM. An Introduction to Clinical Perimetry. St. Louis: Mosby, 1946.

Tyler CW. Analysis of visual modulation sensitivity. II. Peripheral retina and the role of photoreceptor dimensions. J Opt Soc Am A 1985,2:393–398.

Tyler CW. Specific deficits of flicker sensitivity in glaucoma and ocular hypertension. Invest Ophthalmol Vis Sci 1981;20:204–212.

Tyler CW. Two processes control variations in flicker sensitivity over the lifespan. J Opt Soc Am A 1989;6:481–490.

Tyler CW, Hamer RD. Analysis of visual modulation sensitivity. IV. Validity of the Ferry-Porter law. J Opt Soc Am A 1990;7:743–758.

Tyler CW, Hamer RD. Eccentricity and the Ferry-Porter law. J Opt Soc Am A 1993;10:2084–2087.

Tyler CW, Ryu S, Stamper R. The relation between visual sensitivity and intraocular pressure in normal eyes. Invest Ophthalmol Vis Sci 1984;25:103–105.

van Doorn AJ, Koenderink JJ. Spatial properties of the visual detectability of moving spatial white noise. Exp Brain Res 1982a;45:189–195.

van Doorn AJ, Koenderink JJ. Temporal properties of the visual detectability of moving spatial white noise. Exp Brain Res 1982b;45:179–188.

Van Toi V, Grounauer PA, Burckhardt CW. Artificially increasing intraocular pressure causes flicker sensitivity losses. Invest Ophthalmol Vis Sci 1990;31:1567–1574.

Vimal RL. Foveal cone thresholds. Vision Res 1989;29:61–78.

Virsu V, Lehtio P, Rovamo J. Contrast sensitivity in normal and pathological vision. Doc Ophthalmol Proceedings Series 1981;30:263–272.

Volbrecht VJ, Werner JS. Isolation of short-wavelength-sensitive cone photoreceptors in 4–6-week-old human infants. Vision Res 1987;27:469–478.

Wald G. Area and visual threshold. J Gen Physiol 1938;21:269–287

Wald G. Human vision and the spectrum. Science 1945;101:653–658.

Wald G. The receptors of human color vision. Science 1964;145:1007–1016.

Wald G, Clark AB. Visual adaptation and the chemistry of the rods. J Gen Physiol 1937;21:93–105.

Wassle H, Grunert U, Rohrenbeck J, Boycott BB. Cortical magnification factor and the ganglion cell density of the primate retina. Nature 1989;341:643–646.

Watson AB, Ahumada AJ. Model of visual-motion sensing. J Opt Soc Am A 1985;2:322–341.

Watson AB, Ahumada AJ, Farrell JE. Window of visibility: a psychophysical theory of fidelity in time-sampled visual motion displays. J Opt Soc Am A 1986;3:300–307.

Waugh SJ, Levi DM. Visibility and vernier acuity for separated targets. Vision Res 1993;33:539–552.

Wentworth HAA. A quantitative study of achromatic and chromatic sensitivity from center to periphery of the visual field. Psychological Monographs 1930;40:1–189.

Wertheim T. Peripheral visual acuity. Am J Optom Physiol Opt 1980;57:915–924.

Westheimer G. Focusing responses of the human eye. Am J Optom Arch Am Acad Optom 1966;43:221–232.

Westheimer G. Scaling of visual acuity measurements. Arch Ophthalmol 1979a;97:327–330.

Westheimer G. The spatial sense of the eye. Proctor lecture. Invest Ophthalmol Vis Sci 1979b;18:893–912.

Weymouth FW. Visual sensory units and the minimal angle of resolution. Am J Ophthalmol 1958;46:102–113.

Weymouth FW. Effect of Age on Visual Acuity. In MJ Hirsch, RE Wick (eds), Vision of the Aging Patient. Philadelphia: Chilton Co., 1960;37–62.

Weymouth FW, Hines D, Acres L, et al. Visual acuity within the area centralis and its relation to eye movements and fixation. Am J Ophthalmol 1928;11:947–960.

Wilcox WW. The basis of the dependence of visual acuity on illumination. Proc Natl Acad Sci U S A 1932;18:47–56.

Williams RA, Enoch JM, Essock EA. The resistance of selected hyperacuity configurations to retinal image degradation. Invest Ophthalmol Vis Sci 1984;25:389–399.

Williams TD. Aging and central visual area. Am J Optom Physiol Opt 1983;60:888–891.

Wolfe JM. An Introduction to Contrast Sensitivity Testing. In MP Nadler, D Miller, DJ Nadler (eds), Glare and Contrast Sensitivity for Clinicians. New York: Springer-Verlag, 1990;5–23.

Woodhouse JM, Barlow HB. Spatial and Temporal Resolution and Analysis. In HB Barlow, JD Mollon (eds), The Senses. Cambridge, UK: Cambridge University Press, 1982;133–164.

Wright WD. Researches on Normal and Defective Colour Vision. St. Louis: Mosby, 1946.

Wright WD. The Measurement of Colour. New York: Macmillan, 1958.

Wu S, Burns SA, Reeves A, Elsner AE. Flicker brightness enhancement and visual nonlinearity. Vision Res 1996;36:1573–1583.

Wyszecki G, Stiles WS. Color Science: Concepts and Methods, Quantitative Data and Formulae (2nd ed). New York: Wiley, 1982.

Yoshioka T, Dow BM, Vautin RG. Neuronal mechanisms of color categorization in areas V1, V2 and V4 of macaque monkey visual cortex. Behav Brain Res 1996;76:51–70.

Young T. On the theory of light and colours. Philos Trans R Soc Lond 1802;92;12–48.

Yuodelis C, Hendrickson A. A qualitative and quantitative analysis of the human fovea during development. Vision Res 1986;26:847–855.

Zeki S. A century of cerebral achromatopsia. Brain 1990;113:1721–1777.

Index

Note: Page numbers followed by *f* refer to figures; page numbers followed by *t* refer to tables.

Lateral inhibition, 143
    definition of, 175
Letter charts, 114–125. *See also* Spatial
        visual acuity
    confusion letters on, 118
    crowding effect and, 124–125
    letter spacing in, 123–124, 124f, 125f
    for minimum angle of resolution,
        114–116
    relative letter legibility in, 118–119
    single-letter, 119
    stroke width for, 116, 116f, 117, 117f
LGN. *See* Lateral geniculate nucleus
Light
    adapting. *See* Adapting light
    brightness of, 3–4
    detection of. *See* Absolute threshold
        of vision
    intensity of, 3–4. *See also* Intensity
        discrimination; Luminance
    measurement of, 323–330
    photometric units of, 323–324
    photopigment absorption of,
        221–225, 222f
    scatter of, 72–73
Light adaptation, 76, 77. *See also* Dark
        adaptation; Dark adaptation
        curve
    adapting field and, 6–7, 7f
    critical flicker frequency and, 188,
        190–191, 190f
    definition of, 103
    equivalent background theory and,
        93–95
    neural response in, 99–102, 100f, 101f
    photoreceptor response in, 76, 96–99,
        96f, 98f
Likelihood ratio, 27
Limits, Method of. *See* Method of Limits
Localization (Vernier) acuity, 107, 107t,
        110, 110f
    definition of, 136
    in infant, 301, 302f
    optical defocus and, 111
    retinal eccentricity and, 128–130,
        130f, 131f
LogMAR, 114
    definition of, 136
LogMAR scale, 120, 120t, 122f, 123, 124f
    definition of, 136
Low spatial frequency rolloff, 151
    definition of, 175
Low temporal frequency rolloff, 192
    definition of, 214

Lumen, 325, 326f, 330
    definition of, 53
Luminance, 326f, 328, 328t
    background, 9
    critical flicker frequency and, 180,
        183–184, 184f
    definition of, 6, 33
    mean, 149
        definition of, 176
    of reference field, 6–7, 7f, 8f
    relative, 140f
    spatial visual acuity and, 125–127, 126f
    stimulus area and (Ricco's law),
        40–41, 40f
    stimulus duration and (Bloch's law),
        42, 43f
    temporal contrast sensitivity and, 192,
        193f
    temporal summation and, 199–200,
        199f
    of test field, 6–7, 7f, 8f
Luminosity, definition of, 285
Luminous efficiency, 241, 275f
Luminous flux, 325, 326f
Luminous intensity, 326, 326t
Lux, 372t

Mach bands, 143, 144f, 167, 168f
    definition of, 175
Macular degeneration, age-related
        (ARMD), 172
Magnitude Estimation procedure, 29
    definition of, 33
Magnitude of sensation. *See* Sensations,
        magnitude of
Magnitude Production procedure, 29
    definition of, 33
Magnocellular (M) pathway, 158
    in color vision, 263
    definition of, 175, 285
MAR. *See* Minimum angle of resolution
        (MAR)
Masking, 179, 201–204, 202f
    backward, 202, 203
        definition of, 213
    definition of, 214
    dichoptic, 203–204
        definition of, 214
    forward, 201–202
        definition of, 214
    metacontrast, 203
        definition of, 214
    paracontrast, 203
        definition of, 214

in saccadic suppression, 204
simultaneous, 202–203
Maxwell, James Clerk, 235
Mean luminance, 149
definition of, 175
Measurement
of action spectrum, 223
bias and guessing in, 15–18
of dark adaptation in clinic, 89–90
error and visual acuity, 121
fixed parameters and, 36
of intensity discrimination, 56–57
of minimum angle of resolution in
clinic, 172
psychophysical, in elderly, 312
psychophysical, in infants, 293,
301–302
psychophysical methods of, 10–15
psychophysical principles of, 2–34
of sensory magnitude, 29–31
signal detection theory and, 18–28
task complexity and, 4–5
variability in threshold, 8–9
of visual fields, 67–68
of visual thresholds, 4
Membrane potential, and flicker in horizontal cell, 189–190, 190f
Mesopic luminance condition, 76
definition of, 103
Metacontrast, 203
definition of, 214
Metamers, 228
definition of, 285
Method of Adjustment, 14–15, 15f
definition of, 33
Method of Constant Stimuli, 10, 11f
in absolute threshold of vision measurement, 43
definition of, 33
Method of Limits, 11–14, 12t, 13t
definition of, 33
staircase procedure for, 13, 13t
tracking procedure for, 13–14
Michelson contrast, 147f, 148–149, 330
definition of, 175
Middle temporal cortical neurons, in
motion detection, 208–212,
209f, 211f, 212f
Mie scattering, 73
Millilamberts, 330
Minimum angle of resolution (MAR), 111,
114–116. See also LogMAR
contrast sensitivity function and,
171

cutoff high spatial frequency and,
152–153
definition of, 136
Minimum detectable acuity. See Spatial
visual acuity
Minimum discriminable acuity. See
Localization (Vernier) acuity
Minimum recognizable acuity. See Iden-
tification acuity
Minimum separable acuity. See Resolution acuity
Minimum visible (distinguishable) acuity.
See Detection acuity
Miosis, 311–312
definition of, 322
Miss, 20, 21f
definition of, 33
Modulation ratio, 192
definition of, 214
Modulation transfer function, 153–154
Monochromatic light, 221
definition of, 285
Motion, 204–205
apparent, 207, 208f
definition of, 215
Motion aftereffect, 207
definition of, 215
Motion detection, 204–212
direction-selective neurons in, 206–207
middle temporal cortical neurons in,
208–212, 209f, 211f, 212f
neurometric function for, 210–212,
211f, 212f
temporal visual resolution and,
205–206, 206f
Multiple sclerosis, contrast sensitivity in, 173
Munsell Color System, 249

Neural defocus, visual acuity and,
132–134
Neuritis, optic. See Optic neuritis
Neurometric function, definition of, 215
Neutral point, 271, 272f
definition of, 285
Night blindness, 89, 89f
Noise, 9
signal detection and, 18–22, 20f, 21f,
22f, 50
Nonspectral color, 243
definition of, 285

Off-center bipolar cell. See Receptive-field
center
Oguchi's disease, 89, 89f

On-center bipolar cell. *See* Receptive-field center
Optic disk, as absolute scotoma, 71
Optic neuritis, 275–276
  definition of, 285–286
Optical defocus, 111, 113–114, 115f, 153
Opponent color theory. *See* Color opponency
Optotypes, 115
  definition of, 136
Opsin. *See* Cone opsins
Optical density
  of cone photopigments, 224
  definition of, 224

Palmer, George, 234
Paracontrast, 203
  definition of, 214
Parvocellular (P) pathway, 158
  in color vision, 264
  definition of, 175, 286
Payoff matrix, 19–22, 21f
  for bias control, 24, 26–28, 26f
Peak contrast sensitivity, 151
  definition of, 175
Peak temporal frequency, 192
  definition of, 215
Pelli-Robson chart, 171, 171f
  definition of, 175
Percent of "Yes" responses, 10, 10f, 16–17, 17f, 34
Perception, 2
Perceptual response, 2–3
  definition of, 2–3
  probabilistic nature of, 8–10
  variability in, 22–24, 23f, 25f
Perimetry
  kinetic, 70
  static, 70–71
Period, 180
  definition of, 215
Perseveration, 12
Phi phenomenon, 207
  definition of, 215
Photometric units, 323–324, 328–329
Photometry, 324–327, 325f, 326f, 326t, 327t
Photopic luminance condition, 76
  definition of, 103
Photopic luminous efficiency function, 285, 325–326, 326f
  in infant, 306–307
Photopic vision, 325

Photopigment(s), 90–93
  bleached, 76, 91–93, 92f
  concentration of, 77
  light absorption by, 221–225, 222f
  opsins of, 223
  optical density of, 224
  regeneration of, 90–91, 91f
Photoreceptors. *See also* Cone(s); Rod(s)
  age-related changes in, 312
  maturation of, 304
  spacing of, 111, 112f, 153–154
  spatial summation of, 39
  in visual adaptation, 76, 96–99, 96f, 98f
Piper's law, 41
Planckian locus, 246
  definition of, 286
Poisson distribution, 46, 47–48, 48f, 49f
Postnatal vision development, 289–308, 291f
  absolute threshold and, 295
  acuity card procedure and, 301–302
  color vision and, 306
  cone wavelength sensitivity and, 305
  during first year, 292
  forced-choice preferential looking test for, 293–294, 294f
  grating acuity and, 297, 301–302, 301t
  increment threshold functions and, 296–297, 296f
  luminous efficiency function and, 306–307
  photoreceptor maturation and, 304
  rate of, 299–300
  spatial contrast sensitivity function and, 302–303, 303f
  spatial summation and, 295–296, 295f
  swept spatial frequency visual evoked potentials and, 299, 300f
  temporal contrast sensitivity function and, 304–305, 305f
  vernier acuity and, 301, 302f
  vision disorder detection and, 307
  visual evoked potentials and, 297–299, 298f
Presbyopia, 312
  definition of, 322
Primary colors, 234
  definition of, 286
  imaginary, 241
    definition of, 285
Prosopagnosia, 268